COVID CANADA

First Wave, Spring 2020

Robert W. Passfield

Rock's Mills Press

Published by
Rock's Mills Press
www.rocksmillspress.com

For information, including Library and Archives Canada Cataloguing
in Publication data, please contact the publisher at
customer.service@rocksmillspress.com.

Cover Design: Craig Passfield

Second Edition
This book was initially published, by the author, under the title
*Coronavirus Canada, The Politics, Science and Economics of a
Pandemic, Volume One: The Pandemic* (2020), which was to be
followed by a volume on the recovery period. However, the original
book title is no longer appropriate. The pandemic virus is now
universally referred to as COVID, rather than by its original
designation as a coronavirus. Moreover, when first published the book
was regarded as a journal of the pandemic in Canada, but several
subsequent waves of infections rendered it a recording of the impact of
the First Wave of the Spring of 2020. The second edition includes
minor corrections to the text.

Author's website: www.passrob.com

To Susan James

For her understanding and support
as my retirement years continue to be devoted
to a demanding muse – Clio – in the research
and writing of historical works.

Robert W. Passfield

Table of Contents

Preface vii

Acknowledgements ix

Diary Entries:

Chapter One 3
Saturday, March 7th - Wednesday, March 18th

Chapter Two 38
Thursday, March 19th - Wednesday, April 1st

Chapter Three 75
Thursday, April 2nd - Saturday, April 18th

Chapter Four 118
Sunday, April 19th - Friday, April 24th

Chapter Five 147
Friday, April 24th - Thursday, April 30th

Chapter Six 184
Friday, May 1st - Friday, May 8th

Chapter Seven 222
Friday, May 8th - Wednesday, May 13th

Chapter Eight 254
Thursday, May 14th - Tuesday, May 19th

Chapter Nine 289
Wednesday, May 20th - Sunday, May 24th

Retrospective 319

Index 342

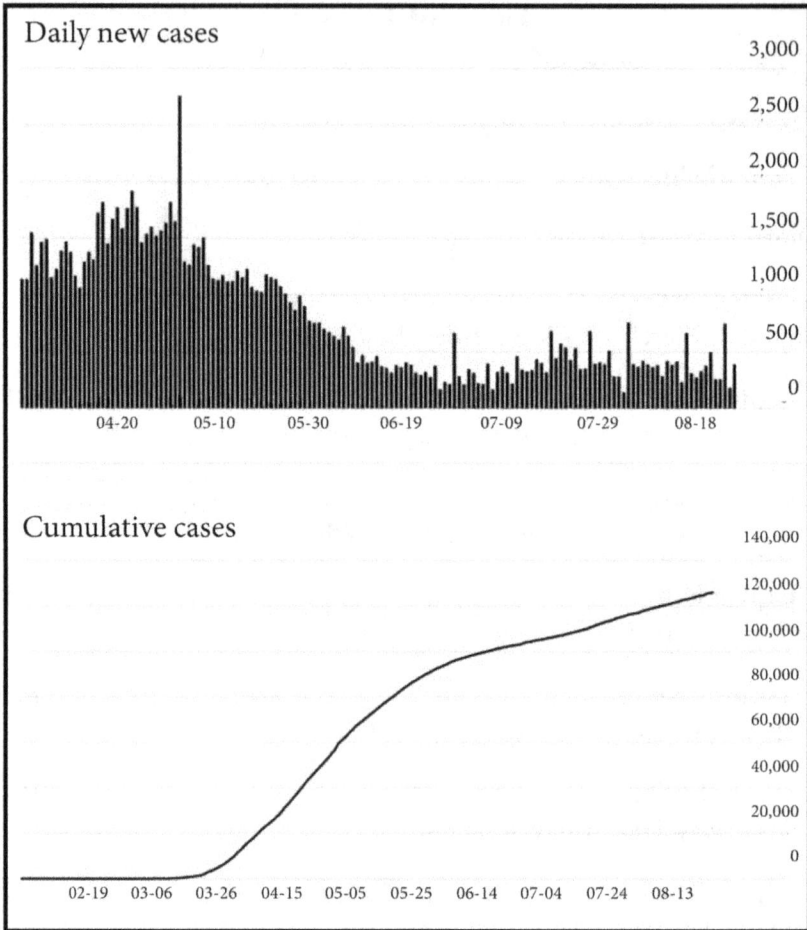

Daily new cases

Cumulative cases

Graph adapted from Global News. In Canada (population 36.5 million), the first presumptive coronavirus case was a Toronto man who became sick on returning from China on January 25th. Thereafter, travellers imported the disease which spread into Canadian communities and by March 21st the number of cases began to soar reaching a record high of 2,760 new daily cases on May 3rd. After that date, the number of new cases gradually declined, with irregular upticks, to a low of 287 daily new cases at the end of May. As of May 24th, Canada had a total of 84,699 confirmed coronavirus cases.

Preface

This book provides an overview of the coronavirus – COVID-19 -- epidemic in Canada in the spring of the year 2020 with a focus on the introduction of the virus, its spread and impact, the response of different levels of government and public health authorities to the virus threat, and the problems encountered in seeking to control its spread and to treat the sick. In addition, the state of the scientific knowledge pertaining to COVID-19, new research advances, the effort to develop a vaccine, and the concept of herd immunity, have been recorded, together with the astounding expenditures that were made by the Liberal government of Prime Minister, Justin Trudeau, in providing financial aid to Canadians who were suffering from the social and economic consequences of provincial lockdowns. A particular attention has been paid to the response of the World Health Organization (WHO) of the United Nations to the threat posed by the coronavirus threat during the initial stages of the outbreak in China, and to the response of the federal Liberal government of Canada to that particular threat, within the context of the close relationship that exists between the WHO and the Public Health Agency of Canada.

The book is written in the form of a daily diary that records significant events and new developments with an on-going analysis and commentary by the author. The entries focus on the period from March 7th through to May 24th, inclusive, which covers the initial surge and the height of the coronavirus epidemic in Canada, with the inclusive references to earlier significant developments. (A second volume of diary entries, analysis, and commentary – to be published separately – covers the period from May 25th to July 31st. It focusses on an initial, rather tentative, recovery phase – following the containment of the virus and the lifting of the provincial lockdowns – with the coronavirus well established within the Canadian community and ever ready to reassert itself in a feared new wave of outbreaks.)

Overall, the two-volume diary comprises an exercise in the writing of a 'present history' of the coronavirus epidemic in Canada as researched, analyzed and interpreted on a daily basis, and written up at it unfolded in the form of a daily diary maintained by an observer. It incorporates insights and observations by the author, as well as re-writes, précises and summaries of published news articles and opinion pieces in newspapers and on the Internet, with an analysis and commentary added by the author. Hence, this is not an original work in terms of research in primary sources. It draws on secondary works -- the research and reporting of others in the news media -- but it is original in the analysis presented, the depth and breadth of the treatment, and the commentary -- from a Tory conservative perspective -- on the course of events and the response of government to a national crisis. Above all, it explains and makes sense of a myriad of different developments during a time of confusion, unease, and fear of the unknown.

———————————————

Acknowledgements

In early March 2020, the author became intrigued by the daily media accounts of a novel deadly virus -- the newly-named COVID-19 -- that originated in Wuhan, China. The unknown virus had caused a widespread sickness and a high death rate in several Chinese cities, was making inroads into Europe, and beginning to surface in North America. It appeared to be 'history in the making', yet another epic struggle of man against the vicissitudes of nature.

In continuing to read about the impact of the COVID-19 virus in the print media and online, the author was struck by the mass of information that was being presented to the Canadian public in a disjointed fashion. Information was being conveyed in news flashes without any orderly analysis of developments, or any presentation of the response of government to a national crisis within a meaningful narrative. The disjointed nature of the news flashes begged for the development of a narrative of developments with an analysis and explanation of what was occurring -- in so far as any understanding was possible. Secondly, the author was struck by the slow, and ad hoc, response of the Liberal government of Prime Minister Justin Trudeau to the threat posed by a deadly virus to Canadians.

The plan adopted was to write a 'present history' of the event in recording, analyzing, and interpreting what promised to be a particularly memorable historical event, and to do so through the recording of the event as it unfolded. At the time, public health authorities in Canada were declaring that Canadians were at a 'low risk' of contacting the coronavirus, but based on media reports of the situation in China and Italy, and the failure of Canada to close it borders to international travellers, the author was convinced that it was just a matter of time until Canadians would suffer the devastating impact of what was becoming a worldwide coronavirus pandemic.

At that point, what came to mind was Daniel Defoe and his *A Journal of the Plague Year* (March 1772) that had recorded the social impact of the Bubonic plague on London in 1665, the plague symptoms and the rising death tolls, inclusive of speculation on how the plague was propagated, and comment on the charity exercised by a Christian people towards their sick brethren. Hence, the author began to think of preparing his historical account, in a diary format, with entries focusing on the daily impact of the coronavirus sickness on Canada, within the broader context of what was becoming a worldwide pandemic. It was a way to make sense of day-to-day developments within a broader context.

To that end, the coronavirus diary would focus on what the author (the diarist) regarded as the critical aspects of a looming public health crisis that needed to be recorded: 1) the politics of the event in recording and analyzing the response of the federal Liberal government and public health authorities in carrying out their duty and responsibility to protect the health and well-being of Canadians, 2) the evolving scientific research pertaining to the nature and contagiousness of the novel coronavirus, and efforts to develop a vaccine, and 3) the financial cost of efforts to mitigate the social and economic impact of the coronavirus on Canadians.

In recording the response of the federal Liberal government of Prime Minister Justin Trudeau to the threat posed to Canada by the coronavirus, the author was surprised by how much the nature of that response revealed about the biases and deficiencies of Modern liberals when faced with a national crisis. In particular, the author was struck by how the response of the federal government to the coronavirus mirrored the globalist values governing the Liberal government establishment under Prime Minister Justin Trudeau. Time and again, the Liberal government acquiesced in the judgements of an international organization, the World Health Organization (WHO), regarding the approach to take to the virus threat when common sense and a concern for the well-being and common good of Canadians would have dictated a different course of action.

It became evident that the Liberal government continually thought in terms of a globalist solution to the virus outbreak, and that initially the federal government was focussed on helping other countries – particularly China, during the initial outbreak in Wuhan – to the neglect of taking any precautions or preparations to protect Canadians from the virus threat. Moreover, political correctness was evident in the original response of the Liberal government to the virus threat in not wanting to appear to discriminate against peoples of any ethnicity or race, or to stigmatize them, by banning the entry of foreign travellers from certain countries as potential carriers of the coronavirus disease. Lastly during the COVID-19 epidemic in Canada, the bias of the Modern liberal mind was quite evident in the focus on grand declarations of policy and globalist values, with a lack of attention to hands-on management and the day-to-day administration of programs.

In retrospect, the COVID-19 epidemic has revealed in stark terms the dangers inherent in globalization, and has highlighted the need for the Nation-State to continue to play a critical role in protecting and promoting the national interest, well-being, and common good of its citizens.

In many ways this diary has evolved into an exercise in the maintenance of a public memory of the COVID-19 epidemic in Canada. It provides a recording and meaningful analysis of developments within a evolving context that transcends the treatment by journalists in the various media who, for the most part, have neglected to provide any on-going historical or background context in their reporting of developments. Journalists have provided little analysis as to whether a program was well designed to achieve its purpose, to whom the monies were being paid, or whether such massive expenditures were necessary. There was little concern that parliamentary oversight of government expenditures was suspended, or that Prime Minister Trudeau continually -- almost daily, in his 'morning show' TV appearances – was introducing grandiose new programs involving the expenditure of massive sums of public monies without much attention to the implementation of the programs. Moreover, there was no analysis of the Modern liberal mindset of Justin Trudeau as reflected in his spending programs and the Liberal government priorities.

Given the large bulk of the coronavirus diary, it was decided to divide the entries into two volumes: a volume one, subtitled 'The Pandemic', which covers the entries from March 7th through to May 24th, and deals with the introduction of the coronavirus and the height of the Canadian epidemic amidst a worldwide pandemic; and volume two, subtitled 'The Continuum', which covers the period of crisis, from May 25th through

July 31st, when tentative steps were being taken to re-open a devastated Canadian economy, supported by massive federal government financial aid programs, amidst the fear of evoking a second wave of coronavirus infections. The fears focussed on the re-opening of retail stores and workplaces, and the projected re-opening of schools, but with some hope provided by the latest scientific advances in treating patients suffering from the disease and by encouraging positive developments in the clinical trials of several potential vaccines.

As a historian, the author is very conscious of the need to provide an attribution for one's sources in a credit line to give a proper acknowledgement of the sources used, as well as credit for the ideas and concepts used in one's writings. However, the drawing on a wide variety of content from different news media -- a variety of newspapers articles on the Internet from different sources presenting the same news item -- made it a hopeless task to provide an attribution referencing each journalist or columnist for a particular news story consulted. The News is the News; and a news story is a news story. Nonetheless, the author readily acknowledges that in producing a diary of the prominent news items, day by day, he relied heavily on collating, summarizing, rewriting, and paraphrasing, news stories reported by newspaper journalists and Internet news sources.

To wit, the author has relied on multiple published sources and posted Internet articles for his news source, but to those reporters and columnists who think they see an element here and there of their news gathering and reporting reproduced in this book, the author can only state in his defence that he could not be present at the briefings given by public authorities, nor was it humanly possible to have access to what will be the future archival record of the historical events. He has had to rely on reports in the press, and a reproduction of the information that the media reporters have gathered, with the addition of his own analysis, after the fact.

In the several instances, where use has been made of a single-sourced news item, or an opinion piece or article produced by a columnist with a particular knowledge of the subject at issue, the source has been cited and the columnist named. That is similarly the case in the rare instances where a contributor to a newspaper has produced an original piece.

In producing a diary of the COVID-19 epidemic in Canada, the author has followed the practice of reading the local *Ottawa Citizen* newspaper early each morning – which contains national news feeds from the *National Post* -- followed by online research on the Internet in the news coverage that is posted from a wide variety of newspapers and TV network news sources. In that pursuit, the author searched out what he regarded as significant and informative reports and observations about the coronavirus, its origins, its spread, and its impact in Canada, as well as general contextual information on developments in scientific research pertaining to the coronavirus, the impact of the pandemic worldwide, and its economic impact. At all times during the research process, the author paid a close attention to the response of the Canadian federal government to the threat that the virus posed to the health and economic well-being of Canadians, and continually sought to discern, and to set forth, the lessons to be learned.

In pursuing Internet research, the author has avoided reading the postings of newspapers that demand payment for access to their news coverage. That was based on a belief that newspaper reporters, as distinct from columnist, furnish the same basic news -- mostly bereft of any intellectual analysis or historical context -- regardless of which newspaper employs them. There was also a vague resentment felt by the author that some newspapers were demanding a payment for access to their news coverage while others were posting their news items for free access. Yet, in taking that stance against paying for news coverage access, the author was being irrational as he strongly believes that newspapers ought to be paid for any of their news content that can be accessed on the Internet through a search engine.

The analysis and judgements present in the diary entries are the product of a Tory Conservative perspective on events, and a firm Tory belief that the Nation-State has a moral duty and responsibility to protect the health, well-being and common good of its citizens by using the power and authority of the State to take command during a national crisis -- under the Emergency Measures Act -- while respecting the traditional rights of parliament to scrutinize and question the actions of government.

This work involved the writing of an instant history, or 'present history' of the coronavirus epidemic as it unfolded in Canada, within a broader world context. It was, and is, a demanding type of history writing that requires a relentless, daily commitment, and the continual exercise of a momentary judgement as to what is truly significant and worthy of being recorded for posterity, as well as an attention to the human cost of the tragedy, and the responses being made to the challenges presented. The all-consuming demands of that commitment were made bearable by the self-isolation demanded during the coronavirus pandemic, and by the abnormally cold, wet, and windy weather during the months of March, April and May in the City of Ottawa that detracted from any desire to be out-of-doors.

The hope is that Canadians, government officials, and public health authorities, will read this account of how the coronavirus was introduced into Canada and how it spread throughout the country to become a full blown epidemic; and that they will learn from the successes achieved elsewhere, and the failures and successes experienced by Canada in seeking to contain the spread of the virus. There are lessons to be learned in combatting future virus threats, or a resurgence of the coronavirus.

All mention of Canadian personages have been linked with an identifier, and the Canadian locations mentioned have been placed within a general geographical reference, to enable non-Canadians to readily read the Canadian narrative without being puzzled by references to unknown personages and places.

To those mild manner Canadians who might object to the acerbic comments and the critique presented herein pertaining to the federal Liberal government, and that embodiment of the Modern liberal mindset, Prime Minister Justin Trudeau, the author can merely respond that the criticism is directed at what they stand for, and for their actions or inactions whatever the case might be. Moreover, after spending a lifetime in reading the highly-biased writings of a Liberal Press that continually disparages, denigrates, and dismisses Conservatives of all types, perhaps the author can be indulged, if not excused, for giving vent to a critique of the Liberal establishment, its Modern liberal mindset as embodied in the beliefs of Prime Minister Justin Trudeau, and its governance of Canada.

The character judgements are based solely on the conduct and pronouncements of the public figures as reported in the press. Readers can form their own personal judgement concerning the character of the public figures so treated.

In preparing this diary on the impact of the coronavirus pandemic on Canada -- with a focus on an analysis and critique of the response of government leaders and government public health authorities to the virus threat -- the author was reminded of an occurrence a good many years earlier during his career as a public historian. In conversation with the Director of Restoration Services, Parks Canada – an architect by profession – the author suggested that Historical Services Branch historians ought to be assigned to produce reports on the restoration projects being undertaken by Restoration Services. The Director replied, "the last thing the engineers want is someone like you recording their mistakes".

On a more personal note, I am indebted to my nephew, Craig Passfield, for the design and preparation of the book covers. The author is solely responsible for the content, inclusive of the judgements and character analyses presented which are based directly on information conveyed in the media.

Robert W. Passfield
Ottawa, ON
September 2020

"that the infection was propagated insensibly,
and by such persons as were not visibly infected,
who neither knew whom they infected,
or who they were infected by."

Daniel Defoe
A Journal of the Plague Year

A Journal of the Plague Year: Being Observations or Memorials of the most Remarkable Occurrences, as well Publick and Private, which happened in London during the last Great Visitation in 1665 (London, 1772), signed H.F. This journal describes the spread of the bubonic plague (y. pestis bacterium) among the districts of London, England, in the plague year, 1665. Although unknown at the time, the bubonic plague bacterium spread from rats to humans through flea bites.

The journal records the soaring death toll from the plague in the districts of London, the suffering of afflicted families, and the efforts of the municipal authorities to remove the dead and isolate the sick in seeking to contain its spread. During the plague, an estimated 100,000 people died, almost one-quarter of the population of London. The 'eye-witness account' is attributed to the writer, Daniel Defoe; yet Defoe was only five years old in 1665! The journal may well have been kept by his uncle, Henry Foe, a saddler, shop keeper, and merchant, who remained in London during the plague year to manage his business interests.

Diary Entries

Chapter One

Background

A Novel Virus Threat: On December 31st, China reported to the World Health Organization that a cluster of 41 patients in the City of Wuhan were sick from a mysterious 'pneumonia' that appeared to have originated in the Wuhan Wet Market; and on January 7th, the novel virus was identified as a new type of coronavirus. The seriousness of the virus outbreak became apparent on January 23rd when the City of Wuhan was quarantined, and the quarantine extended several days later to the entire surrounding Province of Hubei, with bus and rail transport links suspended to the rest of China.

In Hubei Province, as of February 8th, 24,953 coronavirus cases, and 699 coronavirus-related deaths were reported, with an additional 9,923 coronavirus cases, and 35 coronavirus- related deaths reported in the rest of China. The introduction of a lockdown of the City of Wuhan, of Hubei Province, and several other Chinese cities was a radical response to a novel virus threat in enforcing a social spacing on the populace. Clearly, in China a strict quarantine has been effective is preventing a wave of infections beyond Hubei Province and the several isolated Chinese cities were infections were rife in a country with a population of 1.4 billion. However, some spreading of the virus had occurred before the strict quarantine was imposed on Wuhan. On February 11th, the World Health Organization designed the new coronavirus as COVID-19 (SARS-CoV-2).

As of the second and third weeks of February 2020, coronavirus cases were surging in South Korea, Iran, and Italy, and increasing sharply in Spain. By March 6th, China claimed that the number of new coronavirus cases had dropped to less than 100 a day, but with face masks being in short supply – despite China being the primary manufacturer – the Chinese government issued an appeal for medical personal protection equipment to help China deal with the COVID-19 epidemic. (At this point, western news outlets were expressing a suspicion that the Chinese government was under reporting the number of new COVID-19 cases and the death rate)

Saturday, March 7, 2020

Sharon Kirkey, a National Post newspaper columnist, has prepared an interesting survey of the published accounts by medical professionals and epidemiologists on the coronavirus outbreak in China and its implications for other nations. At present, there are over 98,000 confirmed COVID-19 cases, and 3,380 confirmed deaths since the virus outbreak in Wuhan, China, eight weeks ago. Canada has one confirmed case; the U.S. has several dozen cases; and there are thousands of cases in Europe, with Italy reporting 769 new cases in a single day.

The World Health Organization, out of a concern to avoid creating a panic, has refrained from labelling the coronavirus outbreak a 'pandemic', but epidemiologists have concluded that the world is in the early stages of a pandemic. In the United States, modelling suggests that the coronavirus will infect 40 to 60 percent of adults worldwide. In a medical journal article, philanthropist Bill Gates, of the Bill & Melinda Gates Foundation, has surmised that the coronavirus outbreak might be the 'once-in-a-century' pathogen that epidemiologists continually fear will occur.

The World Health Organization is predicting a death rate, among the infected population, of 3.4 percent, which is a higher than the 2.5 percent death rate of the Spanish flu of 1918-1919 which infected over 500 million people and killed over 20 million people worldwide, but lower than the nearly 10 percent death rate of infection cases during the SARS crisis of 2002-2004 which infected 8,095 persons worldwide and caused 774 deaths. One puzzling unknown is why children appear to have an immunity to the disease or are only mildly infected. There is also a concern that children might be super-efficient asymptomatic spreaders of the virus.

Once the virus enters a community, the expectation is that it can spread rapidly. However, unlike the situation in China, it is not expected that a complete lockdown of cities will be required. In Canada, public health authorities are counting on the health care system and the hospitalization of severe cases to minimize the effects of the disease, and the overall number of deaths. It is further expected that social and economic disruptions will be kept to a minimum. The major concern is that a surge in coronavirus cases would put a severe strain on hospital resources, and result in large numbers of people who would need to be tested and treated. However, the assumption is that most people will not be acutely ill.

Public health authorities are recommending that Canada urgently ramp up its ability to test for the virus among the public through setting up special coronavirus clinics, with the goal of identifying the sick to minimize the number of people going to the emergency department of hospitals for a test and potentially infecting hospital staffs. Moreover, testing will enable the infected to be quarantined. It is anticipated that one of the most difficult problems will be to determine who is, and is not, infected because not everyone shows symptoms when infected. That can only be determine by testing.

It is expected that healthy people will subject to only mild infections. It is the population over 65 years old, and individuals with heart disease, asthma, cancer, and other chronic underlying medical conditions, who will run the highest risk -- if infected by the coronavirus -- of suffering from severe pneumonia, acute respiratory distress syndrome, or sepsis. They are groups at the highest risk of death.

What is odd is that the concern to date of the Canada Public Health Agency, with respect to the coronavirus threat, appears to be focussed on preventing the public psyche from succumbing to an irrational fear of the virus. There is stated need to avoid fostering an "epidemic of catastrophizing", and to prevent the arousing of a wide-spread public anxiety, and a blaming of other peoples. One prominent clinical psychologist, who has written on epidemics, expressed his professional judgement that any effort to slow community spread through travel restrictions and quarantines, might lead to a disdain for 'others' and a "war of all against all". He is advising Canadians "not to lose sleep over COVID-19". Furthermore, he is recommending that Canadians 'secure a two-week supply of food and necessary medications, wash their hands frequently, and avoid touching their eyes after touching surfaces'.

Public Health Canada is treating the coronavirus threat in the same vein. Dr. Theresa Tam, the Chief of Public Health Canada, is telling Canadians that the risk is low, and that Canadians need to follow the directives of the World Health Organization (WHO) of the United Nations.

Tuesday, March 10, 2020

In Italy, a lockdown was introduced over the northern provinces on Sunday, March 8th, with the hospitals in Lombardy reaching the point of becoming overwhelmed with what was being described as a 'tsunami of coronavirus patients'. This is the first lockdown outside of China, and the Italian government has just announced that on March 11th, the lockdown will be extended over the entire country of 60 million people. Schools, universities, theatres, cinemas, and nightclubs are to be closed, as well as all non-essential shops and businesses, sports venues, gyms, and swimming pools. Grocery stores, food stores and pharmacies will remain open, and restaurants and cafes between 6am and 6pm, but with a requirement that a one metre spacing be maintained between customers. Travel is restricted except for essential workers and family emergencies, with fines for those who fail to observe the quarantine. Church services, weddings, and funerals will be postponed.

As of March 10th, Italy has a total of 10,156 confirmed coronavirus cases, and a total of 631 coronavirus related deaths, three days later, on March 14th, there were 21,169 cases and 1,441 deaths. Over a month earlier, on January 31st, Italy introduced a ban on travellers from China, following the linking of the two initial clusters of outbreaks in northern Italy to travellers from China. Whether the closing of the Italian border at this date will have a significant impact on curtailing the spread of the coronavirus remains a moot point as the virus is already widespread within the population of Lombardy. However, internal travel restrictions, in conjunction with the border closure, may well impede the spread of the coronavirus to other areas of the country.

Travel Abroad: With the March Break approaching, questions are being raised in the Press as to whether Canadians should avoid foreign travel, and several epidemiologists have warned against travelling abroad for the March Break. At present, it is known that global travel is a major factor in the spread of the coronavirus disease with 110,000 cases reported in up to 100 countries, and 3,800 deaths worldwide. To date, travellers to China, Iran, Italy, and the United States have returned home to Canada infected, and have become sick shortly after their arrival.

Other than advising Canadians to avoid cruise ship travel, and to self-isolate for 14 days upon returning home from abroad, Public Health Canada --

when queried by the Press -- has declined to comment on whether Canadians should stay at home during the Spring Break. The federal government has declared that it will provide 'extra support' to provincial health services, as well as support – as yet unspecified – for Canadians who are self-isolating due to the virus. At present, the federal government is contacting the provinces concerning their "state of readiness".

Health Update: Despite assurance from Public Health Canada that Canadians are at a low risk of contacting the coronavirus, epidemiologists at the University of Toronto have produced a disease-transmission model that surmises the coronavirus could eventually attack anywhere from 35 to 70 percent of Canadians. However, the epidemiologists maintain that the number could be reduced by half through testing and isolating at least 50 percent of those who test positive, and even further by an 'aggressive' social distancing policy, together with large scale quarantines in areas suffering an outbreak. Otherwise, concerns are being expressed by doctors and nurses across Canada that hospitals are already at full capacity, and that supplies of medical personal protective equipment – face shields, respiratory masks, surgical gloves and, gowns – as well as oxygen, drugs, and ventilators, are in short supply. Moreover, the existing laboratory capacity for testing for coronavirus infections is quite limited.

Research in Wuhan, China, published in the *Lancet* medical journal has revealed that older people are most likely to die from a coronavirus infection, as well as younger people with sepsis and other underlying health problems. Up to 80 percent of the virus cases are mild, mostly among the young. The critically ill with severe respiratory problems – lung congestion -- are placed on ventilators to aid them to breath. Those who survive are generally on a ventilator for two weeks, with an additional two week in hospital to recover.

Wednesday, March 11, 2020

Coronavirus Cases: In Canada, there were sixty confirmed cases of the coronavirus as of last Sunday afternoon (March 8th). Most of the cases are in Ontario (26) and British Columbia (29), with four in Quebec, and one in Alberta. By Wednesday, there were three new confirmed cases in Ontario, all three are travel related, and Alberta has four new cases all related to passengers returning from a single cruise ship, which had a coronavirus outbreak. As of today (March 11th), Ontario has 29 confirmed coronavirus cases. The Ontario Public Health Authority announced that "the virus is not circulating locally", but that "given the global circumstances", the provincial health authorities are working with municipal health bodies "to plan for the potential of a local spread".

The Public Health Agency of Canada continues to maintain that the public health risk from the coronavirus is low, but has advised Canadians to avoid large gatherings, such as conferences and festivals, and to avoid eating at buffets, to reduce the health risks. The Canadian government announced that, at the request of the American government, a Canadian Forces plane will be sent to Oakland, California, to retrieve 237 Canadians onboard a cruise ship, the *Grand Princess*, that has had a major coronavirus outbreak on board. The Canadians passengers will be screened for coronavirus symptoms before boarding the plane and will be quarantined for 14 days at the Canadian Forces Base Trenton on their return. This is the second government flight to bring home Canadians from abroad. In February, the federal government flew home 129 Canadians from another cruise ship that had a serious coronavirus outbreak when docked in Japan. The first group of returnees have been released from their 14-day quarantine period.

According to the World Health Organization (WHO), there are over 105,000 confirmed coronavirus cases worldwide, and over 3,500 virus-related deaths to date. In the absence of reliable figures from China and East Asia, the hardest hit country is Italy. In that country over the past 24 hours the number of coronavirus cases has increased by 25 percent to 7,375, and the number of virus-related deaths has increased by 57 percent to 366 new deaths. What is worrying health authorities is that Italy has a death rate of 3.4 percent, which is much higher than other communicable diseases, such as the flu. Speculation is that Italy's high mortality rate from the coronavirus is due to its unique demographics in that 25 percent of the Italian population is 65 years old or older, and hence a high-risk population. [The statistics regarding the number of coronavirus cases and deaths in each country and the WHO totals, vary somewhat owing to the delays in the U.N. tabulating reports from the various countries.]

In the United Kingdom, the number of coronavirus cases increased on Sunday from 64 to 273, the largest single day increase to date in that country, and two patients have died. Most of the cases are concentrated in the London area. In the United States, New York City has thirteen coronavirus cases, with fears being expressed the number of cases in the City might increase to 100 or more "in two to three weeks". (What is clear here is that American health authorities have no knowledge of how contagious the coronavirus can be.)

Public Health Canada: The Canadian federal government has announced a $1 billion spending plan to blunt the negative economic impact of COVID-19. It includes $275 million in new funding for COVID-19 research in Canada, $500 million in health-care financial support for the provinces and territories; and a $50 million contribution to the World Health Organization (WHO). The $275 million for COVID-19 research is intended to promote research on medical countermeasures, inclusive of antivirals, vaccine development, and clinical trials.

(Earlier on March 6th, the Minister of Health, Patty Hajdu announced that the federal government would offer $27 million to research groups at nineteen Canadian universities 'to develop means of managing the outbreak'. As of March 11th, however, there is a clearly a shift in emphasis from the physical managing any outbreak – social spacing, etc. -- to scientific research aimed at developing a vaccine. However, the federal government policy does not include closing the Canadian border to keep out the virus. There is a clearly a passive acceptance that the virus will spread into Canada. However, the federal government has become more proactive. The earlier emphasis on simply controlling the spread of the virus within Canada until a vaccine is developed by the international science community, has shifted with the provision of funding to Canadian research institutions to develop of a vaccine in Canada to stop the spread of the coronavirus within Canada, and to eventually eliminate the virus threat.)

Economic Outlook: In addition to the $1 billion spending plan of the federal government to blunt the negative economic impact of the coronavirus, the Bank of Canada has cut its interest rate by half-a-percent. However, oil prices are falling due to a major reduction in demand during the COVID-19 crisis, and a price war between Saudi Arabia and Russia which has seen the global market flooded with cheap oil. Economists view the $1 billion federal government spending plan as 'far from sizable enough' to have a significant impact in major areas of the economy. Among the suggestions from businesses organizations are that payroll taxes be cut to aid companies; that an investment fund be set up to enable companies to access interest-free loans; that mortgage payments be deferred; that sick pay be provided for those who are diagnosed with the virus or in a self-imposed isolation; and that more cash be pumped by the government into existing federal lending agencies, such as the Business Development Bank of Canada, and Export Development Canada.

Long-Care Homes: Over the weekend, a man in his 80's died in long-care home in British Columbia, the first COVID-19 death in Canada. The Province of Ontario is advising all long-care homes in the province to begin screening staff, volunteers, visitors, and residents for signs of a virus infection. Elderly residents of long-care homes, and individuals with underlying health conditions are viewed as being the most vulnerable to a coronavirus infection. According to Chinese sources, coronavirus patients over 80 years old have a 14.8 percent chance of dying, versus a death rate of but 2.3 percent in the general population.

In Ontario, the Provincial Government has expressed a concern that there is a shortage of staff in long-care homes, and that staff members are working in more than one long-care home which increases the danger of transferring a coronavirus infection from one facility to another. However, Ontarians were assured that long-care homes meet rigorous provincial standards for all public health concerns, and are capable of outbreak management in detecting, curtailing, and controlling any infectious disease outbreaks.

The Ministry of Health is encouraging Ontarians to frequently wash their hands with soap and water, or an ethanol-based hand sanitizer, to sneeze or cough into one's sleeve, and to avoid touching one's eyes and mouth. Ontarians have been warned to avoid contact with people who are sick and are being admonished 'to stay home if you are sick'.

Travel Advisories: On Wednesday (March 11th) the U.N. World Health Organization (WHO) officially declared the novel coronavirus outbreak a pandemic. In Canada, there are 93 confirmed coronavirus cases, and one coronavirus-related death. Public Health Canada has informed Canadians that the public health risk is low for the general population and that the risk to Canadians going abroad is destination dependent. Airline passengers arriving from abroad are asked questions about their health before passing through customs, and anyone arriving from China, Italy and Iran -- where there are major virus outbreaks --- are require to provide contact information upon arrival, are given leaflets advising them to self-isolate for 14 days. They are also advised to contact their local public health authority within 24 hours of their arrival.

Thursday, March 12, 2020

Public Service Planning: With the novel coronavirus continuing to spread to countries around the globe, the Treasury Board Secretariat has been preparing for the possibility that the coronavirus might invade the Canadian Public Service -- 287,000 members --- at some point. At present, Treasury Board is convinced that the COVID-19 poses little health risk to federal government bureaucrats, but there is an immediate concern with respect to foreign service employees of Global Affairs Canada who are serving in countries where there is a high risk of contacting the coronavirus. The concern is particularly acute with respect to foreign service officers over 65 years of age, and those with compromised immune systems and/or underlying medical conditions. These Global Affairs staff working abroad, and their families, have been warned against travelling, and have been encouraged to take 'reasonable precautions', while getting on with their work and their lives.

Public servants have been told that they should "practice hand hygiene regularly", and cough and sneeze etiquette, and that they should notify their supervisor and stay home "if you are becoming sick". However, the Professional Institute of the Public Service union has expressed a concern about the work culture of offices dominated by older males that frown on sick leave. It is one of the 'problems' that the government will need to overcome: to get older male employees to stay home from work when they are not feeling well.

A concern of the two major government unions – the Professional Institute of Public Service (PIPS) and Public Service Alliance of Canada (PSAC) – is whether employees who become sick and are forced to self-isolated at home for two weeks, will be receive their regular pay or will have the quarantine counted against their sick leave entitlement. Treasury Board is requiring managers to prepare contingencies plans for the maintenance of essential frontline services with respect to various scenarios in contemplation where anywhere from 10 to 30 or, at worst, even 50 percent of employees absent with a virus infection. Treasury Board has declared that individual deputy ministers are "accountable for the health and safety of their employees", but that the Treasury Board would be providing policy guidance.

Good Hygiene Practice: A microbiologist at the University of Manitoba was asked by Postmedia News to comment on how to practice good hygiene to prevent the spread of the coronavirus. While recognizing that little is known about the coronavirus, the recommendation focussed on 'the tried and true'. The best defence was judged to be soap and water because "viruses are contained inside a fatty protective membrane that is detergent soluble. Soap breaks apart the outer layer and the virus is split apart". Liquid soap was recommended for surfaces, and bar soap for the skin. All that is required is to "get a good build-up of suds" to inactivate the virus on any surface.

It was also recommended that people avoid touching their face in public after touching common surfaces, that a portable hand-sanitizers – of 60 percent alcohol or higher content – be carried and used, and that hands be washed frequently, whenever possible.

(Health Canada recommends a frequent washing of hands with soap and water "for at least 20 seconds", and especially after using the washroom or before preparing food.)

Public Health Pronouncements: As of yesterday, when the World Health Organization formally declared the COVID-19 virus threat a 'pandemic', 118,000 cases were reported in upwards of 114 countries, with the virus continuing to spread at a surprising rate. In Canada, criticism is growing of the federal Liberal government for its failure to offer business a significant fiscal stimulus amidst business closures, and for its failure to provide public health guidance to Canadians on how best to protect themselves from the threat of a coronavirus infection.

The federal government has yet to provide any advice or guidance as to what activities should be closed down to prevent the spread of the coronavirus, other than to advocate that individuals maintain a social distancing of two metres from others whenever practicable. However, when that social distancing is not possible, then what? When questioned by reporters, the Minister of Health, Patty Hajdu said the decision on closing venues where there are gatherings of people should be made at the provincial or municipal level. Moreover, Hajdu added that people do not need to stay home unless they are sick, and for most people, the COVID-19 is no worse than a cold or catching the flu.

Contrary to the assertions of the Health Minister, it is known that the coronavirus is ten times more deadly than the conventional flu virus. A National Post journalist, Sharon Kirkey, has provided an overview of what is known to date about the coronavirus threat. What epidemiologists are saying is that the key to stopping the spread of the coronavirus is to keep the number of persons infected to an average of less than one for all infected carriers, which will stop the spread of the virus. However, there are several recognized problems: it is clear that infected persons can be asymptomatic as well as symptomatic, which makes it difficult to identify who is spreading the disease; and it appears that infected persons who are pre-symptomatic, can infect others up to three days before they show any symptoms.

There is a general agreement that an aggressive policy of social distancing can achieve what is being called "a flattening of the curve" of new infections. Among the social distancing measures being recommended by public health authorities in many countries are encouraging people to work from home, the closing down of major sport and concert venues, the avoiding of large gatherings, shopping at off-peak hours, and the closing of schools. Few cases of children becoming infected with the coronavirus have been reported, and children appear to be only minimally symptomatic, but it is expected – based on the 'flu' experience -- that children are potentially super spreaders of the coronavirus disease and should be kept at home in isolation.

In Canada, some epidemiologists are claiming that there is 'a low risk of infection in Canada right now'. That statement might be literally true, at this moment, but the statement is disconcerting in its implication for government policy. One of the key principles of the federal pandemic plan is that 'any imposed restrictions on individuals must be proportional to the magnitude of the threat'. Clearly, this principle is inhibiting Canada Public Health from dictating measures to limit the spread of the coronavirus – such as the imposition of a social spacing policy, and mandatory testing of returning travellers at airports – with the coronavirus risk to Canadian held to be 'low'. (Of course, this comment implies that the federal Liberal government would act if the health threat to Canadians were greater, but given its 'hands off approach' in leaving the combatting of the coronavirus to the provinces, it is doubtful that the federal government will take decisive action under any circumstance.)

When questioned further by Opposition MPs -- on March 12th -- as to how many Canadians might become infected with the coronavirus, the Health Minister, Patty Hajdu, refused to speculate, but did mention that modelling suggests that anywhere "from 30 to 70 percent" might become infected. When queried as to whether Canada has sufficient medical supplies to deal with such an epidemic, she replied: "We're planning to buy more supplies", but 'our efforts are about flattening the curve of cases, so that the health system isn't suddenly overwhelmed'. "The intention is to ensure that everyone doesn't get sick at once".

(This is an odd health strategy. There is no emphasis on eliminating the virus, or on completely stopping its spread, but rather the emphasis is on slowing the spread of the virus, and its impact over time, to enable the existing public health resources to dealt with it. In effect, to keep the number of cases from surging out of control until a vaccine can be developed; yet experts are saying it could take anywhere up to three years to develop, test, approve, and distribute a vaccine. At present the federal government health policy is based on calling on Canadians to practice social spacing and a frequent washing of hands, and on advising them to 'stay at home'.)

Sophie Grégoire Trudeau: On Thursday, March 12th, Sophie Trudeau, the wife of Prime Minister Justin Trudeau, returned from a speaking engagement in London on behalf of the WE Charity. She tested positive for a coronavirus infection upon her return. Mrs. Trudeau and the Prime Minister have gone into self-isolation at 'Rideau Cottage' in Ottawa, on the grounds of the Governor-General's residence.

Chinese Lockdown: In China, the coronavirus epidemic has been brought under control with a strict lockdown-quarantine of the City of Wuhan (11 million population), and the surrounding Hubei Province, as well as several other threatened regions of China. A description of the Chinese quarantine in operation has been provided by a Canadian teacher residing in the City of Wuxi (over 6.5 million population), in Jiangsu Province, which has been locked down.

Under the Chinese government lockdown, every person entering the City of Wuxi has to submit to a health screening and an infrared temperature check scan, and anyone with an elevated temperature has to report to a viral treatment centre. Only residents of the city are permitted to enter, and returning citizens are subject to a two-week mandatory quarantine, with regular inspections and temperature checks, and food delivered to the door. Entry to all businesses and public buildings requires a temperature check, and the presentation of a code, issued by the Health Bureau, that the individual is in good health.

Residents of apartment towers need to provide proof of residency, undergo a temperature check in the lobby when entering, and no visitors are allowed into the building. Nothing is touched in the lobby, and elevator buttons are pressed with the apartment door key. Many restaurants have remained open for takeout, and where indoor restaurant service has remained open, diners are seated at least a metre apart with no one opposite them. Curfews keep everyone indoors from 10pm to 5am each day.

Grocery stores remained open, and are busy with customers wearing face masks, but groceries can be ordered, and delivered to the entry gate of a building for pickup. After picking up the groceries, they are washed thoroughly, and hands are washed also. Entertainment for the shut-ins is provided by watching TV, access to the Internet, playing cards, and reading. As reported by the Canadian expatriate, as of March 12th, the Province of Jiangsu has not had a single new coronavirus case for two weeks in a provincial population of over 80 million.

Trump Travel Ban: In the United States, President Donald Trump made a surprise announcement yesterday -- Wednesday, March 11th -- that a 30-day travel ban will be imposed, as of midnight Friday, on European travellers entering the United States. All foreign nationals residing in, or having travelled to, 26 European countries will be banned, with the sole exception of citizens of the United Kingdom -- because of the effectiveness of its National Health Service (NHS). (Earlier, back in February, the United States banned travellers from China and Iran in response to the severe coronavirus outbreaks in those countries.) The new ban on travellers from Europe, does not apply to American citizens and permanent residents returning home, but does apply to tourists, short-term visitors, immigrants, and visa-holders. Flights from overseas will be directed to thirteen American international hub airports where incoming passengers will be visually screened for symptoms of the coronavirus.

Domestically, the Trump administration is being criticized for its failure to follow the example of South Korea, in acquiring testing kits for use at the international airports. In response to the expression of fears by other countries that President Trump intended to impose a trade embargo, the White House later clarified that international trade and commercial traffic would be exempted from the border closure ban.

In Europe, officials of the European Union have strongly condemned the severity of the travel ban imposed by President Trump, and there have been accusations that it was "politically motivated". An official statement issued by the European Union declared that: "The Coronavirus is a global crisis, not limited to any continent, and it requires cooperation rather than unilateral action". In Britain, a high government official was quoted as stating that "scientific evidence does not support travel restrictions", and in the United States, a senior director of the Wilson Center think tank – the Woodrow Wilson International Center -- expressed a concern that 'banning international visitors could have deeper implications for globalization and the unfettered movement of goods and people around the globe'.

(Apparently, according to the Modern liberals who dominate our government institutions, any government that responds to the demands of its people for protection against the importation of a deadly foreign virus, is acting from 'political motives', rather than from an objective, scientifically-sound rationale. Yet, at present, science has provided little reliable information or guidance on how to combat the spread of the coronavirus. To date, it is political action by nation states that has managed to slow the spread of the coronavirus, not science.)

In response to the Trump border closure policy, Canadian business leaders are encouraging Prime Minister Trudeau to keep potential virus carriers out of Canada, but to do so 'without hindering access to the crucial American Market'. Deputy Prime Minister Freeland spoke today with the U.S. Secretary of State, Mike Pompeo, about the efforts that Canada is taking to combat the coronavirus and the strength of the Canadian health-care system. During a subsequent virtual meeting with Prime Minister Trudeau, the Premier of Conservative government of Ontario, Doug Ford, called for Canada to work with the United States to prevent the importation of the coronavirus into North America.

Premier Ford called on the federal government to institute a 'proper screening' – presumably, a testing and quarantining – of foreign nationals entering Canada, while keeping the border with the United States open and "trade flowing back and forth". Alberta Premier Jason Kenney, a former federal Conservative government Immigration Minister, urged the federal government to establish a mandatory quarantine for foreign nationals entering Canada from "countries with a greater risk of infection". The aim is to assure the American government that Canada is doing everything possible to preclude the importation of the coronavirus, and thereby to encourage the American government to refrain from closing their border to Canadians. Such a closure, declared Premier Ford, would be 'the worst blow possible' to the Canadian economy.

Friday, March 13, 2020

Parliament: It was announced early this morning that Parliament will be suspended until April 20th, and that the budget presentation – scheduled for March 30th – will be indefinitely postponed. All parties have agreed that Parliament will be recalled when needed to pass necessary legislation, but with a smaller representation of the parties to preclude all 338 MPs having to fly into Ottawa. The reduced proportional representation of the Members by Party, will also ensure that a physical spacing can be maintained in the Chamber of the House of Commons. Before dissolution, Parliament passed the new NAFTA (USCMA) legislation, and granted the federal Liberal government a needed spending authority.

Trudeau Policy Announcement: To date, the Trudeau government has been widely criticized for its failure to provide leadership and direction in a pending national health crisis. Several newspaper columnists have mentioned that the Canadian public is more aware of the threat posed by the coronavirus than the Liberal government, which to date has rebuffed all demands that the federal government introduce policies to combat the spread of the coronavirus, including the closing of the Canadian border to foreign travellers. However, that perception has now changed somewhat. Today – Friday, March 13th -- Prime Minister Trudeau made a policy announcement that addressed some of the concerns of Canadians.

The Prime Minister revealed that he does not have the coronavirus, but has been in self-isolation with his wife, Sophie, at the 'Rideau Cottage' on the estate of the Governor General in Ottawa. Sophie Grégorie-Trudeau has only a mild coronavirus infection. Then, Trudeau announced new policy initiatives in a TV appearance from a podium in front of the Rideau Cottage, where he stood a good four metres removed from the reporters in attendance. He assured Canadians that he was aware that Canadians are 'worried about their health, about the health of their children, and about their jobs', and he pledged that his government would be taking steps to ensure that "no one would have to worry about paying their rent, buying groceries, or caring for kids or elderly family members".

More immediately, the Prime Minister announced that Canada will be restricting international flights into Canada, will be encouraging all Canadians abroad to return home by commercial carriers, and will be providing financial support for Canadian businesses suffering from the current severe downturn in the financial markets and the dramatic fall in oil prices. Marc Garneau, the Minister of Transport explained further -- in a news release -- that overseas flights to Canada will be limited to landing at a few designated airports; that cruise ships of 500 passengers or more will be banned from Canadian ports; and that no cruise ships will be allowed to stop in the Canadian Arctic this summer, "given the limited health capacity in Canada's northern communities". It was further explained that there will be enhanced screening measures at all ports of entry – land, rail, and marine – which will include a questioning of travellers as to whether they have visited "a high risk country" and a screening for symptoms of COVID-19 . (However, this is simply the visual screening currently applied at Canadian airports. It is not a testing and quarantining program.) No details were provided as to when the new measures will be put in place, or what airports will remain open to foreign travellers entering Canada.

When asked about closing the border, Trudeau responded: that 'at this point', Canada is not closing its borders "with any country", but that could change. "We will make those decisions based on the best science and the best recommendations of our health officials".

Border Closure Issue: Following the new federal government policy announcement by Prime Minister Trudeau, the federal Health Minister, Patty Hajdu, declared that closing the Canadian border could be "counterproductive"; and that "border measures are highly ineffective and, in some cases can create harm". She cited the case of Italy, which shut down its borders at an early date, but now ranks second in the world in the number of confirmed coronavirus cases. (What the Hajdu observation ignores is that the coronavirus was already well established within the population of northern Italy before the border was closed to foreign travellers, and the lockdown implemented.) Furthermore, Hajdu added that when travel bans are enacted "travellers become less honest about where they've come from, where they've travelled to, and what their symptoms may be". (In effect, the argument being presented is that because a travel ban cannot be 100 percent effective, therefore borders should be left open. It is truly unbelievable!) On the other hand, Hajdu exclaimed that the government is well aware that the coronavirus presents "a serious public health threat and a crisis, as well as an emergency, and everybody is working as diligently as possible to contain the spread globally".

The Modern liberals of the Trudeau government have an 'open borders', 'free movement of people and goods', mindset that is overruling common sense and the experience of other countries in closing their borders to foreign travellers to limit the importation of the coronavirus. Earlier, on February 1st, in response to demands by the Opposition parties that a ban be placed on travellers from China to protect Canadians from the importation of the coronavirus, the Liberal government had denounced that demand as being 'discriminatory', and that it would 'stigmatize Chinese people'. Subsequently, on February 3rd, when the United States and Australia acted to ban the entry of foreigner who had travelled to China, Patty Hajdu, the Health Minister, denounced several prominent Conservatives who were calling for a similar ban. She accused them of being guilty of "the spread of misinformation and fear across Canadian society" and demanded that the Opposition parties "not sensationalize the risk to Canadians".

At that time, the Chief of Public Health Canada Agency, Dr. Theresa Tam, publicly endorsed the position of the World Health Organization (WHO), which "advises against any kind of travel and trade restrictions" and said that "they are inappropriate and could actually cause more harm than good in terms of our global effort to contain the disease". (It boggles the mind that a public health authority in Canada, and the WHO, are engaging in such absurd thinking. One suspects that the WHO is more concerned about the economic impact on Third World countries of travel bans by the countries of the developed world. It would be destructive of tourism -- the life blood of the economy of many Third World countries.)

With respect to the upcoming Spring Break, the federal government has been silent as to what Canadians ought to do. However, Patty Hajdu has suggested that Canadians consider "a staycation" -- a vacation at home. In the strongest statement made to date, she advised Canadians that for Public Health Canada, all travel outside of Canada is "considered a high-risk for Canadians right now". Canadians returning from abroad, and visitors, were advised to self-isolate for 14-days following their arrival in Canada.

The Conservative Opposition in Parliament has been criticizing the Liberal government for failing to test people who arrive in Canada from the three countries that have a major coronavirus outbreak: China, Iran, and Italy. The Conservatives are arguing that the current Liberal government policy of providing new arrivals with a pamphlet advocating self-isolation for 14-days, and screening out the travellers who have visual symptoms of an coronavirus infection, does little to protect Canadians from asymptomatic carriers who neglect to self-quarantine.

(At present, it is known that many individuals infected with COVID-19 are asymptomatic and can spread the virus in circulating within the community, which undermine all efforts to flatten the curve of new infections. It is not known what percentage of infected persons are asymptomatic, or how contagious an asymptomatic person may be, but it is a matter of serious concern or ought to be.)

At present, Public Health Canada has revealed that out of 103 confirmed cases of COVID-19 in Canada, 79 percent were travellers from abroad, and a further 12 percent were in close contact with travellers from abroad. Only 9 percent of new cases are currently attributable to an in-community infection transmission.

U.S. National Emergency: On Friday, with the ban coming into effect of foreign nationals travelling to the United States from Europe, President Trump declared a state of national emergency which enables the Federal Emergency Management Agency (FEMA) to provide $50 billion in disaster relief funds to state and local governments, and to deploy support teams, in the effort to combat the spread of the coronavirus. The President also stated that the federal government was partnering with private companies to accelerate the production of testing kits; and that initially five million testing kits would be produced. However, Americans were cautioned not to seek to be tested unless they were experiencing symptoms. It was also announced that Walmart Inc. will be setting up drive-thru testing centres in their store parking lots, and that Google Inc. had agreed to create a website portal that will enable individuals to determine – through answering a series of health questions -- whether they need to be tested.

Saturday, March 14, 2020

Coronavirus Threat: In Europe, epidemiologists are worried that the coronavirus may sweep northward and westward from Italy. Mathematical modelling of the virus infections spread has revealed the potential of a sharp upwards trajectory of infections in Spain, France, Germany, and Britain. If unchecked, the number of infections more than doubles -- at a contagion increase rate of 2.5 on average -- every five days. In the case of Spain, which currently has 3,000 coronavirus cases, the number of cases could reach 250,000 in a month, based on the current unrestrained rate of new infections. Epidemiologists are denouncing the lack of urgency on the part of European governments in wasting valuable time that is needed to confront the coronavirus threat.

In defiance of the European Union leadership, on Friday Denmark announced that it would unilaterally close its borders the next day (Saturday) – the second European country to do so, after Italy. All travellers, vacationers, and foreigners, who "cannot demonstrate a creditable reason' for entering the country will be turned away at the border. Danish citizens and foreign workers will be able to enter and leave the country, as well as all essential transport goods, inclusive of foods, medicines, and industrial products. Denmark (5.7 million population) has 801 confirmed coronavirus cases to date, and no deaths.

Sunday, March 15, 2020

Personal Protective Equipment: A website portal of the Department of Public Services and Procurement has a request for proposals posted for Canadians companies that can manufacture surgical face masks, N-95 respiratory masks, surgical gloves, hand-sanitizers and other medical supplies.

Travel Ban Demand: For a week or more, the Trudeau government has been under pressure from the Opposition parties in Parliament, and a growing public opinion, to close Canada's border to foreign travellers to prevent any further introduction of the coronavirus from abroad. In particular, the Health Minister of British Columbia has sent a strong message to the federal Liberal government urging a border closure with the United States. American visitors are pouring over the border from

Washington State – an area with a high coronavirus infection rate --to shop and bar hop in Vancouver and take to advantage of the low 70-cent Canadian dollar.

To date, the Liberal government has done nothing beyond a visual screening of new arrivals for coronavirus symptoms, and the placing of signs and the distribution of pamphlets at airports and border entry points to advise anyone entering Canada that they must self-isolate for 14 days. After resisting all demands to close the Canadian border, today -- Sunday, March 15th -- Prime Minister Trudeau commented in an interview that the question of whether to close the border to foreign travellers was "up for discussion" in Cabinet. He added that "things are changing fast"; and that the action of President Donald Trump in closing the American border "gives us things to think about".

On her part, Dr. Theresa Tam, the Chief Public Health Officer Canada, continues to be opposed to a border closure. She maintains that Canada must maintain an "essential movement of people and services", and that the closure of borders "has not worked in other countries" in limiting the spread of the coronavirus. For Dr. Tam, the coronavirus pandemic is "a societal phenomenon" that requires people to be personally socially responsible in their actions; that travellers arriving in Canada cannot be forced to self-isolate; and that public health authorities cannot monitor every traveller. "Public Health is going to do what it can".

(Here is a complete abdication of authority and responsibility on the part of the federal Liberal government and the federal public health authority. There is no commitment to closing the border to minimize the importation of the coronavirus, no commitment to taking action to keep the coronavirus from spreading within Canada, and no commitment to use the emergency powers of the federal government -- in a national health emergency -- to impose a compulsory testing and mandatory quarantine on anyone who tests positive with an especial focus on any travellers entering Canada, inclusive of returning Canadians and permanent residents. The federal Liberal government has a rather passive view of the role of public health authorities, and is leaving it up foreign travellers, Canadians, and permanent residents, to do the right thing in self-isolating on entering Canada from abroad, and/or when feeling ill.)

Monday, March 16, 2020

Canadian Travel Ban: This afternoon, March 16th, Prime Minister Trudeau reversed the earlier position of his government and announced a decision to partially close the border. The federal government will impose a ban on foreign travellers entering Canada, effective on March 18th, inclusive of a ban on sick people travelling into the country. Canadians are being encouraged to cancel all non-essential travel outside of the country, and Canadians abroad are being encouraged to return home.

Travellers from the United States are exempt from the border crossing ban. Otherwise, Canada will refuse entry to all international visitors, except for diplomats and flight crews. Only Canadian citizens and permanent residents, and their families, will be allowed to enter the country, and they are being advised to self-isolate for fourteen days following their return.

The Trudeau government has stated its intention to mandate that airlines must apply 'a basic health test' to assess whether returning Canadian citizens and American visitors might be infected. Americans who test positive will not be permitted to enter Canada, and Canadians who are infected will be encouraged to seek health care in the United States rather than returning to Canada. How such a mandate is to be enforced, and what particular 'basic health test' is to be applied, remains unspecified. At the same time, the Trudeau government has announced that all international flights from overseas bringing Canadians home, will be redirected to just four airports: Montreal, Toronto, Calgary, and Vancouver, to ensure passenger screening. Within Canada, Canadians are being advised to "stay at home" as much as possible to avoid spreading the disease.

Prime Minister, Justin Trudeau, declared that Canada is taking a 'step by step approach' to the coronavirus crisis as it developed. However, every day his government has proven itself incapable of taking control of the situation. There is a lack of follow up to enforce new requirements on travellers, a reliance on the provincial and municipal governments to deal with the public health crisis, and a dependence on the willingness of Canadians to self-isolate to contain the spread of the virus within Canada.

Today, the Public Safety Minister, Bill Blair, declared that the four airports were ready to inform Canadians arriving from overseas that they need to self-quarantine for 14 days; yet, there are reports that passengers arriving at the Toronto Pearson Airport are not being screened or informed of the necessity to self-quarantine. In Montreal, the Quebec provincial government has sent provincial public servants to the international airport to distribute leaflets to inform incoming passengers of the need to self-quarantine for 14 days. A letter to the editor in the Ottawa Citizen newspaper has asked: 'Are the over 300,000 immigrants who enter Canada each year being tested at the border?' If not, how many more Canadians will become infected from carries of the virus within these new arrivals?'

(Why the Trudeau government is leaving the U.S.-Canadian border fully open and encouraging some 430,000 Canadians travelling abroad who have entered their names in the Registration of Canadians Abroad database, or the three million Canadian expatriates who are living and working abroad, to return home from foreign countries currently in the grip of a widespread coronavirus pandemic is beyond comprehension.

It will facilitate the further conveyance of the coronavirus into Canada, and will result in the four airports that are open to receiving overseas flights, being jammed with returning Canadians who will be put at risk to catch the virus; it will further overload Canadians hospitals and the provincial health care systems; and it will introduce and spread the coronavirus among Canadian communities. It would be far better for expatriate Canadians to stay in the countries where they are settled, and Canadians visitors abroad to stay there, and to practice social distancing. One approach might be to insist that no Canadian abroad can access an airline flight home unless they are tested for the virus and wearing a proper face mask to prevent any transfer of a coronavirus infection by an asymptomatic carrier to others in the close confines of an aircraft cabin.)

There are currently 324 Canadians infected with COVID-19 – mostly in Ontario and British Columbia, with a smaller number of cases in Alberta and Quebec. There have been eight confirmed deaths.

In the Middle East and Europe, the countries suffering the most from a major wave of coronavirus infections are Iran (Tehran), Italy (northern

Italy), and France (Paris). France is the latest European country to impose a national lockdown to control the spread of the coronavirus. Restaurants, cafes, bars, and cinemas are now closed, as well as libraries, shopping malls, and sports venues, with only essential businesses – primarily food stores and gas stations – remaining open. However, in European countries there is no enforce quarantine of residents, in contrast to the situation in China. In Europe, the emphasis is on individuals to self-isolate once the public facilities are locked down with the people being encouraged by government to 'stay home'.

Initial Virus Threat Response: To date, the federal government has taken no particular action to combat the spread of the coronavirus, other than an ineffectual effort to visually screen passengers arriving at the four designated airports. The federal Chief Medical Officer of Health, Dr. Theresa Tam, has stated that the Public Health Agency of Canada provides guidance to the provinces, but that it is up to each province to decide how to respond to the coronavirus crisis. In effect, the federal government has taken the stand that public health is a provincial responsibility under the Constitution. Yet, over past decades, federal governments have continually intervened in public health issues, and the federal government is able to readily take control of the national health crisis by enacting the Emergency Measures Act (the former War Measures Act). What Dr. Tam is ignoring is that international airports are under federal government jurisdiction.

Tuesday, March 17, 2020

The Province of Ontario has declared a State of Emergency and has ordered the closing of indoor recreational programs, public libraries, theatres, cinemas, private schools – public schools were closed earlier, on March 14th – and daycares. Bars and restaurants can remain open, but only for takeout services. Gatherings of more than 50 persons are banned. Moreover, Ontarians are being encouraged to stay home to avoid contacting or spreading the virus. Ontario has begun testing for the coronavirus, with a focus on individuals who are exhibiting severe symptoms of illness, the aged, and those with underlying health problems who are deemed most at risk. However, testing in Ontario is reportedly quite limited owing to a shortage of the nasal swabs used in the coronavirus testing kits. (On March 28th, the ban on large public gatherings was extended to forbid gatherings of over five persons.)

Quebec was the first province to declare a State of Emergency and to introduce a provincial lockdown to impose a physical spacing, which it did on March 15th.

Wednesday, March 18, 2020

Coronavirus Update: Today, Public Health Canada reported that there were 690 confirmed cases of the coronavirus in Canada, of which 69 percent could be traced directly to infection by someone who had travelled outside of Canada and conveyed the virus home, and a further 13 percent were infected by someone who had been in close contact with a recent traveller from abroad. In effect, 82 percent of the COVID-19 infections are traceable directly to travellers returning home to Canada, which means that the imported virus has already spread within Canadian communities. Local community transmission is currently accounting for 18 percent of the individuals infected with the virus. To date, there are nine deaths attributable to the coronavirus in Canada. Most of the travellers, who have conveyed the virus to Canada, are known to have visited China or, in a substantial number of cases, had visited Italy which is another country that is being ravaged by a widespread coronavirus outbreak.

U.S. Border Closure: Common sense has finally prevailed within the federal Liberal government. Canada and the United States have agreed to close their common border to non-essential travel as of Saturday, March 21st. Canadians will still be able to return home, but only commercial traffic would be allowed to cross the border to keep open critical supply chains. Why the government finally took such an obvious and sensible step, after the Liberal Health Minister, Patty Hajdu, had unequivocally rejected a border closure as an "ineffective" response to limiting the spread of the virus, remains unexplained. Two days earlier, on March 16th, Prime Minister Trudeau had finally announced that Canada was closing its border to international travellers as of March 18th. However, at that time he had made an exception in keeping the American border open. Now, Americans visitors will be banned as well.

When he announced two-days earlier that the Canadian border would be closed to international travellers on March 18th, with the exemption of Americans, Prime Minister Trudeau failed to explain to Canadians why refugees from all over the world were continuing to enter Canada during the coronavirus pandemic in the weeks prior to the planned closure of the border to international travellers. The Liberal government had asserted that any refugees arriving in Canada who tested positive for the coronavirus would be placed in quarantine for fourteen days, but with apparently no follow up to ensure that there was actually a testing system in place at the international airports. Moreover, there was no recognition that the existing testing system – taking nasal swabs for analysis in a laboratory -- takes several days to attain results. The exposure of Canadians to the coronavirus, and doctors, nurses, and hospital personnel to the virus through the arrival of infected refugees, is apparently not a concern of the Liberal government.

Thursday, March 19, 2020

Illegal Migrants: It has become known also that the federal Liberal government has not taken any steps to block the entry of illegal migrants into Canada through the Roxham Road crossing on the Quebec/New York border. Apparently, the Liberal government has no concern about illegal migrants continuing to enter Canada who have not, and will not be, screened for coronavirus symptoms or tested for the virus.

That situation changed today in response to public criticism. Prime Minister Trudeau was asked by reporters to explain why the 'irregular border crossing' on Roxham Road near Saint-Bernard-de-Lacolle, Quebec, had not been closed to stop illegal migrants entering Canada. He declared that anyone entering Canada at the Roxham Road crossing -- whom he referred to as "asylum seekers" -- will be placed in quarantine for 14-days upon entry into Canada. Apparently, the fact that these so-called "asylum seekers" are law breakers and queue jumpers who are entering Canada illegally without undergoing any health screening, or check for a criminal record, is not an issue for young Trudeau. To date, while the coronavirus is raging in China and western Europe, the number of illegal migrants entering Canada at the Roxham Road crossing is now about 80 peoples per day, which is a significant increase from the 50 to 60 average number of daily crossings two weeks ago.

Friday, March 20, 2020

Illegal Migrants: Today, Prime Minister Trudeau in continuing his ad hoc, seat-of-the-pants response of the federal Liberal government to the coronavirus epidemic, reversed himself at the podium. He declared that the "irregular border crossers" are going to be treated the same as all foreign travellers. They would be turned away at the border. It boggles the mind. How could Prime Minister Trudeau not have seen earlier that allowing illegal migrants, whom he calls "asylum seekers" and "irregular border-crossers" to enter Canada in a clear violation of our immigration laws, and pose a serious threat to the health of Canadians in the absence of any screening or testing? Thankfully, a modicum of common sense has finally prevailed in Liberal La La Land.

Treating illegal migrants entering Canada as immigrants or "irregular asylum seekers" is a travesty that is insulting to legitimate refugees and immigrants who come to Canada legally in respecting Canada's immigration laws and immigration regulations. The Liberal government under Prime Minister Trudeau ignores Canadian law, and the well-being of Canadians in letting illegal migrants enter Canada without impediment, and then treats the illegal migrant as refugees, rather than illegal migrants. They have already passed through a so-called third country, the United States, where they could have made a refugee claim and hence, they are not legitimate refugees in entering Canada under the United Nations regulations.

What is particularly galling is that the illegal migrants are not only allowed to stay in Canada, but legal council is provided by Canada for the individual to challenge Canada's immigration laws and regulations in claiming that they do not apply to them. This situation is beyond belief. If Canadian laws declare that anyone who just shows up at the border is ineligible to enter Canada, then that person is ineligible, and should be refused entry. Moreover, migrants who cross the border illegally should be immediately apprehended and summarily deported back to their home country.,

What is equally disconcerting, is how can our federal Liberal government be so detached from the reality of the threat of the coronavirus being transmitted from country to country, to have neglected to take steps, weeks ago, to close the border to all foreign travellers. Unfortunately, the spread of the virus in Canada has now reached the stage where a growing number of Canadians are becoming infected through local community transmission, in having no apparent contact with a traveller from overseas.

As for the Liberal Press, columnists are praising Justin Trudeau for 'getting it right' in closing Canada's borders to foreign travellers, and for supposedly being prepared 'to do what it takes' to combat the spread of the Coronavirus. What the Liberal Press is neglecting to mention is that for well over a month the Conservative Party opposition has been calling for the federal government to close the border to foreign travellers, and has been demanding that the federal government take decisive actions to curb the spread of the coronavirus among Canadians, while the Liberal federal government has continued to dither.

Peter MacKay, a leading contender for the Conservative Party leadership, has demanded: that Canada close its borders to all non-essential travel – no tourists or cruise ship dockings; that only returning Canadians and necessary goods be allowed to enter the country; that there be a mandatory 14-day isolation period for Canadians returning home; that Employment Insurance benefits be made available immediately for anyone who was forced to stay off work to prevent the virus transmission; that zero-interest loans be provided to businesses negatively affected by the Coronavirus crisis; that the federal government doubling of the carbon tax on April 1st be aborted to help restraint any rise in prices; and that the tax filing deadline be extended.

Erin O'Toole, another leading contender for the Conservative party leadership, has been advocating that the Trudeau government invoke the Emergency Measures Act (former War Measures Act) to empower the government to prohibit foreign travel, enforce self-isolation of Canadians returning home and to control assemblies; that the Canadian Armed Forces be mobilized to assist in the health care sector and in other areas – presumably employing military medical personnel in testing and treating the sick, in establishing and manning quarantine stations, and in conveying sick travellers to quarantine stations -- and that Canadian industry be mobilized to ramp up the production of ventilators to meet that critical shortage, as well as government financial support be provided to research scientists to speed work on the development of an antidote.

Derek Sloan, another Conservative leadership contender, has been calling for weeks for the federal Liberal government to immediate close Canada's border to foreign travellers, for the imposing of a testing system to detect the presence of the coronavirus among returning Canadians, and for the immediate closure of the 'Roxham Road' crossing by which illegal migrants were entering Canada.

Dr. Leslyn Lewis (Juris Doctorate), another contender for the Conservative Party leadership, has criticized the Trudeau government for failing to show leadership during the coronavirus crisis, and has been questioning why the government neglected to impose a quarantine on travel to and from China -- "on day one" -- as soon as it became known that China was the source of the Coronavirus outbreak and the critical threat that the virus posed to the health and life of anyone contacting it.

Taiwan Response: In Taiwan, with a population of over 23 million and close travel ties with China, the coronavirus spread has been contained by an activist government that established a centralize command centre in late December, on first learning of the seriousness of the coronavirus outbreak in China. The command centre was in operation before even the first COVID-19 infection was reported in Taiwan on January 23rd. As early as late December, health officials began boarding and inspecting passengers on incoming flights from Wuhan for signs of a fever or pneumonia symptoms. Individuals who appeared ill were isolated and tested for the virus while being held in isolation.

Among the general population, anyone using their health card to obtain health care for any illness was screened for symptoms of the coronavirus, their travel history was gathered; and those with severe respiratory symptoms were tested for the coronavirus. Those who tested positive for the virus were put into a mandatory 14-day quarantine, with officials, wearing protective gear, responsible for checking on them and providing any assistance required and the contacts of quarantined persons were tracked down and tested. Quarantined individuals were given a government-issue cell phone with an app that enabled officials to employ cell phone tracking to ensure that the sick and asymptomatic carriers of the virus remained in quarantine, with heavy fines being imposed on anyone breaking the quarantine.

The Taiwanese were told to refrain from going abroad, unless it was absolutely necessary; and residents returning home from high-risk areas, who showed no visible signs of flu or pneumonia-like symptoms were required to self-isolate for 14-days. As soon as it was ascertained that some visitors to Taiwan from China, Europe and Africa were testing positive for the coronavirus, the government banned all foreigners from flying into the country.

Later, it was revealed that the Taiwanese had developed a simple, but effective method of detecting individual infected with the coronavirus. Individuals were told to hold their breathe for ten seconds without coughing. Anyone with the virus in their lungs could not do so. The Taiwanese were also using hand-held temperature screening devices to assist in identifying the sick during their initial screening of passengers on incoming planes.

Through such prompt and decisive measures, the government of Taiwan managed to contain and almost completely prevent the spread of the coronavirus into that country. As of March 15th, there were only 48 confirmed cases of coronavirus in Taiwan, and only one death due to the virus. Life in Taiwan has remained completely normal with schools, offices, and factories remaining open, as well as restaurants, recreation facilities, and cafés. Patrons entering public places are simply required to have their temperature taken and to disinfect their hands with a sanitizer before being granted entry.

In Taiwan, there is a government in power with traditional conservative values – in Canada, Tory conservatives values -- prepared to use the authority of the state for the protection of the general population by taking charge -- in the face of a threat of the importation of a foreign virus -- to install controls over the lives and travel of its citizens through initiating mandatory testing and quarantining, and ultimately a total ban on foreigners entering the country. In contrast, the discipline adverse Modern liberal government of Justin Trudeau has appealed to Canadians to self-isolate, has called on Canadians to get themselves tested –how that is to be done given the severe shortage of testing kits remains unexplained – and has rather belatedly ordered Canada's airports to be close to foreign visitors with no follow up to ensure that the order is being strictly enforced. Moreover, Canadians returning home are not being tested for the virus. Prime Minster Trudeau has simply advised Canadians to "Go Home. Stay Home".

Liberal Press Bias: The contrast between the success of the Taiwanese government in containing the Coronavirus and the abject failure of the Liberal government of Canada to take positive action at an early date to prevent, or to limit in so far as possible, the entry of the coronavirus into Canada and to contain the spread of the Coronavirus once present, is readily apparent. Yet, the International Liberal Press is praising young Trudeau for his courage in finally closing Canada's borders, and is touting his ad hoc responses to the coronavirus crisis as being admirable.

"Closing borders and banning foreigners is deeply contrary to Trudeau's brand as a champion of progressive globalism, and he deserves credit for subordinating his ideological considerations to rational crisis management – even if the piecemeal ways such policies have been rolled out will continue to invite criticism." (J.J. McCullough, *The Washington Post*, March 18, 2020.)

Financial Aid Packages: At the same time as the Trudeau government finally acted to close the borders of Canada to foreign travellers, the economic cost to Canadians of the failure to quarantine China during the early stages of the outbreak in that country -- back in late January-February 2020 – is becoming apparent. On March 18th, the Trudeau government announced an $82-billion financial aid package for Canadians. It augments the $1 billion promised earlier to combat the spread of the coronavirus, fifty percent of which was intended to support provincial health care efforts.

The greatly expanded economic aid package is intended to support Canadians suffering from the negative economic impact of the shutdowns that are being imposed by the provinces in seeking to stave off a coronavirus epidemic. Already manufacturers, tourism, airlines, retail stores, restaurants, theatres, and hotels, and their employees, have been extremely hard hit by the provincial shutdowns, as well as the oil and natural gas industries which were already suffering from cripplingly low crude oil prices owing to the actions of OPEC in flooding the market with oil in its production limits dispute with Russia.

The new economic aid package of the Liberal government will include increases in the Canada Child Benefit payments to families of $300 per child per month ($2 billion cost), the establishing of an Emergency Support Benefit for laid-off workers who do not qualify for employment insurance (cost $5 billion), an Emergency Care Benefit to provide quarantined workers with $900 weekly for up to 15 weeks (cost $10 billion), a one-time Goods and Services Tax credit to low income families worth $400 to eligible individuals and $600 per couple, subsidies to small businesses covering ten percent of payroll costs and a partial payment of ten percent of the wages of employees, up to $1,375 per month maximum, for four months to encourage employers to keep their staff on the payroll during closures, and a six-month pause in student loan repayments.

In addition, the Business Development Bank of Canada and Export Development Canada will extend credit to businesses in need of financial aid (cost $5 billion), and $300-million in new funding is to be made available to First Nation communities to address their 'immediate needs'. Lastly, the deadline for filing income tax returns will be postponed until June 1st, and the paying of any taxes owed will be deferred until August 31st to ease the immediate financial burden on taxpayers.

Whether the federal government financial aid package will prove anywhere near adequate to keep the Canadian economy from totally collapsing during the lockdown period, remains to be seen. What is evident is that the closure of businesses and industries is imposing a far higher cost on the economy than the actual health care costs involved in treating patients sick with the Coronavirus.

Indigenous Financial Aid: As part of the $82 billion financial aid package, the federal government will provide $305 million in support of an Indigenous Communities Support Fund. At present, there are no cases of the COVID-19 among Indigenous communities. The monies are to enable the communities to prepare to manage any future outbreaks. Some far northern and fly-in First Nations are considered high risk for major outbreaks because of residential overcrowding, the prevalence of diabetes and other medical conditions, and a shortage of nurses. In Ontario, a Grand Chief has called for the government to conduct on-reserve testing because of many people on the reserves find it difficult to get to urban centers. There are drivers, but the concern is that they might not want to expose themselves to the virus by driving to urban centres during the COVID-19 epidemic.

How the $305 million in funding will be distributed remains unclear. The Finance Minister, Bill Morneau, stated that the intention is to have funds 'in place to respond to any situation faced by Indigenous communities, as the pandemic unfolds across the country'; and that the federal government intends to work with Indigenous communities "to figure out the details".

Additional financial support is also available to Indigenous communities across Canada. Last week, Prime Minister Trudeau announced that Indigenous communities will be able to draw from a $100 million envelope that is part of a $1 billion federal government investment to enhance public health measures.

Border Closures: As of March 18th, the European Union leadership began to discuss whether to shut Europe's external borders to travellers. The problem is that what was once a sensible and practical policy to prevent the Coronavirus entering Europe, is now no longer a viable option for stemming the spread of the virus. Travellers from foreign countries have already conveyed the virus into Europe where it is now well established and is spreading locally. The financial costs involved in the effort to offset the negative economic impact of the shutdowns imposed to contain the spread of the Coronavirus within each country, is staggering. It is evidenced by the national financial aid packages proposed by various countries: Spain, $150 billion; Britain, $584 billion; Italy, $39 billion; and France, $545 billion; as well as the United States, $850 billion.

The lesson that the spread of the Coronavirus teaches is the dangers inherent in the Modern liberal concept of 'open borders' and the 'free movement of peoples' in the current global mindset of our governing establishment. Countries need to maintain their traditional border services to screen returning residents, permanent residents, immigrants, refugees, and foreign travellers who seek to enter the country; and countries need to maintain their capacity to restrict or refuse access to foreigners when deemed necessary for the protection of the health and safety of the citizens of one's own country.

Chinese Virus Threat: Secondarily, countries need to be aware of the risk that China poses as a potential source of virulent viruses: viz. the SARS pandemic (Severe Acute Respiratory Syndrome, March 2003-2004); and the related Coronavirus pandemic (COVID-19, Dec. 2019-2020). Medical researchers have not yet identified the precise genesis of the disease, but believe that the virus originated in bats, and then jumped to animals sold at the market in Wuhan, China. The culprit is the Chinese wet market culture. In local wet markets (farmers' markets) in China, wild animals and domestic fowl are kept in open-wire cages, stacked up one on top of another, in fetid conditions, in close contact with humans, and the animals are slaughtered for food under unsanitary conditions in the open stalls in the local marketplace.

Such conditions are ripe for the transfer of virulent viruses from wildlife to humans who consume them. (It is suspected that the coronavirus passed from bats, through other animals, to humans.) China has tried to put an end to the sale of wild animals for food and medicine, but it is difficult as the practice is well-established in the Chinese culture. Hence, there is a critical need for other countries to quarantine China as soon as a virulent virus makes it appearance in any Chinese city. That is similarly the case with several African countries where Ebola outbreaks are a constant threat.

To its credit, the Chinese government was able to contain the Coronavirus within China itself in taking decisive action as early as January 23rd to enforce a strict quarantine around Wuhan at the epicenter of an epidemic. Similarly, Taiwan successfully limited and contained the virus by taking decisive government action. However, Canada took no action to quarantine China at that early date, or to stop the Coronavirus at our borders by immediately banning flights from countries suffering a Coronavirus epidemic. The first case of the Cornavirus in Canada was reported on January 26th in a Canadian who had returned home from visiting Wuhan.

Where China is concerned, the Canadian government should have imposed a quarantine on all flights to and from China in late January or early February, when the Wuhan situation was becoming well known. Canadian visitors to China ought to have been told to self-quarantine in airport hotels for at least two-weeks to determine if they had any coronavirus symptoms, and to be tested, before boarding a plane to fly to Canada. The Canadian government could have arranged with the national banks to remove the credit card limits of the individuals concerned, with the government agreeing to reimburse the said individuals to enable them to finance their enforced extended stay.

In wartime, young Canadian military personnel are sent overseas for years on end to risk their lives to safeguard the interests of the nation, and the security and well-being of our people. Canadian tourists and business travelers, if forced to stay at an airport hotel in China during a quarantine, would similarly be serving their country through protecting the health of 36.5 million of their fellow Canadians. Moreover, all Canadians returning from countries that were not yet suffering from an outbreak of the disease should have been screened and tested for the COVID-19 virus at the airports on their return, and held in designated hotels until the test results became known. Those who tested positive could than have been compelled to go into quarantine for treatment by medical personnel.

Federal Government Failures: At present, with Canada in the grips of a potential coronavirus epidemic, and with a now stagnant Canadian economy, Canadians are paying the price for the failure of the Justin Trudeau government to show leadership, decisiveness, and a take-charge mentality at critical points during the early stages of the international Coronavirus pandemic. The number of Canadians infected with the virus has increased from one on January 26th – the first confirmed case in Canada, an isolate case – to 646 as of March 18th , and the number of deaths has increased from one on March 8th to nine as of March 18th. During that time, the federal Liberal government has followed an ad hoc, day-to-day, approach to dealing with the coronavirus threat. Although the border has finally been closed to foreign travellers, the government has called only for a 14-day voluntary self-isolation for Canadians and permanent residents returning to Canada. The irony is that the returnees are not even being informed of the federal government self-isolation health policy upon their arrival at airports in Canada.

The laxity of the federal Liberal government in failing to provide the administrative and policing support needed to carry out its policies, such as they were; its unwillingness to use the authority and emergency powers of the national government to actively combat the introduction and spread of the Coronavirus; and its failure to immediately mobilize Canadians industries and laboratories to produce personal protective equipment, ventilators and testing kits, and the slowness in providing government funding for vaccine research, is beyond belief. Were it not for willingness of Canadians to self-isolate, and the initiatives of the provincial and territorial governments and private companies to protect the health of Canadians, and the heroic efforts of medical practitioners, frontline responders, and personal care workers, the COVID-19 virus would have swept across Canada with a far more devastating impact than it has had to date

Chapter Two

Thursday, March 19, 2020

COVID-19: The coronavirus, or COVID-19, is a respiratory virus that spreads primarily via droplets when an infected person coughs, sneezes, or breathes out, or through droplets of saliva or discharge from the nose. The virus can infect people through being breathed in, or through touching an infected surface and conveying the virus by touch to one's eyes, nose or mouth. The virus can remain active on different types of surfaces anywhere from three hours to three days. It has been conveyed from Wuhan, China -- the source of the original outbreak -- to different countries by travellers who were sick or were asymptomatic carriers of the virus in exhibiting no visible symptoms.

There is no vaccine for Coronavirus: COVID-19. It is a respiratory virus of which the symptoms are a high fever/high temperature, persistent coughing, and a severe shortness of breath. In severe cases, patients develop Acute Respiratory Distress Syndrome -- generally among the elderly and those with a suppressed immune system – in which the virus spreads into the lungs, develops into pneumonia, and fills the lungs with fluids that make breathing very difficult, if not impossible. Individuals who develop pneumonia need to be placed in Intensive Care and, in the most severe cases, connected to a mechanical ventilator to push oxygenated air into their lungs. In addition to respiratory failures, it can cause blood clots, strokes, and cardiac issues in some patients.

On their own initiative, laboratories across Canada are working on the development of a vaccine, but that can take at least twelve months, and several months more to conduct clinical tests, get public health approval for marketing any new vaccine that might be developed, and to manufacture and distribute it. Moreover, initially a priority would be given to protecting hospital medical personnel, first-responders, and personal care workers.

In the absence of a vaccine, the only truly effective means of preventing the spread of the Coronavirus is a complete quarantine of the people in the local outbreak areas to prevent residents travelling and transmitting the virus to others. China has done that, rather belatedly, in instituting a strict quarantine of the City of Wuhan and environs, the epicentre of the Coronavirus infections in that country. In the West, the opportunity to impose a quarantine to restrict travel out of China, on the outbreak of the epidemic there, was lost. All air travel to and from China ought to have been banned immediately by the western countries as soon as the severity of the COVID-19 epidemic became known, in January, or very early in February. Now, the only hope for an eradication of the Coronavirus, which is spreading exponentially in areas of new outbreaks in Europe and the United States, is that it will burn itself out.

In China, as of mid-March 2020, there were 82,000 people who have been infested with the Coronavirus, and 2,788 have died. However, the rate of increase, which on several days had reached as high as 15,000 new cases daily in mid-February, has fallen off by mid-March to practically nothing. On March 18th and 19th, China reported no new cases of the Coronavirus which appears to be a product of the virus burning itself out in the epicentre in Wuhan, as well as the result of the containment of the virus by the enforcement of a strict local quarantine to prevent its spread into new areas.

Health authorities consider that an outbreak cannot be considered ended until the affected area goes 28 days – two 14-day incubation periods – without any new cases. In Canada, the number of confirmed Coronavirus cases has increased from two on January 27th to 773 on March 19th. The number of deaths from the virus infection has increased from a single death on March 8th to nine known deaths.

Friday, March 20, 2020

Testing Kits: Today, it was reported in the media that a private Canadian company, Spartan Bioscience of Ottawa is in the final stages of developing a hand-held coronavirus testing kit that can identify the coronavirus on site in less than 45 minutes from a DNA cheek swab. If approved by government regulators, the company projects a weekly manufacturing run of 9,000 test cartridges for the kit. Last month, a Korean Company, Kogen Biotech, produced a readably portable Coronavirus testing kit, but the final analysis needs to be done in a laboratory over a period of several days.

Hand-sanitizers: In Nova Scotia and Ontario, several craft breweries have begun producing virus-killing hand sanitizers and cleaning sanitizers which they are shipping initially to health clinics and hospitals, and providing to local police, health workers and long-term care homes for free, with plans to sell the product to the general public. The hand sanitizers are produced from alcohol and glycerol (an ingredient of soap) with a bittering agent added to discourage ingestion.

Ventilators: While the federal Health Department has focussed on searching for existing inventories of ventilators and building up its inventory of N-95 respiratory masks to supply any province faced with a surge in demand, the Ontario Health Ministry has been meeting with automobile manufacturers and auto-parts companies to encourage them to 'change gears' in their closed plants to produce medical equipment: primarily ventilators. Several of the industries are willing to do so, but they need to secure agreements with the company holding the product patent. Had the federal government taken action to declare that the coronavirus threat constituted a national emergency -- under the Emergency Measures Act (1985) -- it would have enabled the manufacture of ventilators to proceed immediately as an 'essential service', with a financial compensation to be worked out later through an agreement with the patent holder. However, at present (March 20th), the Trudeau administration is reportedly just 'looking at the Emergencies Act' which, if enacted, would provide the federal government with sweeping powers, for a ninety-day emergency period, to deal with the Coronavirus epidemic.

Prime Minister Trudeau did announce that his government would support auto-parts manufacturers 'gearing up' to produce medical equipment. There was no mention that it was an initiative of the Conservative Government of the Province of Ontario.

Seasonal Workers: On Friday, the Prime Minister announced that temporary seasonal workers and international students will be given exemptions to the ban on international travellers entering Canada. Farm organization have been calling for the government to admit temporary seasonal workers as they are held to be essential workers in maintaining the food supply chain. Each year, under the Seasonal Agricultural Workers Program (SAWP), upwards of 50,000 to 60,000 foreign workers are permitted to enter Canada for up to eight months to work in agriculture and food processing plants. Men, and a significant number of women, from the Philippines, Mexico, Guatemala, and the Caribbean are employed in the planting, maintenance and harvesting of crops and in livestock operations, and in food processing plants, inclusive of meat packing and seafood processing plants.

On March 24th, the Minister of Immigration, Refugees and Citizenship, Marco Mendicino, announced that temporary seasonal workers will be allowed to enter Canada for 'up to two years', will undergo a health screening and will be isolated for 14 days upon arrival. In addition, the seasonal workers will be screened for symptoms of illness before being allowed to board the planes. How that is to be done, by whom, and how that requirement will be enforced, remains unexplained.

Where the travel ban exemptions are concerned, there are questions that need to be posed. How will seasonal workers managed to get to Canada when their home countries have a ban on international travel? (Some farm organizations have suggested that the government send planes to fly the migrant workers to Canada, but at what cost?) Who will be responsible for organizing and administering a screening system for season workers at their point of arrival in Canada? Who will be responsible for paying the seasonal workers, and for the cost of their room and board while they are in isolation, and not working, for 14 days following their arrival? Why is the Liberal government stating that it is going to allow temporary seasonal workers to stay in Canada for two years when the Seasonal Agricultural Workers Program (SAWP) -- as enacted by parliament -- only allows seasonal workers to remain in Canada for a maximum period of eight months? Why are international students being exempted from the ban on foreign nationals entering this country? These exemptions run counter to the whole concept of closing the borders to foreign nationals as a means of drastically limiting the potential importation of the coronavirus into Canada.

Saturday, March 21, 2020

Ventilators: The morning newspaper is reporting that the federal government has ordered a total of 550 ventilators to date. However, there is a supply problem. Only one Canadian company, Thornhill Medical of Toronto, manufactures ventilators in Canada, and manufacturers in the United States, the United Kingdom, Germany, and Ireland are currently overwhelmed with orders from their own countries.

The Thornhill company has been approached by the federal government to ramp up production, but it is a small company that requires two weeks to produce a single ventilator. Nonetheless, Canadians were assured by Navdeep Bains, the Minister of Innovation, Science and Economic Development, that talks were underway with four auto-parts companies to retool to produce ventilators. Given that there have been reports for weeks past about a life and death crisis in Italy over a shortage of ventilators during the coronavirus epidemic, it is unbelievable that the federal government has not addressed, until now, the potential critical shortage of ventilators in Canada.

Respiratory Masks: It has also been reported that the federal government has been stocking N-95 respiratory masks that have air filters capable of blocking 95% of airborne particles and are fully capable of providing a secure protection against the rather large infectious droplets of the Coronavirus. The N-95 mask is distributed by a Montreal company, Medicom. The federal government apparently has already issued purchase orders for 11.3 million N-95 respiratory masks. Canadian medical doctors, dentists, nurses and hygienists, and health care workers with a heavy exposure to the COVID-19 virus, have been calling for such masks for weeks past; yet there was no explanation offered by the Liberal government as to why the N-95 masks have not already been distributed from the national stockpile depots.

Why wait until a province has a major outbreak of coronavirus cases before distributing the masks, when the masks, if distributed, could prevent such an outbreak. The respiratory masks ought to be distributed to front line medical health workers, to those who test positive for the COVID-19 virus (including both the sick and the asymptomatic who test positive), to the elderly, to the chronically ill, and to individuals with an immune deficiency. Given the number of masks ordered by the federal government, it appears that the intention is to supply as many Canadians as possible with the N-95 mask in areas of major outbreaks across Canada, but why the delay?

Testing kits: As for Minister Bains, he expressed the government's interest in acquiring the new diagnostic test kits being developed by Spartan Bioscience Inc. of Ottawa to screen for the Coronavirus at Canada's four major airports. Such testing kits are acutely needed, but the DNA swab technology has not yet been approved by Public Health Canada.

Screening & Testing: The News media has reported that the screening of returning Canadians and permanent residents is rather simplistic prior to their boarding a flight to Canada. Airline staff are responsible for questioning returnees as to their health and the countries visited, and the Airline staff are required to look for flu-like symptoms. Anyone who displays obvious flu-like symptoms is barred from flying to Canada for 14-days, or until a medical certificate is obtained confirming that there is no infection. This impromptu process does nothing to protect Canadians against asymptomatic carriers who are conveying the virus but show no signs of illness, and apparently is not even effective in stopping the visibly ill from flying to Canada. A 72-year old woman, who was clearly sick with the COVID-19 virus -- with a constant cough and shortness of breath symptoms -- was allowed to fly from Los Angeles to Toronto on Saturday, after having travelled from China, and she passed though the Toronto airport without being detained. She died of the coronavirus disease within a few hours of arriving home. Calls by Conservative parliamentarians for a tighter screening process at airports, land border entry points, and ports, have been ignored by the federal Liberal government.

In Ontario, the provincial government has been testing individuals with flu-like symptoms to identify and isolate coronavirus cases. Now, owing to a shortage of swabs used in testing, the province has shifted its focus to testing front-line workers in the health industry to prevent institutional spread by quarantining the sick and self-isolating the asymptomatic carriers among the medical staffs. However, the Ontario effort has been hamstrung by a severe shortage of testing kits, and the inability to acquire them on the open market.

Government Lack of Direction: Information is totally lacking from the federal government with respect to what should Canadians do after the 14-day period of self-isolation expires. Canadians cannot stay at home indefinitely. Would it not be better to focus isolation, containment, and medical care on those who are sick, as well as encouraging the high at-risk population – the elderly, those suffering from a serious pre-existing health problem, and those with an immune system deficiency -- to completely self-isolate?

At present, the federal Liberal government is encouraging Canadians to "Go Home. Stay Home", and when outside the home to practice social distancing – at least six feet – and to disinfect one's hands after contact with any surface outside the home through washing frequently with soap and water and the use of hand sanitizers. However, if the plan is to have Canadians isolate themselves until the COVID-19 epidemic burns itself out several months from now, the repercussions of such a shutdown of the Canadian economy will be disastrous. It might well trigger a full-scale economic depression.

Respiratory Masks: The millions of N-95 respiratory masks purchased by the federal government, ought to be immediately widely distributed, and fitted, to health care professionals and workers, the sick and high at-risk individuals, as well as to Canadians returning from abroad at the four airports, land border crossings, and ports. The N-95 respiratory masks also ought to be distributed, and fitted, to Canadian workers more generally to enable healthy Canadians to get back to work, and to get businesses, stores, and industries back in operation. It would enable Canadians to get on with their lives without fear of contacting the virus, or of spreading the virus if an infected person is asymptomatic.

(Later, it was revealed that the federal government has been experiencing insurmountable difficulties in getting its orders for the N-95 respiratory masks filled from China and the United States and, to date, has been unsuccessful in acquiring the 11.3 million masks on order.)

European Border Closures: The failure of the Modern liberal politicians of the European Union to abandon their open borders mantra and to close the borders of Europe to foreign travellers immediately upon the Chinese epidemic becoming known, is writ large in the coronavirus pandemic now raging in Europe. In northern Italy, the epicentre in Europe, there are over 53,000 infected persons, 4,800 have died of complications caused by the Coronavirus, and in but one day 793 new cases were reported. Italy is now in a total lockdown, but with the COVID-19 virus already present in local communities, it is now too late to effectively contain the spread of the imported virus. Various countries in Europe are instituting border entry restrictions in attempting to control the spread of the coronavirus. In doing so, they are ignoring calls by the European Union leadership that member nations refrain from imposing border restrictions within the Union.

Monday, March 23, 2020

Emergencies Measure Act: For weeks now prominent Conservatives and medical practitioners have been calling on the federal Liberal government to implement the Emergency Measures Act to take control of all efforts to contain the coronavirus, and to provide a unity of direction to Canadians as to how to respond to the crisis. At present, the Canadian provincial governments and the territories have enacted emergency legislation and, among various efforts, have closed large public venues, restaurants, theatres, and sporting events, and have banned public gatherings of various sizes -- 5, 20, or 50 persons, depending on the province. Fines are being levied against those who ignore the regulations. The Northwest Territories and Nunavut governments have even closed its borders to entry by Canadians from elsewhere in the country, to prevent the virus being imported into the North. However, there is no uniformity in the provincial bans and regulations in force across Canada. What is lacking is the enforcement of a standard set of regulations on nation-wide basis under the leadership and direction of the federal government, with more cohesion and consistency in the messaging that Canadians are receiving.

At present, the Prime Minister, Justin Trudeau, and his Cabinet Ministers are resisting all calls for the enacting of the Emergency Measures Act. They are doing so out of an ideological belief that civil rights – our basic political and social freedoms -- are universal human rights that should not be violated by a national government. Under the Emergency Measures Act, the federal government would have the power -- for a period of ninety days -- to temporarily restrict travel within Canada, to ignore property rights, and to impose restraints and fines on anyone contravening any order or regulation issued under the Emergencies Act. In calling on Canadians to voluntarily obey the calls of public health agencies for self-isolation, the Public Health Minister, Patty Hajdu, declared that if the federal government were forced to enact the Emergency Measures Act, it would constitute "an assault on the civil liberties" of Canadians. Such is the reasoning of our Modern liberal establishment.

In contrast, Tory Conservatives believe that the civil rights of Canadians are established and guaranteed by the Constitution of Canada, inclusive of the Canadian Charter of Rights and Freedoms, and by the Canadian common law tradition; that civil rights are liberties established under the law for the benefit, well-being and common good of Canadians; and that whenever the life, health or well-being of Canadians is under threat in wartime or during an epidemic, the common good of the people might well require government to temporarily suspend civil liberties. In effect, the Emergency Measures Act is framed within that context. If enacted, it would empower the Government in Council (the Cabinet) of the federal government to act to meet any threat that endangers the lives, health and safety of Canadians by introducing temporary measures that go beyond what would be acceptable otherwise under the rule of law and civil rights legislation.

Screening & Testing: Recently, Ontario, Alberta, and Saskatchewan, and presumably the other provinces, have posted a self-assessment tool online to allow individuals to test – self-diagnosis – whether they have contacted the COVID-19 virus. The federal government has done the same on its Public Health website. It is a preliminary screening process to enable individuals to determine whether they need to consult a medical practitioner for a coronavirus nasal swab/PCR laboratory analysis test.

Coronavirus Impact: The impact of the coronavirus on the Canadian economy is yet to be fully determined, but what we are witnessing is bordering on the catastrophic. During the first week after the introduction of the new economic package, 500,000 claims were submitted to the Employment Insurance office by laid off workers seeking employment insurance payments.

Tuesday, March 24, 2020

Ontario Response: Premier Doug Ford of Ontario, under the provincial Emergency Management and Civil Protection Act, has announced that schools will remain closed beyond the initial three-week period specified earlier, and he has ordered the shutting down of all non-essential businesses in the province. Only grocery stores, pharmacies, restaurant takeout and delivery services, liquor and beer stores, and essential supply chain suppliers, some manufacturing industries, and some vital public transportation services, would be allowed to remain open. Among the essential workers are truck drivers, food supply personal, takeout food preparers, delivery drivers, personal support workers, and grocery and pharmacy store employees.

Nationally, it was reported that there were upwards of 4,000 Canadians infected with the coronavirus, with 39 deaths in Canada attributed directly to the virus. Funeral services were declared to be an essential service and limited to ten persons – exclusive of staff – with an advisory to maintain social distancing and to staff to wear personal protective equipment. The Office of the Chief Coroner for Ontario set up a system whereby death certificates can be secured electronically by funeral homes to enable burials, entombments, and cremations to proceed without delay.

Returning Travellers: The Canadian Border Services Agency reported that over one million people returned to Canada from abroad in the week between March 14th and 20th, of whom 96 percent were Canadians and four percent were permanent residents. (These figures are misleading, as prior to March 18th, foreigners were permitted to enter Canada without any restrictions and many have done so, and American visitors were able to freely cross the border until March 21st.) Presumably, a large majority of the Canadians returning home were snowbirds returning to Canada from Florida and the southern United States, which has greatly complicated the task of Airline personnel, and the Canada Border Services Agency, to conduct visual screenings of the arrivals for coronavirus symptoms.

Initial Financial Aid Package: To avoid having to recall all 338 members of the House of Commons back to Ottawa during the coronavirus epidemic, it has been arranged by the parliamentary parties that when parliament reconvenes on March 24th only 32 MPs will attend the session of the House to permit social spacing in the legislative chamber. The members present will represent their respective parties, with the representation based proportionally on the comparative number of elected MPs of each Party. It was also agreed the members present would unanimously assent to the $82 billion financial aid bill that Prime Minister Trudeau had previously announced. The intention was to secure the enactment of the legislation through an unanimous consent which allows the requisite three readings to be held on one day, to speed the passage of the legislation for approval by the Senate and its signing into law by the Governor General. The intent is to rapidly distribute the financial aid to the businesses and workers impacted negatively by the impact of the COVID-19 virus. The arranged unanimity soon dissipated.

Liberal Power Grab: When the draft bill was circulated to the opposition parties, it was found to contain a clause that gave the Finance Minister an unlimited power to raise taxes, borrow and spend monies, without parliamentary approval, until December 31, 2021 – a period of twenty-one months. The Conservative Party objected that the length of the supposedly temporary suspension of parliamentary oversight was far too long; that it was "a power grab"; and that it was unprecedented in constitutional history and constituted a threat to the 'political liberties' of Canadians. The NDP joined the Conservative in refusing unanimous assent to the bill.

Had the members of parliament known their history, they would have noted that the Liberal government effort to seize an absolute power to tax, borrow and spend monies without the consent of parliament, was exactly what the royal absolutism of King James II embodied in Great Britain, before he was deposed in the Glorious Revolution of 1688. Indeed, in the fundamental constitutional document the "Bill of Rights" (1689) -- enacted by parliament during the subsequent revolution settlement -- there was a vital clause that 'the levying of taxes without the consent of parliament was illegal'; and yet another clause stipulated that parliament 'ought to be recalled frequently' to deal with government measures. In seeking to by-pass parliament, and usurp an absolute power to tax, borrow and spend, the Liberal government of Justin Trudeau was attempting to stage a political revolution through establishing an absolutist form of government for a period of almost two years.

Emergencies Measures Act: In contrast, the extraordinary powers that would be gained by the government through the evoking of the Emergency Measures Act (1985) to meet a national crisis, are strictly limited in their scope. The Emergency Measures Act conveyed only a temporary, 90-day, authority to the Governor General – in effect, the Cabinet – to impose orders and regulations required to deal with a national emergency. Moreover, the Emergencies Act specifies the areas where the extraordinary powers could be applied: in the prohibiting of travel; in ordering evacuations; in property requisitions; the distribution of essential goods and services; the making of emergency payments; the erection of shelters and hospitals; and the imposition of fines up to $5,000 or six months in jail, or both, to anyone violating any emergency order or regulation. Moreover, the rights, powers and privileges of parliament would remain undiminished following the passage of the Emergencies Act, and parliament could rescind the Emergency Measures Act at any time.

Liberal Power Grab: What Canadians are seeing is a Prime Minister, Justin Trudeau, is a man who has no respect for Canada's tradition of parliamentary government, and who craves power to implement his political agenda, like all zealots for a cause which is his case are the causes of Modern liberalism and environmentalism. He has declared repeatedly that his Liberal government sees no need to invoke the Emergencies Act; and yet his government has submitted to parliament a draft bill that will grant his Liberal Party government an arbitrary and absolute power to govern without any oversight or consent from parliament for almost two years.

The predilection of Modern liberals for absolute power, and their lack of respect for the common people and their representatives in Parliament, is well-illustrated by this political episode. The Liberal attempt to seize an absolute power to tax, borrow and spend without the assent of parliament is a clear violation of what has become recognized as two parliamentary axioms: 'no taxation without representation' in parliament, and all money bill must originate in the House of Commons and require the assent of Parliament.

In the past, Justin Trudeau, has declared his admiration for the absolute authority wielded by the Communist Party government of China. His lack of respect for Parliament, for parliamentary rules and procedures, and for parliamentary traditions, has now become quite clear. It is a barefaced attempt to take advantage of the good will and willingness of the opposition parties to quickly, and unanimously, pass a financial aid package. The opposition parties are anxious to get government monies flowing to working Canadians who are losing their jobs in large numbers with the closing down of businesses and industries during the coronavirus epidemic, and who are lacking any income to pay their rent or mortgage, and to purchase basic necessities.

(On April 24th, a month after this was written, Ken Rubin -- an Ottawa freelance researcher who specializing in Access to Information retrievals -- pointed out that if the Liberal Party had secured its freedom to 'tax, borrow and spend monies' without parliamentary approval until the end of December 2021, "any associated background records would be excluded from public scrutiny as so-called 'cabinet confidences' under the Access to Information Act for 20 years, until 2041". What we have here is still another indication that the Liberal government does not want its response to the coronavirus threat to be scrutinized by parliament.)

What is equally appalling is that when Modern liberals, such as Justin Trudeau, seek absolute power, it is not to promote the national interest and common good of their own people and to build much needed infrastructure within their own country – witness the poor record of the Trudeau Liberals is undertaking infrastructure projects in Canada. What the Modern liberals want is an absolute power to tax and spend hundreds of millions of dollars on social transformation projects and programs to promote social equality, diversity, and egalitarianism, both within the nation and worldwide. In effect, Modern liberals want to take multiple billions of dollars -- through taxation -- from the citizens of the developed countries to support United Nations efforts to effect social change in the Third World and supposedly achieve a prosperous and egalitarian world society. Such aspirations may be praiseworthy in theory – to those who do not think too deeply on the nature of society. Such a commitment is utterly futile and foolish in practice in ignoring human nature, deep-seated cultural values and traditions, market principles, and historic realities.

All too often U.N. financial assistance, through the International Monetary Fund, is coupled with an insistence that the recipient countries adopt Modern liberal cultural values and free trade economics -- a new form of Imperialism that is destructive of native cultures and economies. Given the fact that the opposition parties in parliament had already express their willingness to quickly pass the Liberal financial package to deal with the devastating economic impact of the Coronavirus epidemic, what was the motive of the Liberal government in seeking to grasp an absolute power to tax, borrow, and spend uncheck by parliament? One suspects an ulterior motive. That it was motivated by a perceived need to avoid having to secure the support of parliament for the financing of social transformation projects, both within Canada and abroad. What it amounted to was a recognition on the part of the Liberal Government that it is Canadians who will be heavily taxed to pay for the desired 'social and economic transformation of society', and the 'save the world aspirations' of the Modern liberal elite; and that Canadians might well not support such social projects if the projected expenditures were presented to the representatives of the people in parliament for approval.

Canadians have already seen the unrestrained spending of the federal Liberal government before Canada was struck by the coronavirus epidemic, and now the Liberal government is trying to use the crisis in an attempt to hoodwink the opposition parties into giving it unlimited taxing, borrowing and spending powers. This is a government that has declined to enact the Emergency Measures Act to enable it to temporarily take control, on a national scale, of efforts to contain the COVID-19 virus, and has defended its inaction by arguing that the invoking of the Emergencies Act would constitute an 'assault on the civil liberties of Canadians'. Yet, the Liberal government has no compunction about taking away the constitutional and traditional political right of Canadians to control 'the public purse' through their parliamentary representatives.

Wednesday, March 25, 2020

Financial Aid Package (March 25th): Fortunately, the Liberal Party, in being in a minority government position, did not have the votes to push through the draft bill. The Conservative Party, supported by the New Democratic Party, objected to the clause of the draft bill giving the government an absolute power to tax, borrow, and spend without the approval of parliament. After an all-night session, and further negotiations with the opposition parties, the Liberal government removed the contentious power grab component of the Bill. The financial aid package then received unanimous consent from the House of Commons early on Wednesday morning, was quickly passed by the Senate in the afternoon, and immediately signed by the Governor General into law.

As enacted, the Bill comprised the $72 billion financial aid package announced earlier by Prime Minister Trudeau with the removal of the last-minute addition of the clause granting the government an absolute power to 'tax, borrow and spend'. Any additional financial aid required by Canadians during the coronavirus epidemic will have to be voted by parliament, if, and when, needed, and the expanded financial powers were granted for only six months, until September 30, 2020. Moreover, the Act specified that consultations were required with the provinces and territories on some spending initiatives, and that the Minister of Finance must appear before the House Finance Committee every two weeks to update Parliament, and the Canadian people, on the monies expended to date. What this episode teaches is that members of parliament, and the opposition parties, must always be vigilant in defending the rights and privileges of parliament against any government that might be tempted -- in taking advantage of a crisis situation -- to seize absolute political power. Such is the long history of the struggle to attain and maintain parliamentary government by the representatives of the people, against the common bias of governments in wanting absolute power in any democracy, whether under a monarchical or republican form of government.

Canada Emergency Response Benefit: The financial aid package passed by Parliament includes a major change in the scope of the payments to laid off workers, and the administration of the program. The new Canada Emergency Response Benefit (CERB) is to be administered by the Canada Revenue Agency (CRA). It will provide a $2,000 per month taxable benefit to any worker who earned $5,000 or more in the previous year, and now has no income because a loss of employment due to the Coronavirus epidemic. The new CERB program is intended to relieve the Employment Insurance system from being overwhelmed by claims, which had soared to 1,500,000 claimants over the previous week. The new bill effectively almost doubles the previous payment that the government had declared it would provide for those forced into unemployment by the coronavirus epidemic. Moreover, it covers a broader field of claimants in having been extended to cover the self-employed and workers who lack the number of weeks of employment needed to qualify to receive Employment Insurance payments. Laid off workers can apply online at the CRA portal, or by telephone.

Several economists have predicted that the expanded financial aid package, in its entirety, will push the federal deficit to over $82 billion for this fiscal year. Moreover, the Minister of Finance, Bill Morneau, announced that a further financial aid package, targeted for small businesses, will be brought forward within several days.

In Canada, the number of confirmed cases of the COVID-19 virus has reached 3,409.

The Bauer Sports company has volunteered to produce plastic face masks for medical personnel. Why the production capacity of such a company was not mobilized a month ago, remains unanswered.

Illegal Migrants: The American government has revealed that, several days earlier, the United States, Mexico, and Canada signed an agreement to close their borders to illegal migrants and to return them to their country of arrival. At the same time, it was revealed that Canada had objected "in the strongest diplomatic language" to an American proposal to station troops on the U.S.-Canadian border to enforce the agreement. Deputy Prime Minister, Chrystia Freeland, has publicly objected, in strident terms in declaring the opposition of the Canadian government to "the militarization of the border". Prime Minister Trudeau declared that it was in the interests of both Canada and the United States to maintain: "the longest unmilitarized border in the world". Other than in the Liberal Government rhetoric, the proposed deployment of 1,000 American troops along a 6,415 km (3,987 mile) border -- at crossing points -- in no way constitutes a 'militarization' of the border. Apparently, the Liberal Government wants to uphold the old liberal-Whig history myth of 'the undefended border'.

Here was an opportunity, at American expense, to effectively stop illegal migrants – bogus refugees -- from third party countries from using the United States as a stop off to enter Canada in violation of Canada's immigration laws and, in doing so, to prevent any illegals who might be infected with the COVID-19 virus from entering the country. However, once again the Liberal Government of Justin Trudeau has revealed a reticence to effectively close the border to foreigners. One suspects that a blind adherence to United Nations refugee policies, and to the Modern liberal ideology of 'open borders' and the 'free movement of peoples', is taking precedence over common sense and the rule of law despite public assurances -- given to Canadians several days earlier -- that the border would be closed to illegal migrants. One wonders whether the Trudeau

Government had any real intention of ever enforcing the proclaimed border closure against foreigners seeking to enter Canada illegally, whom Trudeau regards as 'irregular border crossers' and 'irregular asylum-seekers'.

The Canadian Press has reported that 'a foreign policy expert' is worried that the positioning of American troops on the border will initiate "a diplomatic crisis", and a retired naval Vice-Admiral has been quoted to the effect that the positioning of a thousand American troops on the border "makes no military sense". What such nonsense ignores is that the United States has the right to deploy its troops wherever it wants within its own borders; that the Americans are not engaging in a hostile act in sending small detachments of troops to border posts; and that Canada and the United States have already signed an agreement to close the border. Moreover, during the past year, the United States apprehended 1,185 people who were trying to enter Canada illegally from the United States – principally on Washington State- British Columbia border -- of whom a significant number were from China and Iran, which are currently epicentres of the COVID-19 pandemic. In contrast, the eastern New York State-Quebec border remained open, to the passage of illegal migrants, principally from west Africa. It is time to get real, people!

Thursday, March 26, 2020

Canada Emergency Wage Subsidy: Prime Minister Trudeau announced that his government plans to introduce a payroll wage subsidy program – later designated the Canada Emergency Wage Subsidy (CEWS) program -- which will provide financial support for the owners of small- and medium-sized businesses to keep workers on their payroll. The payroll wage subsidy for businesses will cover 75 percent of the wages of each surplus worker, up to a maximum of $847 per worker per week for four months, during the COVID-19 epidemic, and will be back dated to March 15th. (The new payroll wage subsidy greatly exceeds the 10 percent coverage of wages legislated earlier.) The intention is to encourage businesses to keep their employees on the payroll rather than lay them off as revenues decline so that businesses will be able to start up quickly when the lockdown is lifted. The payroll wage subsidy program (CEWS) for small- and medium-sized business will be backdated to March 15th and will end on June 6th. In addition, business owners will be allowed to defer their GST and HST payments, as well as duties and taxes owed on imports, until June 2020, to provide them with immediate extra monies – liquidity -- during the shutdown or slowdown of their businesses.

(How the program is to ensure that companies do not simply put their entire workforce on the CEWS payroll subsidy plan whether they were to be laid off or not, remains unexplained.)

Business Credit Availability Program: Export Development Canada and the Business Development Bank, will make up to $12.5 billion available for loans to small- and medium-sized business owners through an enterprise loan and guarantee program – later designated the Business Credit Availability Program (BCAP). To be eligible small and medium-sized businesses must have been in business by March 1st, 2020, must have been financially viable, and must have been negatively impacted financially by events related to COVID-19. In addition, businesses must have an annual payroll between $50,000 and $1 million to qualify for an emergency loan.

Under the BCAP umbrella, there are two lending streams. There is a 'Co-Lending Program' where the Business Development Bank of Canada and a lending institution co-lend loans to provide small and medium-sized businesses with cash flow – 80 percent of the loan from BDC, 20 percent from the lending institution – up to a maximum of $6.25 million in incremental credit. The second lending stream involves the Export Development Bank of Canada (EDC) providing immediate funding to financial institutions to enable them to participate in loaning monies to small and medium-sized businesses, with the loans to the financial institutions being 80 percent guaranteed by the EDC, and repayable within one year.

Canada Emergency Business Account: Subsequently, a $25 billion Canada Emergency Business Account (CEBA) program was established for small businesses and not-for-profits that provides a $40,000 interest-free emergency loan to enable them to meet operating expenses during a temporary reduction in revenues owing to the impact of the COVID-19 virus. If the loan is repaid before December 31, 2020, the government will forgive 25 percent of the loan -- $10,000.)

Financial Aid Package (March 24ᵗʰ): The new financial aid package will cost, in total, an estimated $71 billion, inclusive of the payroll wage subsidy program and the loan programs in support of small and medium-sized businesses. The $71 billion in projected new expenditures in conjunction with the $82 billion projected cost of the earlier financial aid package, and the sharp drop expected in federal government revenues as the economy contracts, may well result in a federal deficit of upwards of $200 billion for the current fiscal year. Such a massive deficit equates to about ten percent of the GNP. It is a startling figure, but what Canadians need to fear is that expenditures will get out of control in the dispensing of such large sums of money in so many different programs. Corruption might well flourish with false claims being submitted for payments.

We are under the governance of a Liberal government dominated by Modern liberal zealots who have proven inept in controlling spending and who are discipline adverse, uninterested in day-to-day management issues, and far from detail oriented. To wit, the earlier gross incompetence, and soaring costs of the mismanagement of the inauguration of the computerized Phoenix pay system by the Liberal government of Justin Trudeau, and the soaring national debt before the onset of the coronavirus crisis.

What is curious about the pronouncements of government policies being made by Prime Minister Trudeau at his residence, is that the Press has not picked up on a remark by Andrew Scheer, the Conservative Party leader, that government policy pronouncements ought to be made in the House of Commons where members can respond and question the government. Granted there was a need for Trudeau to self-isolate while his wife was infected with the virus, but she has fully recovered, and the Prime Minister has remained free of any infection. The proper place for announcing government policies is in Parliament, rather than the Prime Minister addressing the Press, in a presidential manner, from a podium at his residence before TV cameras and the national press.

Manitoba Testing: The Province of Manitoba -- 1.34 million population – is focusing its publish health team testing on individuals who are showing symptoms of the coronavirus in remote communities, and in shelters, jails, long-care homes, and workcamps, where there are vulnerable people living in close association. A Health Links phone line has been set up to provide a self-analysis to members of the publish to whom a number of questions are posed to determine whether the caller needs to be tested. If so, the caller is directed to the nearest testing site, based on the caller's postal code. There are twelve testing sites in the province. They are drive-ins where the driver can have a nasal swab taken while seated in the vehicle. There are also testing centres with a waiting room where social spacing is practiced. It takes 24 to 48 hours to complete the laboratory test with a central lab having a capacity of 500 tests per day. Both the negative and positive tests are conveyed by phone, with public health workers dispatched to provide medical aid and assistance to the individuals testing positive. To date, there have been four coronavirus-related deaths in Manitoba.

Friday, March 27, 2020

Illegal Migrants: It was reported that the Deputy Prime Minister, Chrystia Freeland, is alarmed at reports that the U.S. Customs and Border Protection plans to deport illegal migrants -- who are caught trying to enter Canada -- back to their native countries in the shortest possible time. When Freeland was questioned by reporters about whether Canada is thinking of re-opening its borders to illegal migrants to preclude them being caught and deported to their country of origin by the Americans, she would not say. After publicly expressing the indignation of the Trudeau government at the American proposal to position troops on the border to apprehend illegal migrants attempting to cross the border, Freeland now says negotiations on the subject of what is to be done with illegal migrants will be conducted in private with the United States. Freeland did mention that Canada must honour its international obligations, under the United Nations, to ensure that refugees are not returned to countries "where they might face violence or persecution". Why illegal migrants are being classed as 'refugees' and treated as if they have the same rights as refugees under international agreements, was not explained by Freeland.

At a time when Canada is in the grips of a deathly virus epidemic, with its economy closing down, with unemployment levels and the national debt soaring, why the Deputy Prime Minister of Canada is fixated on granting asylum to illegal migrants who are exploiting both the American and Canadian immigration systems, and entering Canada illegally, is beyond belief. Moreover, that is especially so as only a handful of illegal migrants are turning up at irregular border crossing owing to the March 13th ban by President Trump of flights to the United States from overseas countries. The fixation of Chrystia Freeland on illegal migrants at such a critical time bespeaks an unwavering commitment to U.N. dictates, and the La La Land mentality of the Modern liberal.

Personal Protective Equipment: In Ottawa, Algonquin College, which teaches health care courses in respiratory therapy, announced that it has loaned its school equipment for distribution to Ottawa hospitals. Included in the loan package are nine ventilators, 125,000 gloves, over 7,000 respiratory masks, and 100 protective gowns. Presumably, the Canadian military medical corps has similar virus protection equipment for combatting pandemics. Why has the Trudeau government failed to mobilize the military to furnish virus protection equipment, as well as virus screening and medical support? Being Liberals, do they dislike the appearance of military personnel among our frontline medical personnel at airports?

What is even more disturbing, while doctors and nurses are expressing their worries and anguish about a critical shortage of the N-95 respiratory mask, surgical gloves and gowns, and medical plastic face shields, was the revelation on March 25th -- in the national press -- that the federal Liberal Government sent sixteen tonnes of protective medical equipment from Canada's National Stockpile to China between February 4th and 9th. The shipments, which depleted Canada's National Stockpile, comprised N-95 respiratory masks, medical plastic face shields, medical gowns, goggles, and several hundred thousand pairs of surgical gloves. Earlier, on February 9th, a brief public announcement of the "gift to China" had been made by Foreign Affairs Minister Francois Philippe Champagne, but the negative implications of that gift for the health of Canadians, was not picked up on by the national press. At the time, Champagne declared: "Our deepest thoughts are with all those affected by this outbreak".

When Canada's national stockpile of personal protection equipment was shipped to China, there were only a few isolated coronavirus case in Canada -- the first, a traveller who had returned home to Toronto from Wuhan on January 26th. However, upon hearing of the rapid spread of the coronavirus in China, the quarantine of Wuhan on January 23rd and the severity of the virus infections, common sense should have dictated the exercise of caution, and the keeping of the medical personal protection equipment for the protection of Canadians. Even the World Health Organization, for all its faults, had declared earlier, on January 30th, that "it is expected that further international exportation of cases [from China] may appear in any country".

Moreover, while the personal protective equipment was being shipped to China – through the Canadian Red Cross -- the World Health Organization predicted, on February 7th, that there will be "severe coronavirus-related disruptions" in the supply of personal protective equipment. In sum, how was Canada to readily replace the equipment that was 'gifted' to China? When questioned as to why the personal protective equipment was shipped to China from the national stockpile, the Deputy-Directory of Communications for Global Affairs, responded: "Global pandemics require global co-operation. After all, pandemics know no borders. Co-operation is vital to ensuring the health and safety of people around the world. This includes protecting people here in Canada, as support of this kind can help to slow the spread of the virus".

This is the height of naivety. What the WHO has predicted on February 7th was a fact by mid-March with shortages of personal protective equipment and global markets unable to fulfill orders. On March 15th, the European Union had new rules in place requiring that the export of personal protection equipment had to be authorized by government, and as of March 21st, 54 governments worldwide had restrictions on the export of medical supplies. Moreover, India placed a ban on the export of 26 pharmaceutical ingredients, some of which were used in treating coronavirus patients. The vaunted globalist approach of the federal Liberal government to the coronavirus threat is a farce. Yesterday, the Globe and Mail reported that hospitals in Ontario are rationing personal protective equipment. In Parliament, the Conservative Opposition Leader, Andrew Scheer, declared it "outrageous" that the Liberal government had shipped the PPEs to China, and demanded to know the extent to which the national stockpile of PPEs had been depleted. No answer was forthcoming from the government.

Within two weeks of sending the shipments of personal protection equipment to China in early February, there was a real and obvious prospect of the coronavirus spreading to Canada and causing an epidemic here. Professor Amir Attaran, School of Epidemiology and Public Health, University of Ottawa, expressed his surprise on learning that Global Affairs had shipped personal protection equipment to China. He commented: "It was absolutely certain in early February that we would need this equipment. This decision went beyond altruism into high negligence and incompetence because Canada did not, and does not, have surplus equipment to spare".

Government Policy: As of March 27th, Dr. Theresa Tam, the Chief Public Health Officer for Canada, assured Canadians that the fact Canada's fatality rate is currently less than one percent of infected patients, indicates that the health system is coping, and is not being overwhelmed. There was no mention of the critical shortage of the N-95 respiratory mask, plastic face shields, face masks, surgical gloves, and squabs for testing kits, as well as ventilators. Dr. Tam repeated the federal government admonition to practice social spacing, to avoid large gatherings, and to wash one's hands frequently. She threatened that fines or jail time might be imposed on those who failed to self-isolate. Dr. Tam also announced a new government policy. A mandatory 14-day quarantine was being imposed on Canadians returning home from overseas, and anyone who violated the quarantine would face a stiff fine or six months in jail. Random checks, including home visits, would be done to ensure that returnees were abiding by what Dr. Tam was quoted as having referred to as "the quarantine law".

It sounded good, but there was no follow up by the Liberal government to establish an administrative or policing system to enforce 'the quarantine law': the Quarantine Act (2005). Under the terms of the Quarantine Act, the Minister of Health may designate individuals, or a class of persons, as health officers "to protect public health by taking comprehensive measures to prevent the introduction and spread of communicable diseases". The designated health officers are authorized to screen travellers entering or leaving Canada, and may isolate an infected person, or persons suspected of having been in close contact with an infected person, and transfer them to a quarantine officer for a medical examination. If an infected person refused to isolate, a health officer could apply to a provincial court judge to issue an arrest warrant, with the peace officer authorized to use force to apprehend the individual. Individuals convicted of a summary offence can receive a fine of up to $500,000 or six months in jail, or both and if convicted of an indictable offence, can receive a fine of up to $1million or three years in jail, or both.

(Twelve days later, on April 11th, it was announced that the RCMP has been given new powers to visit homes to ensure that individuals who are under a mandatory 14-day quarantine remain at home, and to make arrests in situations where the quarantine order was being ignored. Individuals who violate a quarantine order can be fined up to $750,000 and imprisoned for six months. Presumably the new RCMP powers were granted under the Quarantine Act. However, why the Liberal government took twelve days to authorize the RCMP to enforce the new quarantine policy remains unexplained, nor is there any explanation for setting the maximum fine at $750,000 rather than in accordance with fine structure established in the Quarantine Act.)

Canadian Banks: The big six Canadian banks have announced a new coronavirus-related mortgage payments relief plan in response to the receipt of over 230,000 requests from mortgage holders for a deferment of mortgage payments. The banks will defer mortgage payments for an indefinite time, depending on the individual situation, with the accrued interest to be added to the outstanding balance of the mortgage. In effect, once mortgages payments resume, the mortgagee will have the back interest added to the monthly payments or added to the end of the mortgage term. (In such a time of crisis, one might ask: Why are the big banks not sharing the pain of the COVID-19 crisis by waiving the interest accruing on a mortgage during the duration of the deferred payments period?) The banks are expecting earnings to fall drastically on loan-losses through the unemployed being unable to service their credit card debt and other unsecured loans.

Saturday, March 28, 2020

GAVI: Epidemiologists working for an international vaccine organization, GAVI, are calling for a global effort to develop a COVID-19 vaccine, and are predicting that it could well take 18 to 24 months to develop a vaccine, and that public monies will be needed to support the effort. A major concern of GAVI is that when a proven vaccine is developed, it will be distributed equally to poorer countries rather than just sold to countries that can afford it. GAVI is an alliance of public and private donors, associated with the World Health Organization (WHO) and the United Nations International Children's Emergency Fund (UNICEF), that brings together the technical expertise of the developed world, donor nations and private funding, and private companies, for the implementation of vaccination programs worldwide. It has a commitment to ensure "the equitable use of vaccines" in the poorer countries of Asia, Africa, Latin America and South America. GAVI holds periodic donor conferences, hosted by different nations, and raises billions of dollars to support its vaccination work. Canada contributed $500 million to GAVI for the past five year, and GAVI is currently seeking a $600 million commitment from Canada for the next five years.

Canadian Military: In Canada, the Chief of the Defence Staff, General Jon Vance, announced that the Canadian military is assessing how it can lend support to the federal government, the provinces, and territories, in the current medical crisis. He confirmed that the military is well equipped to set up mobile shelters and medical facilities; and that it has an extensive logistical capacity to provide support to vulnerable populations anywhere in Canada. However, to date, neither the federal government nor any province or territory has requested the assistance of the military during the coronavirus epidemic. In fact, any deployment of the military would have to be made by the Governor-General, the Commander of the Forces, on the recommendation of the federal government. Why the federal Liberal government has neglected to call for medical aid and assistance from the military remains a mystery. In China, hundreds of military doctors, and nurses, and tonnes of military medical supplies, were fully employed in the struggle to bring the Coronavirus epidemic under control and to provide medical care for the sick.

Government Policy: It was announced by the federal Liberal government that China will be donating 30,000 face masks, 1,000 sets of protective clothing, 10,000 goggles and 50,000 pair of surgical gloves, and a further shipment of N-95 respiratory masks, to Canada. At the same time, Prime Minister Trudeau announced that "the federal stockpile of medical equipment is sufficient to meet the needs of the provinces". That statement is totally absurd. It is unbelievable that the Prime Minister thinks that a promised donation from China will meet the need of Canada's medical personal, frontline responders and personal care workers for personal protective equipment, when and if the Chinese medical protection equipment arrives? It appears that Prime Minister Trudeau is completely out of touch of the situation on the ground. While the Chinese donation is greatly needed, and much appreciated, there is some cause for apprehension. The Netherlands government just announced the recall of 600,000 face masks imported from China. They did not fit properly, and do not prevent the coronavirus from passing through!

Coronavirus Response: Three of Canada's largest auto parts manufacturers are now working with the Province of Ontario to produce several thousand ventilators for use in hospitals. The Bank of Canada announced that it will commence the purchase of up to $5 billion of provincial government bonds per week to help stabilize the economy. Moreover, economists have expressed their approval of the financial aid package of the Liberal Government. The magnitude of the financial aid has finally brought Canada's efforts to support the economy closer to the level of expenditures that the European countries have been making – on a per capita basis relative to their respective populations -- during the coronavirus epidemic.

Testing Kits: In the United States, an American company, United Biomedical, has developed an antibody testing kit which can detect COVID-10 infections within hours, rather than in the two days to a week required to obtain laboratory results from a nasal swab (nasophyngeal swab) or throat swab (sputum swab). The test kits, which are being manufactured by a subsidiary Covaxx, are now being tested in China and Colorado.

In Europe, the failure to introduce a widespread testing for the coronavirus at an early date is attributable to problems with the testing kits that governments purchased in the millions from China. When testing commenced, Spain, the Czech Republic, Slovakia, and Turkey reported that the testing kits that had been purchased from China gave 'inaccurate results', 'wrong results', 'incorrect results' and 'too high an error rate to be usable", respectively. The United Kingdom ordered 3.5 million testing kits from China, but the kits were found to be unusable when they arrived. In the United States, the Center for Disease Control developed its own testing kit, which proved unreliable and set back testing for the better part of a month or more in that country. Only recently have China and the United States, and several European countries, developed testing kits that appear to provide a reliable test for the COVID-19 virus in the traditional manner of taking a nasal swab for analysis in a PCR (polymerase chain reaction) machine in a laboratory. The PCR machine identifies pathogens in the swab secretions by detecting their DNA (deoxyribonucleic acid), in a laboratory process that can take one to three days.

Saturday, March 28, 2020 (continued)

Government Policy: Prime Minister Trudeau announced that, effective as of next Monday, anyone showing COVID-19 symptoms will be banned from domestic flights and trains. Why the federal government neglected to impose such a ban a month or more earlier, was not explained. Surely, the basic principle in containing an epidemic is to prevent travellers from spreading it from one community to another.

The provincial governments have not hesitated to declare a state of emergency, and to use their emergency powers to combat the spread of the Coronavirus in closing down non-essential businesses, stores, and schools, in prohibiting large gatherings of people, in introducing testing to identify the sick and the carriers of the virus, and in taking steps to enforce a self-isolation policy. In Ontario, gatherings of more than fifty persons have been banned, and a broad testing program has been introduced. However, the testing program has been of a limited extent owing to a shortage of the nasal swabs used in the testing kits.

Today, Premier Doug Ford of Ontario announced the immediate introduction of a further limit on public gatherings -- to no more than five persons – and that legislation has been enacted to provide severe penalties for price gouging. Individuals who engage in price gouging in the hoarding and sale of essential medical supplies needed for combatting the spread of the COVID-19 virus and the treatment of its symptoms -- such as masks and gloves, disinfectants, and non-prescription medications – are to be fined and/or jailed. Individuals can be ticketed and fined $750 or, if summoned and convicted in court, can be fined a maximum of $100,000 or jailed for a year. Directors and officers of offending companies can be fined up to $500,000 and sentenced to up to a year in jail, and corporations can be fined up to $10 million.

Coronavirus Status: In Ontario, there are 1,444 confirmed Coronavirus cases, with 63 patients in intensive care and 19 on ventilators. To date, the province has experience 19 virus-related deaths out of a provincial population of 14 million.

More generally in Canada, the COVID-19 virus is already well established domestically with 65 percent of the infections now reported as related to community transmission. Currently Canada has 4,700 coronavirus cases with a total of 61 related deaths out of a population of 36.5 million people. In China, the COVID-19 epidemic has been brought under control, but in the two currently worst cases, Italy and the United States, the virus has been spreading rapidly. In Italy, there are over 92,400 confirmed cases of the Coronavirus disease, and over 10,000 deaths have been recorded to date. In the United States, the virus has spread to every state on the mainland, with 123,600 infections, and 2,100 deaths. In both countries, as well as in Canada, there is a critical shortage of medical face masks, plastic face shields, and ventilators. How, and when, the COVID-19 crisis will end is the great unknown. However, China is presenting a cause for hope.

Sunday, March 29, 2020

Recovery in China: In China, the COVID-19 virus epidemic appears to be have almost burnt itself out. Beginning back on January 23rd, the Chinese government imposed a strict quarantine on the City of Wuhan -- the epicentre of the Coronavirus disease in China – and around other areas of infection, which eventually effectively confined over 800 million Chinese to their homes. The general lockdown was lifted on March 23rd. Now, the strict quarantine that was imposed on Wuhan, is being lifted after a two-month period of isolation.

As a first step in reviving the national economy, the Chinese government has allowed stores, businesses, and industries to re-open, as well as the operation of trains, subways and airports, and shopping malls, with employees wearing face masks and encouraging shopper and travellers to maintain a safe distance. However, with the opening of airports, it was found that some of the Chinese nationals, who were returning home to Beijing from abroad, were carriers of the COVID-19 virus. Hence, international travel controls were re-imposed, as well as a strict testing at airports. Returnees testing negative are ordered to self-isolate at home for 14-days; while returnees who test positive are immediately quarantined in one of five hotels that have been designated as quarantine stations with medical personnel in attendance. Not only are asymptomatic carriers of the virus a source of contagion to others, but the Chinese have discovered that asymptomatic carriers of the virus will develop the disease themselves in 75 percent of the cases.

Face Masks: The Dalian Institute of Chemical Physics in China has announced that a nanomaterial has been developed that can absorb and deactivate up to 99.9 percent of the COVID-19, the coronavirus. The Institute is seeking to work with companies to apply the technology in the manufacture of face masks and air purifiers. One presumes that the intention is to replace the faulty material used in some of the face masks currently being produced in China.

Monday, March 30, 2020

CEWS Extension: Prime Minister Trudeau has elaborated on the company payroll wage subsidy plan (CEWS) for small and medium sized businesses. It will now be made universal to cover all companies and business, both large and small, and will be extended to cover non-profits and charities. To qualify for the payroll wage subsidy, which covers 75 percent of the wages of their workers to a maximum of $847 per week for four months, the companies must maintain their employees on the payroll and recall any employees who have been laid off. The intention is to keep workers on the job and businesses ready to open as soon as the lockdown is lifted, even though there may well be nothing for workers to do in the interim while the lockdown remains in effect. Workers who are recalled by a company – or, more realistically, are put back on the payroll while they self-isolate at home – will not be eligible for the Canada Emergency Response Benefit (CERB) wage subsidy to avoid double dipping.

Businesses, companies, non-profits and charities that want to apply for the company payroll wage subsidy, will have to show that their revenues have declined by at least 30 percent under the impact of the Coronavirus epidemic; and that they have hired back any employees laid off in the two weeks since March 15th, when the Coronavirus first struck Canadians in force. Moreover, the government will require assurances that the 75 percent payroll wage subsidy payment will go directly to the employees.

The Canadian Federation of Independent Business (CFIB) has declared that the payroll wage subsidy will not help small businesses that have been forced to close completely. Their major fixed cost is the monthly rent payment due to a landlord, which cannot be made with no revenue to draw on. Yet, no level of government has offered any program of rent relief, or a rent moratorium for businesses that are closed. The Ontario government has partially addressed the situation in stating that the province will not authorize any eviction orders during the coronavirus epidemic. However, the payroll wage subsidy initiative of the federal government will greatly help the small businesses that are struggling to remain open. Small businesses are the backbone of the Canadian economy. A total of over a million small independent businesses, mostly in the service industry, employ upwards of ten million Canadians. There have been fears expressed that, in a worst case scenario, upwards of thirty percent of the small business operators might not have the financial means to re-open, if they are forced to stay closed for any extended period of time.

U.N. Security Council: As of March 30th, the Global Affairs Minister, François-Philippe Champagne confirmed that the Liberal government is continuing its campaign to obtain a seat on the United Nations Security Council – for a two-year term -- in competition with Norway and Ireland. With African countries holding 54 of the 193 seats in the U.N. General Assembly, Canada has been advised -- by U.N. supporters -- that it will need to provide "several hundred million" dollars of financial aid to the African Union to have any hope of securing the votes of the African nations for its Security Council seat bid. The money would supposedly support peace keeping, as well as used to combat the COVID-19 threat. Canada has already pledged $50 million, but apparently that is not enough.

The Liberal Government ought to reject outright this sordid blackmail attempt and should abandon any further pursuit of a Security Council seat. It is an ephemeral source of prestige on the world stage that ought not to be purchased at the cost of Canada's dignity, honour, and moral character. At this moment, there are critical, literally life and death, concerns that demand the attention of the Canadian Government. It is doubtful whether any Canadians, other than Prime Minister Trudeau and his inner Cabinet of Modern liberal globalists, currently gives a tinker's damn about securing a Security Council Seat for Canada at the United Nations. Presumably either Norway or Ireland will be a suitable representative of traditional western values at the U.N Security Council; although not necessarily representative of the Modern liberal values of the Trudeau government.

Screening & Testing: A rural county -- Renfrew County in Ontario – has introduced an innovative way of limiting the spread of the coronavirus while relieving the stressful demands being placed on the medical staff at hospitals. Individuals who are sick with flu like symptoms are encouraged to call a hotline to undergo a medical assessment of their condition over the phone, rather than going to an assessment centre or hospital emergency department where they would mix with others who may be seriously ill with the virus. If the symptoms diagnosed over the phone conform to the coronavirus symptoms, paramedics equipped with protective equipment are dispatched to the home to do a clinical assessment and testing in taking nasal swabs. Patients with mild symptoms are encouraged to stay in self-isolation in their homes, with only the seriously ill being removed to hospital. The intent is to discourage individuals with minor symptoms from descending on hospital emergency departments, which burdens hospital medical staff who need to be free to focus their medical interventions and care on the seriously ill.

Coronavirus Response: Elsewhere in Canada, hospitals have sought to curb the spread of the virus, and reduce pressures on medical staff, by cancelling elective surgeries. Moreover, hospitals are setting up temporary, makeshift medical ward centres in other buildings off-site to accommodate non-COVID patients to preclude their being exposed to the virus.

Tuesday, March 31, 2019

Liberal Government Deficiencies: A spokesperson for the Canadian Association of Emergency Physicians has criticized the federal Liberal government response to the coronavirus threat as being: "desultory, incremental [and] reactive" with "little dribs and drabs of information" forthcoming from time to time. He accused the federal government of focusing on "trying not to provoke mass panic" rather than "preparing for a national disaster". He characterized the federal government role in the crisis as "leadership by news conferences". Another frontline emergency medicine doctor lamented the shortage of personal protective equipment for medical staff, declared that the federal government should have 'declared war' on the virus in taking whatever measures were required to mobilize industry "to make the equipment that is required to protect the frontline health care providers." Yet, to date the Liberal Government has rejected all calls to enact the Emergency Measures Act, which would enable it to take direct action in ordering industries to produce what is needed.

A newspaper columnist has reported that Justin Trudeau made an absurd claim, on behalf of his government. In addressing Canadians yesterday. Young Trudeau claimed that:

> "We've been making sure we have money set aside for a rainy day. Well, it's raining, and we are now able to invest in Canadians".

The reality is that the free-spending Liberal government was facing the prospect of a record $27 billion deficit for this fiscal year before the coronavirus impacted Canada. In Liberal La La Land, the truth is apparently expendable when appealing to the public for support.

According to Keynesian economic theory, governments should decrease spending and save monies when the economy is booming, and should spend monies when the economy is contracting -- in times of an economic recession or a depression – to stimulate growth and increase consumer demand which is the driving force of the national economy. In contrast, the federal Liberal government spent freely during a period of economic prosperity. It ran up massive deficits each year during its first term of office: $19.0 billion (2016); $19.0 billion (2017); $14.0 billion (2018); and $19.8 billion (2019). Now, the Trudeau government is in the process of imposing a truly colossal multi-generational national debt on Canadians – a projected $200 billion deficit for 2020 -- in addressing what has become a severe national economic crisis with the federal government bereft of any substantial financial reserves to draw on. It will have to resort to heavy borrowing in international money markets.

Personal Protective Equipment: After receiving what was described as "a flood of offers" from Canadian industries offering to produce badly needed medical equipment, the Trudeau government has signed letters of intent with several companies for the manufacture of ventilators, personal protection medical equipment, and coronavirus testing kits. Thornhill Medical is working with a manufacturer to produce an initial order of 500 ventilators which will be ready to begin distribution to hospitals by early April; Medicom of Montreal has been engaged to acquire the N-95 respiratory face masks; and Spartan Bioscience Inc. has succeed in producing a COVID-19 testing kit capable of quickly identifying the presence of the virus. The Stanfield's Limited company of Truro, Nova Scotia, has also received a letter of intent from the federal government for converting its production line to produce surgical gowns. The company states that it will be able to produce 2,000 gowns daily. Moreover, the Canada Goose company has switching its production line from making parkas to manufacturing medical gowns and has the potential to produce 100,000 gowns per week.

The government is contributing funding for the re-tooling of existing facilities that are being converted to the manufacture of the requisite medical equipment. The government has now pledged to order 157 million plastic shield surgical masks, 60 million N-95 respiratory masks, and 1,570 ventilators at a cost of $2 billion. The number of surgical gowns to be ordered remains unspecified.

Initially, it appeared that the over the top reaction of the Liberal government -- in purchasing such an absurd amount of medical personnel protective equipment -- was the product of minds not well grounded in a sound common sense: viz. the ignoring of critical shortages for upwards of a month, followed by a panic mode purchase of protective medical equipment on a scale far in excess of any possible Canadian needs. However, an explanation was provided by Prime Minister Trudeau: "The goal is not only to meet domestic capacity requirements, but ultimately to produce masks for other jurisdictions in the future". Whether the 'other jurisdictions' will pay Canada for the medical personal protective equipment and ventilators that are to be supplied to them, remains to be seen.

(Two weeks later, the Minister of Public Services and Procurement, Anita Anand, explained that the department was "ordering everything that it can, recognizing that not everything will be delivered", and confirmed the Prime Minister's statement that the government was 'buying both for now and the future'. As of that later date, April 17th, the government had ordered 290 million plastic shield surgical masks, including 100 million from two Canadian companies, and had received 17 million to date. Of a total of 130 million N95 respiratory masks on order, two million were about to be delivered for distribution to the provinces. It appears that the federal government after ordering a phenomenon number of the various personal protective equipment items from foreign sources, is now ordering an equally phenomenal number from new domestic suppliers. Has the government given up on ever seeing its global orders filled, or is it a case of no one paying any attention to what, and how many, items are being ordered on the spur of the moment?)

One presumes that the gargantuan oversupply of medical protective equipment, ordered by the Trudeau government at a cost of hundreds of millions of dollars, is to be shipped to Africa in support of an ongoing United Nations initiative to combat and contain the coronavirus threat to that continent. If so, a cynic could find an ulterior motive in speculating that the Liberal government might be motivated to pursue such a course -- at least in part – out of a desire to secure support among African nations for the upcoming June 2020 vote at the United Nations that will determine which two of the three candidates -- Canada, Ireland and Norway – will gain the two open Security Council seats to be filled by a vote of the General Assembly. To date, the number of confirmed coronavirus cases is quite low in the various sub-Saharan African nations, although the virus poses an ominous threat of passing into the general population of 1.09 billion peoples. In all of Africa, inclusive of northern Africa, there are currently 5,559 confirmed cases of Coronavirus, with 532 cases resolved, and a total of 221 deaths.

Second Financial Aid Package: Service Canada of the department of Employment and Social Development Canada -- which handles employment insurance applications and benefits among other services -- has closed its offices in response to staff refusing to report to work out of fear of contacting the coronavirus while interacting with the public. Service Canada is now operating exclusively online with its staff working from home. Canada's Finance Minister, Bill Morneau, announced a major delay in the approval and issuing of the payroll wage subsidy benefits. He maintained that it would take a projected three to six weeks to set up the online portal needed for employers to access the payroll wage subsidy program for small- and medium-sized businesses. Moreover, the government needs to recall parliament to pass legislation to authorize the $71 billon payroll wage subsidy program. (The earlier $82 billion financial aid package approved by parliament, included a wage subsidy for workers who have lost their job through the coronavirus epidemic lockdown.)

Oil & Gas Sector: As of March 31st, the federal government has neglected to provide any financial aid to the energy sector which is suffering the double blow of the coronavirus shutdowns and a severe drop in heavy crude oil prices caused by Saudi Arabia flooding the market with oil in its price war with Russia. In the face of that double blow to the Canadian economy, the loonie has fallen to as low as 70 cents against the American dollars, equity stocks have currently fallen 22 percent, and over a million Canadians have been laid off to date. There are rumours of a split in

Cabinet between ministers who want to prepare a financial aid package for the oil and gas industry companies, and the environmentalist zealots among the ministers who are opposed to any direct financial aid and want to see a phasing out of the oil industry in Canada.

One wonders why western governments have not acted to resolve one major economic problem that is susceptible to being immediately resolved by government action. Why the United States and the western powers are not intervening to bring an end to the oil prices crisis by putting pressure on Saudi Arabia to reduce its oil production to pre-crisis levels, is beyond belief. Presumably the 'great powers' of the West have the power, the leverage, or a creditable threat, that can be used against an irresponsible foreign government to force it to do the right thing in reducing its oil production to let prices recover in the world oil market?

Liberal Press: When the coronavirus crisis is finally surmounted, and Canadians are back to work, there is one certainty as sure as death and taxes. The Liberal Press will praise Justin Trudeau and his Liberal Government for their 'heroic efforts' in combatting the coronavirus epidemic. Yet, the reality is that the drastic actions needed to stop the spread of the virus were taken by the Canadian provinces and territories and by local municipal public health authorities and medical personnel; that the federal Liberal government was very reluctant and slow to close the borders of Canada to travellers from infected countries who were importing the virus into Canada and transmitting it among Canadians; and that the federal Liberal government failed to take command of a worsening health crisis in continuing to follow an ad hoc, day to day, crisis mode approach that was reactive rather than proactive.

The federal government does deserve credit for finally realizing the seriousness of the economic impact of the coronavirus epidemic on Canadians, and for responding in introducing two major financial aid packages. However, it remains to be seen whether the Modern liberal ideologues of the Trudeau government are capable of administering such complex major government financial aid programs efficiently, responsibly and effectively, given their abysmal past record in failing to control government expenditures, and their penchant for announcing dramatic initiatives and failing to follow through with a 'hands-on' management of their implementation and administration.

March 15th – March 31st

Workforce Situation: Statistics Canada has reported on the impact of the coronavirus epidemic on the Canadian labour market. To date, the professional class has been comparatively little effected by layoffs. It appears that employees of government, and of major companies and institutions, have retained their employment, with many employees working from home on their laptops during the lockdown. However, professionals in small firms or private practices – lawyers, doctors, dentists, and physiotherapists, etc. -- have had to close their businesses.

With the closure of retail stores in mid-March, Canadian retail sales -- which were strong earlier in the month -- dropped 10 percent to $47 billion for the month. Sales decline by 50 percent for clothing, shoes, and luxury items; whereas the essential stores that stayed open – grocery, beer and liquor, and pharmacies – increased their sales by 20 to 30 percent. Convenience stores that stayed open experienced only a slight decline during the first two weeks of the provincial lockdowns. (Statistics Canada, April 26, 2020.)

Chapter Three

Wednesday, April 1, 2020

Coronavirus Status: In China, eight days after the ending of the lockdowns, the national economy is recovering strongly with over ninety percent of the major manufacturers and two-thirds of the small manufacturers back in production and shipping goods. The Chinese economy is reportedly well on its way to returning to its former level of activity prior to the COVID-19 epidemic.

Elsewhere, the public health situation remains rather grim, and particularly so in Italy and the United States, the worst hit among western countries. Italy has reached a total of 105,792 confirmed virus cases, with 75,528 active cases, 14,620 resolved cases, and a total of 12,428 deaths -- a death rate of eleven percent. The United States has 174,467 confirmed cases, and over 3, 416 deaths nationwide since the first infections were detected in early March. Worldwide, a total of 803,650 Coronavirus cases have been confirmed, with 39,000 coronavirus-related deaths to date.

In Canada, as of the end of March, there were 7,448 Coronavirus cases, 925 resolved cases, and 90 deaths. Ontario reported its highest single day increase in infections; there is a high rate of COVID-19 infections in Quebec and British Columbia; and several western provinces have seen a minor increase in infections. Across Canada, seven percent of the virus infection cases have required hospitalization of which three percent were critical cases, with a 1.2 percent death rate nationwide. In round terms, upwards of 220,000 Canadians have been tested for the virus with three percent confirmed as positive, and 93 percent negative. Canada is still in the throes of the coronavirus epidemic but so far the actions of the provincial and municipal health authorities have been successful in preventing any mass outbreak of virus infections, despite a critical shortage of medical personal protective equipment, and the lack of any firm direction or major interventions by the federal Liberal government. Moreover, the death rate has been kept quite low by the work of our severely stressed hospitals and medical care personnel, and by Canadians in self-isolating.

CERB & EI Payments: On April 1st, the federal public service opened a new website portal for the payment of CERB claims, together with a streamlined payments system for the existing EI (Employment Insurance) program. The new, fully automated computer processing systems were designed to efficiently process an expected flood of millions of claims from Canadians who were being forced into unemployment by the provincial coronavirus lockdowns.

Columnists writing for the Financial Post and the National Post have praised the outstanding achievement of computer programmers and staff employed by the CRA in setting up a computer system online to quickly process the new Canadian Emergency Response Benefit (CERB) payments which will be made to Canadians who have been laid off, or had their pay reduced by more than 15 percent because of the coronavirus epidemic. High praise was bestowed as well on the programmers and staff at Services Canada who streamlined an existing computer system to quickly process applications for Employment Insurance payments to Canadians who were laid off previous to the Coronavirus provincial lockdowns – which is generally dated from March 15th -- and are now unable to find work.

Following the March 25th enacting of the major financial aid package for Canadians -- inclusive of the new CERB wage subsidy program -- the federal government received a combined total of 3.7 million claims for either Employment Insurance (EI) or the new CERB wage subsidy payments. That total comprised over 18 percent of the Canadian workforce who were without any income in having lost their job on the imposing of the coronavirus lockdowns, or who were reduced to working part time and were in receipt of an income of over 15% less than previously.

At the CRA, the new web portal was able to quickly process CERB payments online. After filling out a short form, applicants were informed that the initial payment of the $2,000 monthly wage subsidy would be deposited in their account within three to five days. The speed of payment was possible because of the flat rate of $2,000 being paid, and the employment of the honours system which eliminate upfront delays in verifying the information being submitted. Applicants did not, and do not, need to provide proof of their job loss or proof of a 15% or more reduction in income.

When processing such a stupendous number of submissions, the key was to keep the inputs and outputs straight forward and simple. The earlier financial aid package of March 18th , which had provided for a wage subsidy equal to ten percent of the wages of each individual up to a maximum of $1,375 per month to encourage employers to maintain workers on their payroll, would have proved a nightmare to process with all of the different wage rates in various occupations and variations in wage levels across Canada, and over a million applications to process and issue differing payments. One need only the recall the earlier Phoenix Pay System fiasco of the federal Liberal government to understand the problems that might have occurred in setting up a computerized pay system.

Earlier Phoenix Pay System Fiasco: In 2009, the Conservative government of Prime Minister Stephen Harper initiated a plan to replace the 40-year old decentralized federal pay system with a centralized pay system that was envisaged as eliminating duplications, saving costs, and improving efficiency. A contract for $5.7 million was let to IBM Canada to set up an off-the-shelf payroll software program to administer and process the pay of a total of 101 government departments, comprising almost 300,000 employees. At total of $320 million was approved for the entire project, which was to be online by 2015. However, in May 2015, IBM reported there were critical problems with the project and advocated a delay in its implementation. That advice was ignored, and subsequently, the department of Public Services and Procurement Canada cancelled a pilot project to test the Phoenix system in processing the payroll of a single department.

When the Liberal government of Prime Minister Justin Trudeau came to power, following the October 2015 general election, there was no re-appraisal of the centralized payroll project; it was pushed forward aggressively. As of February 2016, the new centralized pay centre was launched in Miramichi, New Brunswick. The centralized pay centre was responsibility initially for processing the payroll of 34 departments, comprising 120,000 employees. In early April, complaints began to emerge that some employees were being underpaid, but the complaints were ignored by the Liberal government. As of April 21, 2016, the rest of the 67 departments of the federal government were added to the centralized payroll system and the old payroll processing systems were decommissioned in the various departments.

During 2016 and 2017, continuous complaints were raised that thousands of federal government employees were being underpaid, overpaid, or not paid at all, as the monies expended in investigating and correcting the sources of error escalated to $400 million as of May 2017, and $540 million as of November 2017. (IBM would receive $185 million in total for its services, with the federal government saddled with paying the cost overruns to IBM and the addition costs of trying to fix the problems with the Phoenix system.) To complicate matters, as of May 2018 there was a backlog of 600,000 pay requests that needed to be addressed. Decisive action was taken only after the Senate Standing Committee on Finance reported in July 2018 that the Phoenix system costs had risen to $954 million, and that the expenditures in trying to operate and fix the system would soar to $2.2 billion by 2023, if the system were not scrapped.

In May 2019, the federal Liberal government announced a competition to replace the Phoenix pay system. Hopefully, with simpler inputs and outputs. What is obvious is that the Phoenix system was overwhelmed by all the variables in processing the payroll of upwards of 300,000 employees at 101 government departments with different job categories, pay levels, pay increment periods, and overtime pay provisions, inclusive of seasonal workers under a wide variety of different contract terms governing their pay. Moreover, the information was being input by new employees who were not highly trained.

CERB Payments System: In contrast to the Phoenix Pay System , when the Canadian Emergency Response Benefit (CERB) was established in March 2020, within the Canada Revenue Agency, the managers and software personnel were given an immense, but straight-forward task: to process a flat-rate $2,000 monthly payment to upwards of millions of applicants, without a lot of parameters to factor in regarding eligibility. The project was pursued aggressively, and it was up and running successfully in a remarkably short period of time. It is a credit to the Public Service managers, programmers, and support staff of the CRA.

It is not clear whether it was the government or the Public Services who realized the critical necessity of not clogging up a computer program with too many variable and variant factors when inputting millions of files for processing. However, what is evident is that the decision to change the initial CERB system of calculating the among of the wage subsidy on the income of the unemployed individual to a uniform flat-rate of $2,000 per month for every applicant, was critical to the successful operation of the CERB payments program and the speedy distribution of the benefit to several million newly unemployed or underemployed Canadians impacted by the coronavirus lockdowns.

At Employment Canada, the impact of the closing of all non-essential business and industries by the provincial governments as of mid-March, resulted in the receipt of upwards of 2.23 million Employment Insurance claims in the following two weeks. Despite adding staff from other departments and re-engaging former EI processors who volunteered their services, the department managed to process but 560,000 claims during that period and there was a growing backlog. However, in late March, the government decided to go with the flat-rate unemployment insurance payment of $2,000 per month – matching the payments under the CERB – and the requirements that the claimants provide a record of employment and an explanation of why he or she was unable to find work, were dispensed with. At that point, the departmental tech team modified the software program to fool the computer into thinking that the claims had already been processed and approved, and that only the payment needed to be issued to the claimant.

On April 1, 2020, the new system was activated with all claims switched to the fully automated system. The streamlined EI payments system managed to clear 500,000 claims for payment in just 24 hours. (By Monday, April 6th, a total of 2.24 million claims would be processed with either electronic or paper cheques issued or in the mail.) Once again, Public Service managers, technical support personnel and staff did a superb job, in a time of crisis, to ensure that funds were quickly forwarded to Canadians in dire need.

To preclude a possible fraud with an individual applying for both a CERB payment and an Employment Insurance payment, the names of the recipients of benefits under each program will be compared to discern any double-dipping, and the 2020 Income Tax returns of the recipients will be reviewed.

(Subsequently, the integrity of the CERB system was compromised when the Liberal government introduced a policy of granting payments to anyone who applied to the CERB program. The government deliberately abandon any flagging of suspicious submissions, any cross checking, and any investigation of false claims. The new policy was justified on the grounds of necessity -- to get payments to unemployed Canadians with no source of income. It was a false argument that ignored the fact that payments were being rapidly processed from the very establishment of the CERB payment processing system.)

Thursday, April 2, 2020

N-95 Respiratory Mask: It was revealed today that the Liberal federal government thinks that the COVD-19 shutdown may need to be continued until July – three months hence. That is preposterous. It will destroy the Canadian economy and social cohesion. What needs to be done – now that the manufacture of respiratory masks is finally underway in Canada -- is to issue Canadians of all ages with a N-95 respiratory mask, and face shields for those with breathing problems, as soon as they are available, so that Canadians can go out in public, go to school, and go to work, without any danger of being infected by the COVID-19 virus or, if asymptomatic, of infecting others. Simply staying at home for an indefinite period, is not a viable long-term strategy.

The current drastic shortage of N-95 respiratory masks for Canadian medical personnel and front-line responders is deeply lamented. It is the direct result of the asinine decision by the Liberal government -- in early February -- to ship Canada's stockpile of surgical masks, N-95 masks and other medical personal protective equipment to China, without taking potential Canadian needs into consideration. One presumes that the decision was made by the Trudeau government in haste and in response to the World Health Organization request that the western nations provide medical personal protective equipment and ventilators to China to aid that country in combatting its coronavirus outbreak. Such appeals are laudatory, but the primary duty and responsibility of the Trudeau government was to protect the health and well-being of the Canadian people, which it has failed to do. The needs and welfare of the Canadian people ought to be the first thought and priority of any, and every Canadian government.

Rapid Blood Testing: To date, the only testing method in use in Canada for detecting a coronavirus infection, is one that employs the taking of a nasal swab to secure secretions -- deep in the nose -- from the upper throat cavity, which sample is then analyzed in a P C R (polymerase chain reaction) machine in a laboratory to detect whether the secretions contain genetic material from the Coronavirus DNA. The process can take anywhere from one to three days. However, there is a shortage of swabs which are imported from Italy, and of the testing chemicals which are imported from China. Consequently, in Ontario, health authorities are only able to test individuals who show symptoms of the disease, and the recommendation by several doctors that everyone in long-care homes should be tested for the presence of the coronavirus, cannot be carried out. However, there is one testing method that is not being used in Canada: viz. a rapid blood test that can detect a coronavirus infection within fifteen minutes.

Blood tests are unable to detect the coronavirus during the first five to seven days of infection, which is the time required for the immune system to produce antibodies in the blood. However, thereafter the blood test is totally accurate in detecting the coronavirus antibodies in the blood. Hence, the rapid blood test is highly valuable in detecting individuals with mild symptoms, and in identifying asymptomatic carriers of the virus. It is being widely used in Europe, Asia, and Australia, as well as in American hospitals. In Canada, no rapid blood test kit has been approved by Health Canada, which is ironic given that a Canadian company is a major producer of the rapid blood testing kit.

At present, BTNX Inc. of Markham, Ontario, has shipped 20,000 rapid blood testing kits to American hospitals, where it has been approved by the American government for use, and is preparing to ship a further 200,000 kits that are on order and sell for $10 U.S. each. The test is relatively simple. A drop of blood is taken from a finger prick, and placed in a well, followed by two droplets of a buffer, and after 15 minutes there is a reaction. If COVID-19 antibodies are present, red lines appear on a test paper. If not, the test paper remains clear. The test is highly sensitive test, specifically for the coronavirus.

Another company, Healgen Scientific Inc. of Houston, Texas, has also developed a rapid blood testing kit, and has a capacity to produce over 500,000 testing kits per day. The Healgen rapid blood testing kit has been approved for use in the United Kingdom, France, and Italy in early February, and in the United States for use by health care professionals only. However, both companies have submitted their testing kit to Health Canada for approval, and they have been informed that Health Canada is consulting with the National Microbiology Laboratory for validation testing and research before the rapid blood testing kits can be approved. Then the kicker. Health Canada informed the companies that "the World Health Organization does not currently recommend serological tests for clinical diagnosis, and Health Canada is following this advice". To which was added, Health Canada is giving the traditional PCR testing kits priority for testing. Why Health Canada officials cannot think for themselves and are wedded to the pronouncements of the WHO is beyond belief. Perhaps it starts at the top with the Chief, Public Health Officer for Canada, Dr. Theresa Tam.

Elsewhere, epidemiologists are expressing the view that the use of population-wide rapid blood tests can be an important tool in the eventual recovery process -- from the coronavirus pandemic -- in determining how many have been exposed to the virus, and to what extent a community has acquired some form of immunity to the virus.

Friday, April 3, 2020

Ontario Virus Impact Modelling: The Conservative Premier of Ontario, Doug Ford, revealed to Ontarians the modelling on which the Province is basing its policy decisions in its efforts to stop the spread of the Coronavirus. It is the first government in Canada to do so. In a worst-case scenario, based on the current trajectory, Ontario expects an upsurge in infections -- through community transfer -- to upwards of 80,000 COVID-19 cases and 1600 deaths in the month of April. However, in a best-case scenario, with new "enhanced measures" being introduced by the Ontario government, the projection is for a total of about 12,500 COVID-19 cases and 200 deaths in the month of April.

The modelling projection indicates that had the Province of Ontario failed to institute a shut down of non-essential services, the number of Coronavirus cases would have soared to 300,000, with a total of 6,000 deaths. However, with the closing of all non-essential businesses, schools, day-care centres, movie cinemas, theatres, and recreational facilities, the banning of large public gatherings, and the introduction of a self-isolation policy, the number of Coronavirus cases and deaths in Ontario -- as of April 3rd – reached only 3,255 and 67, respectively.

To prevent, the projected April surge in cases and deaths, Premier Ford announced that the list of essential businesses allowed to stay open, would be reduced still further. Pet supply stores, hardware stores and office supplies – except for delivery or curbside pickups – are being closed down; a so-called 'ring of steel' is to be placed around long-term care facilities to prevent the importation of the virus among the vulnerable elderly; teams are being established to implement an aggressive tracking system to identify and isolate anyone having been in contact with a person testing positive for the virus; all manufacturing companies have been closed down -- with the exception of companies producing medical supplies and equipment; new residential construction projects will not be authorized; and stiff fines will be given to anyone who neglects to maintain a two-metre physical distancing in public.

According to the modelling, the enhanced measures will greatly flatten the curve of new Coronavirus cases in Ontario and will prevent the projected surge in new cases and deaths during April. However, it is being admitted that modelling is not an exact science. It is based on data accumulated on the infection and death rates in other countries and in Canada to date and assumes a general fatality rate of 2.1 percent overall. What it fails to take into account are factors such as how many victims to date were already suffering from a debilitating disease or serious health problems, how crowded the cities were in the outbreak centres, and the general comparative health of the population of the different countries.

Saturday, April 4, 2020

Procuring Personal Protective Equipment: Canada's Health Minister, Patty Hajdu, revealed that Canada is paying inflated prices for medical personal protection equipment because of 'the extreme competition in the global market for the limited supply'. What was left unsaid was that if the federal government had invoked the Emergency Measures Act at the beginning of the coronavirus epidemic, it could have avoided the current crisis in struggling to purchase the needed medical personal protection equipment in the global market at exorbitant prices. The Canadian government would have had the authority to direct Canadian companies to manufacture the needed medical personal protection equipment and ventilators, to set a fair-market price for the medical equipment being manufactured in Canada, and to ban the export of medical equipment from Canada to the global market during the coronavirus epidemic. What is particularly galling to a Canadian nationalist is that the Liberal government is still placing massive orders for Medical personal protective equipment with Chinese companies, paying exorbitant prices, and organizing transport by cargo planes to get the supplies to Canada, when Canadian companies are starting up production runs that will be quickly meet Canada's real needs. Moreover, the quality of the Canadian manufactured equipment is uniformly good.

China is also an unreliable source of medical supplies of any sort. A Toronto doctor took the initiative, back in early March, to order 500,000 face masks from a Chinese company. The masks were packaged and ready for loading on a plane at the Shanghai airport, when the shipment was taken and loaded on another plane. The explanation offered by the company was that another customer had offered a higher price.

Sunday, April 5, 2020

Supply-Chain Problems: On April 4th, Premier Ford of Ontario condemned President Trump for banning the export of N-95 respiratory masks to Canada by an American company – the 3 M Company of Minnesota – which manufacturers the masks in its plants in China. Ford concluded: 'Never again in the history of Canada, should we be beholden to another country for the safety and well-being of the people of Canada". Premier Ford emphasized that Ontario was the manufacturing heartland of Canada; that the Province had the capacity to produce the needed medical supplies; and that he wanted to ensure that in future all such strategic supplies would be manufactured within Canada. Also, Ford pointed out that Canada could take a hard line with the United States, if need be. A significant number of Canadian doctors, nurses and health care workers were crossing the border each day from Windsor to Detroit to aid the Americans in combatting the COVID-19 epidemic in that City, and were sorely needed during the coronavirus epidemic raging in Detroit. (It was later reported that 1600 medical personnel who live in Windsor, cross the border every day to work in hospitals and health care facilities in the Detroit area.)

Subsequently, Prime Minister Trudeau denounced the action of President Trump, and Canada complained through diplomatic channels as well. The American government responded by allowing a shipment 500,000 of the N-95 respiratory masks to be shipped to Canada by the 3M Company.

What Premier Ford was advocating concerning establishing a domestic security of strategic medical supplies, fits well with the Tory Conservative belief that Canada ought to establish a national policy of strategic economic development to ensure that country has the production capacity to be self-sufficient in strategic goods and services, as well as in basic foods.

Premier Ford complained that his provincial government had been trying for several days to get approval from Health Canada regulators for a Mississauga company, Woodbridge Group, to manufacture a respiratory mask, similar in purpose and capacity to the N-95 mask. Why the delay? It is not rocket science. Surely, a respiratory mask mock-up can be quickly evaluated and approved based on the efficiency of the material used in blocking the passages of viruses, and the quality of the product. It does not require extensive testing in a laboratory. Such a lack of urgency and action on the part of a department of the federal government is inexcusable in a situation where there is a critical shortage of supplies amidst a coronavirus epidemic.

A cynic might conclude that the Liberal government does not want Canadians manufacturers of respiratory masks to spring up when it has already made a major commitment to purchase over 157 million N-95 respiratory masks on the global market: from the Medicom company of Montreal, which is currently manufacturing the respiratory masks in China. Moreover, the federal government has already placed a major order an American company – the 3M Company -- which has a manufacturing facility in China. Apparently, additional major orders have been placed by Public Services and Procurement Canada directly with Chinese companies. The expressed intent of the Trudeau government to purchase such a stupendous number of respiratory masks, is to not only meet Canadians needs but to have a surplus for distribution to Third World countries threatened by the COVID-19 virus. The unreality of the magnitude of the purchase orders submitted for respiratory masks by the federal Liberal government, is mind boggling. It defies belief. One can only conclude that it is the product of the La La Land mentality of Modern liberals.

What is equally off putting is that the federal Liberal government is reportedly already involved in negotiations with the Chinese government to maintain a free trade in medical supplies to ensure that Canada receives the N-95 respiratory masks that have been ordered. China is always quick to promote its national interest by taking steps to extend its hegemony in various fields and markets. To date, the Chinese have experienced no difficulty in doing so. They have found it easy to take advantage of the naivety of Modern liberals with their blind faith in universal free trade in keeping with their mantra of the 'free movement of goods and people, services and capital'. Having a free trade in medical supplies with China will make it difficult, if not impossible, to develop a viable domestic medical supply industry with Canadian laboratories and manufacturers having a capacity to supply Canadian needs during any future epidemic.

Monday, April 6, 2020

Personal Protective Equipment: Prime Minister Trudeau admitted today that Canada has been plagued by a non-fulfillment, or only partial fulfillment, of orders placed in other countries for critically needed medical personal protection equipment. He singled out the United States for blame for blocking an order for N-95 respirator masks from being shipped to Canada. In effect, President Trump has invoked the Defence Production Act which compels American manufactures of the medical personal protection equipment – principally the 3M Company -- to give a priority to the filling of domestic American orders. However, such a policy is readily understandable for any national government to adopt. In the face of the impact of a virus pandemic, a government ought to focus first on the critical needs of its own people. Such a stance should have been expected amidst a pandemic.

Rather than trying to deflect blame onto the United States government for the critical shortages of medical personal protection equipment in Canada, young Trudeau should look in the mirror for the culprit. It was his shipping of Canada's entire national stockpile of medical personal protective equipment and ventilators to China in early February -- to combat the coronavirus epidemic in that country -- that caused the shortages crisis in Canada. And it was his failure to enact the Emergency Measures Act to marshal Canadian manufacturers to produce the needed medical personal protection equipment that let a growing shortage evolve into a critical national health crisis.

Tuesday, April 7, 2020

Ventilators: In his TV 'Morning show' announcement of the day, Prime Minister Trudeau revealed that orders had been placed with Canadian companies for the manufacture of 30,000 ventilators. The companies were later fully identified as: Thornhill Medical of Toronto in association with Linamar Corp., a major auto-parts manufacturer in Guelph, Ontario; StarFish Medical of Victoria, a major medical devices design company; and CAE Inc. of Montreal (formerly Canada Aviation Electronics), a manufacturer of flight simulators.

What was not said is that there is a production problem. It will take upwards of three months for each company to produce 10,000 units, and several of the key ventilator parts will need to be purchased abroad as the suppliers are situated in China, the United States, and Europe. With other countries competing for the same components, there is potentially a nine-week lead time for parts orders to be filled. As of mid-April, Canada has 5,000 ventilators in total, and Canadian health authorities are relying on the stay-at-home/self-isolating policy, and the practice of social distancing, to prevent a surge in Coronavirus infections that might result in multiple thousands of critically ill patients needing ventilators before they can be produced in large quantities in Canada. It is a rather sorry comment on the free trade policies that have enabled Canada's manufacturing base to be depleted through the moving of production offshore. There are even mentions in the press that if hospitals become overwhelmed with patients in need of a ventilator for life support that hard decision might have to be made as to who would have access to the limited number of units available, with a preference being given to youth over the elderly.

Trudeau admitted that the purchase orders for such a vast number of ventilators was based on "a worst-case scenario", and that 30,000 ventilators would probably not be needed in Canada. In which case, the surplus would be shipped to other countries that might have a critical need for ventilators. Whether the other countries will be required to pay for the ventilators, or whether they will be donated gratis, was not specified. Once again, the Liberal government revealed its commitment to globalism. With Canada in the throes of an economic crisis, and the national debt soaring, the Liberal federal government is expending millions of dollars ordering the manufacture of ventilators far in excess of any potential Canadian need, for the benefit of other countries, yet to be determined.

Wednesday, April 8, 2020

Canadian Suppliers: As of early April, as an awareness of the critical shortage of medical personnel protective equipment became known among the Canadian public, more and more Canadian companies are voluntarily gearing up to produce the needed equipment. Stanfield's Limited of Truro, Nova Scotia,, a manufacturer of long john underwear, jockey and boxer shorts, and fleece clothing items, has announced that the company intends to re-establish and maintain a domestic supply line of surgical gowns which was wiped out earlier by free trade and offshore production. In Ottawa, a high-tech firm, B-Con Engineering – a developer and producer of optical systems for NASA – has started, on its own initiative, to produce plastic medical face shields. It is immediately shipping 150 medical face shields to frontline medical personnel, with 400 face shields to follow next week.

It was also announced that the CHEO Research Institute of the Children's Hospital of Eastern Ontario is combatting a potential shortage of N-95 respirator masks for its medical personnel by introducing an ultraviolet germicidal irradiation (UVGI) sterilization process employing ultraviolet light. It is a process that was developed by the University of Nebraska Medical Centre in the United States, where masks with the wearer's name on them are collected, decontaminated by the ultraviolet light treatment, and returned to the original user.

What these situations highlight is a further failing of the federal Liberal government. The Trudeau government ignored the early complaints by medical personnel of a developing shortage of ventilators and personnel protective equipment for medical personnel and health care workers, neglected to appeal directly and immediately to Canadian companies to produce the needed supplies, and then once the shortage became critical, the government panicked and ordered a massive number of ventilators and an excessively large volume of personal protective equipment supplies on the international market and has paid exorbitant prices for what it seeks to acquire.

Finally, the federal Liberal government is doing one thing right. It is following the initiative of the Province of Ontario, in approaching Canadian companies to produce ventilators, and the needed personal protective equipment, to produce the quantity of equipment needed for frontline medical personnel, health care workers, and personal support workers. Canadian companies have responded admirably, but given the immediate critical need, in the midst of fears that coronavirus cases might surge upwards, the federal government has been forced to make purchases in the global market. It is a market where other countries are competing to purchase the same equipment for the protection of their own medical personnel and health care workers.

Canadian companies must be encouraged to keep their new product lines in operation after the ending of the coronavirus pandemic, to provide a domestic source of critical medical protective equipment and ventilators, once they re-open their factories to produce auto parts, motor vehicles, other high tech components, and clothing. Moderate tariffs, with regulations and fines against foreign dumping and domestic price gouging, would suffice. The Province of Ontario has already introduced legislation to prevent price gouging in the marketing of medical protective equipment and disinfectants during the coronavirus epidemic.

Thursday, April 9, 2020

Global Supply Chain Problems: Yet another problem in purchasing critical supplies directly from China is that there is no assurance of any quality control when dealing with Chinese companies. On March 28th, the Netherlands announced a recall of six hundred thousand face masks manufactured in China that do not fit properly and do not prevent the coronavirus from passing through. On April 7th, it was reported that the City of Toronto has had to recall 62,000 "poor quality" face masks that had been distributed to long-care homes in the City. The masks were purchased from a Chinese company at a cost of $200,000.

The height of incongruity was reached on Tuesday, April 7th when Prime Minister Trudeau did an about face in his response to the coronavirus crisis. In commenting on the purchase of ventilators and personal protective equipment for medical personnel, Prime Minister Trudeau declared: "We need a stable supply of these products and that means making them at home". Yes, Prime Minister, that is what is needed: a Canadian manufacturing base for the supply of medical equipment. A Canadian manufacturing base is critical not only to meet any future need during a virus epidemic, but to ensure the supplies can be purchased at a fair market price, and that they will be manufactured in keeping with quality control standards set by the Canadian government.

It is obvious why the Liberal government of Justin Trudeau has abandoned its belief, at least temporarily, in global markets. Deputy Prime Minister, Chrystia Freeland, described the global market in medical supplies and ventilators, as being a "Wild West". It is a situation where purchase orders might not be fulfilled, or are being only partially fulfilled, where exorbitant prices are being demanded, and the securing of air transport of equipment and medical supplies to Canada is a vexing and costly problem. Out of 230 million face masks reputedly ordered by the Canadian government from China, only 16 million had been delivered to Canada as of April 7th. Moreover, earlier China placed a temporary ban on the export of the face masks and the N-95 respiratory masks to meet the critical need of its own people during the height of the Coronavirus epidemic in that country.

Friday, April 10, 2020

Rejection of Globalism: What is heartening for a Canadian Tory conservative is to see that, as of mid-April 2020, articles are beginning to appear in the press that are questioning the Modern liberal commitment to globalization – universal free trade and the free movement of goods, people, services, and capital; and policy wonks are speculating about the need for a "global decoupling" to ensure that supply chains are no longer "centralized around hubs like China". There is a growing belief countries will adopt a new industrial strategy that will see governments intervening in critical areas of the economy to protect the national interest and well-being of their country with an emphasis on having a domestic supply base to provide basic necessities to the nation in times of a world crisis.

Given the shortages of medical supplies being experienced during the coronavirus epidemic – with China being the source of needed medical personal protection equipment, antibiotics, enzymes for analyzing swab secretions, and raw materials needed for the development of vaccines -- it is evident that countries cannot continue to rely on global markets and free trade for their supply, regardless of the lower prices and production efficiencies that it may yield to the benefit of the international corporations. Yet another problem revealed during the coronavirus epidemic is that India is the source of upwards of 70 percent or more of the generic drugs needed by Canadians, the supply of which was cut off when India put restrictions on drug exports to maintain a supply for its own people during the coronavirus pandemic.

Canadian government policy should favour the manufacture of generic drugs in Canada, and if Canadian entrepreneurs are not up to the task, the government ought to establish laboratories and a Crown corporation to produce and market generic drugs at cost plus a modest profit. It would greatly relieve provincial health insurance plans of the burden of paying exorbitant prices for the generic drugs needed by Canadians.

Following the discovery of insulin at the University of Toronto laboratories (1920) – by Frederick Banting, and its purification by Charles Best and James Collip, and its refinement by J.J. R. Macleod -- the insulin was manufactured and sold in Canada and abroad at cost, for the treatment of diabetes, by the Connaught Medical Research Laboratories, a wartime public health agency in Toronto that was established to produce diphtheria antitoxin. The insulin was further licensed, under a non-exclusive licensing contract to the Eli Lilly and Company in the United States.

There is no reason, other than a lack of will, why Canadian laboratories and Canadian generic drug manufacturers cannot be similarly organized to produce and market the generic drugs needed by Canadians on a cost-plus basis. Moreover, pharmaceutical companies that are manufacturing patented drugs ought to be directed to establish branch plants to produce their patented drugs in Canada for the Canadian market, if they want to have the purchase of their drugs covered by the provincial health plans. It can be done, but what it takes is a Tory conservative frame of mind to engage government to play an active role in the establishment of strategic industries that are in the national interest and for the public good.

Saturday, April 11, 2020

Recall of Parliament: A special session of parliament, with a reduced 32-member representation from all parties, was called to enact legislation to authorize the business payroll wage subsidy benefit that the federal government had promised earlier – which is being called the Canada Emergency Wage Subsidy (CEWS) program. Prime Minister Trudeau announced earlier, on March 26th, that a business payroll wage subsidy benefit would be provided for small- and medium-sized businesses. Thereafter, on March 30th, he had announced further that the benefit would be expanded to cover all businesses that met the access criteria. Ten days later, on April 9th, the Conservative financial critic, Pierre Poilievre, complained that no government monies were being provided to Canadian businesses. The Liberal government had neglected to recall parliament to authorize the spending. The announcement of new policies and the lack of any immediate follow-up action to implement them has become an all-too-common failing of the Justin Trudeau Liberal government.

Financial Aid Package (April 11th): During the Saturday session on Easter weekend, a bill was passed authorizing the government to pay companies and businesses a payroll wage subsidy equivalent to 75 percent of the first $58,700 earned by each employee, up to a maximum of $847 per week for twelve weeks (reduced from 16 weeks in the original announcement). To be eligible to access the program, a business must have experienced a revenue drop of 15 percent in March, or 30 percent in April or May (a change from the flat 30 percent criterion announced earlier). An expenditure of $83 billion was authorized to cover the cost of the business payroll wage subsidy program, which all Canadian businesses, who meet the criteria, are eligible to access.

In addition, during a six-hour session of speeches and debate, the House supported a motion that the government provide non-repayable loans for small- and medium-sized businesses who have fixed costs, such as rent, that needed to be paid. An NDP/Bloc Quebecois motion was also adopted that called for the government to provide assistance to seasonal workers and owner-operators of small businesses who cannot meet the established criterion for financial assistance under the earlier wage subsidy benefit for workers: the Canadian Emergency Response Benefit (CERB).

The business payroll wage subsidy bill (CEWS) was passed by the House of Commons 'on division' with several members dissenting; it passed the Senate on Saturday evening; and it received the royal assent immediately from the Governor-General. The government announced that it would need two to five weeks to get the financial aid program in operation. Apparently, nothing much had been accomplished since the Prime Minister announced the intention of his government to introduce such a program on March 26th.

Sunday, April 12, 2020

Easter Sunday: a day of relaxation and contemplation in self-isolation.

Monday, April 13, 2020

Testing Kits: Spartan Bioscience Inc. of Ottawa announced that it has received Health Canada approval to market its portable testing kit which is capable providing test results for the coronavirus on site, from a DNA mouth swab. The so-called "Spartan Cube" kit – about the size of a coffee cup – is highly portable and uses a patented swab and a cartridge manufactured by the company in Ottawa. It permits a rapid testing with the test results obtainable within an hour by non-laboratory personnel, and can be readily used at airports, border points, or remote locations, as well as in hospitals and long-term care centres. It has a 100 percent accuracy rate in detecting the presence of the coronavirus. The process is quite simple. A cartridge with the DNA swab is inserted into the cube, a button is pressed, the analysis commences, and the test result is generated.

The new testing kit technology was developed with funding from the National Research Council of Canada. As early as April 2nd, the Province of Alberta ordered 100,000 of the coronavirus testing kits, and the Province of Ontario ordered 900,000 texting kits, with both orders dependent upon approval being received from Health Canada for the testing kit. Now, that the new technology has been approved by Health Canada, Quebec has ordered 200,000 Spartan testing kits. The initial production capacity of Spartan Bioscience is only 14,000 testing cubes per month, and efforts are underway to ramp up production.

In Canada, the existing virus testing kits system requires a long nasopharyngeal swab to be inserted up into the nose to collect secretions from the uppermost part of the throat, behind the nose. The swab containing the secretions, is then sent to a hospital or a public health laboratory for processing in a machine that conducts a polymerase chain reaction (PCR) test to determine whether the COVED-19 virus DNA is present. That process can take several days to a week, depending on the demands put on the laboratory. To date, use of the nasal swab testing for coronavirus infections has been quite limited in Canada, owing to a shortage of the nasal swabs which are produced primarily in Italy, but also in China, and testing chemicals which are produced in China. (Two days later, the House of Commons Health Committee was informed that 100,000 testing swabs imported by the Canadian government from China -- in early April -- had arrived contaminated and were discarded.) Testing will be on a far too-limited scale in Canada until the Spartan cube can be produced in mass production runs.

(The U.S. efforts to test for the COVID-19 virus have also been equally hamstrung by a reliance on Italy for swabs and on China for the enzyme needed for the chemical reaction in the laboratory analysis of the swab samples collected with the conventional nasal testing kits. As of mid-April, 147,000 coronavirus tests were being administered each day in the United States, which is far too low to get the epidemic under control there. However, as of April 17th, U.S. Cotton, the largest American manufacturer of cotton swabs, announced that the company had developed a polyester-based Q-tip-type swab that is fully compatible with COVID-19 testing standards. It has been approved by the Food and Drug Administration (FDA) for use in the United States. Several days later, on April 21st, it was reported that another company, the Laboratory Corporation of America (Lab Corp), has developed a COVID-19 testing kit, called the Pixel. It has been approved by the FDA for commercial sale to individuals to use for home testing through collecting a nasal swab sample and placing it in an insulated package for mailing to a Lab Corp laboratory for diagnosis. Whether the Pixel kit uses the new polyester-based Q-tip-type of swab was not reported.)

Tuesday, April 14, 2020

Oil Industry: Jason Kenny, the Premier of Alberta, declared the Canadian oil and gas sector, inclusive of the service sector and the drillers, will need $20 billion to $30 billion in federal government financial aid to survive the current economic crisis. The Alberta industry has suffered a double blow: a thirty percent drop in demand owing to the impact of the Coronavirus epidemic in Canada; and the drastic fall in the price of Western Canadian Select crude from $40 US per barrel to as low as $4.42 US per barrel on the global market, owing to the flooding of the oil market by Saudi Arabia in its price dispute with Russia. Canadian oil producers have been saved from bankruptcy only by the banks refraining from calling in loans. The banks are not interested in acquiring oil industry assets from loan defaulters.

It is a real travesty that the federal Liberal government has delayed providing sorely needed federal financial aid to the Canadian oil and gas sector, which is centred on Alberta. The Fraser Institute has calculated that between 2007 and 2015, Alberta contributed over $221.4 billion more to Canada through tax revenues raised by the federal government in Alberta -- which was prospering from the oil and gas industry – than the $92 million it received in federal government services. That money was used to finance equalization payments to the 'have not provinces' -- Quebec, Manitoba, Newfoundland-Labrador, Nova Scotia, New Brunswick, and Prince Edward Island -- to aid them to maintain their social and health programs and a equitable standard of living. Now, is the time for the federal government to come to the aid of Alberta.

The one good bit of news is that President Trump intervened last week in the oil price crisis with a threat to impose "very substantial tariffs" on Saudi Arabian oil imports to the United States. In response, an agreement was reached on Sunday among Saudi Arabia, the other OPEC members, and Russia, to reduce global oil production by 9.7 million barrels per day, which represents the equivalent of ten percent of the current global production. The other oil producing countries of the G20 energy nations agreed to cut their production by 3.7 million barrels per day. Canada was not requested to cut its production. However, due to a lack of pipelines Canada is not a significant contributor to the global oil market, and oil production has already been drastically curtailed owing to the dismal American market price for Canadian crude oil. The hope is that oil prices will rebound to relieve some of the severe economic distress being suffered by the North American oil and gas industry, and particularly in Alberta where the price of Canadian crude oil per barrel is at less than half the cost of production.

One would hope that when the coronavirus epidemic has run its cycle, when industries are ready to re-open, and when foreign investors have massive amounts of capital in hand looking for safe investments, that the federal government will throw its power and legislative authority behind the construction of oil and gas pipelines and LNG projects to enable Canadian oil and gas to reach export markets and to provide a secure energy supply for Canada. Planning for a number of these massive projects is already completed, and such projects are labour intensive, are a great stimulus to manufacturing, are a potential source of major tax revenues, and when protected from endless court challenges by over-zealous environmentalists and illegal blockades by malcontents, can be, and have been, a major driver of the Canadian economy. Indeed, there is little hope for Canada experiencing a reasonably quick recovery from the current economic recession without a prosperous oil and gas industry attracting multi-billions of dollars of foreign investment. The demand for oil energy is growing rapidly as the world's population moves into urban areas, and oil prices will rapidly recover once the lockdowns are lifted, international travel restrictions are relaxed, and factories re-open.

Wednesday, April 15, 2020

Self-Isolation Policy: Deputy Prime Minister, Chrystia Freeland, announced that all Canadians returning to Canada will be required to explain where and how they plan to self-isolate for 14-days, and face masks will be given to all returnees regardless of whether they are exhibiting any sickness symptoms. Those who do not have an acceptable place to self-isolate, will be quarantined 'in a location, such as a hotel, agreeable to Canada's chief public health officer'. Given that phraseology, it is apparent that quarantine stations have yet to be established for the four airports that remain open to Canadians returning from abroad. Furthermore, under new regulations introduced under the Quarantine Act, anyone causing a risk of death or serious harm to another person by spreading the virus can be fined up to $1 million dollars or three years in jail; and the police have been given the authority to issue tickets to people who fail to comply with orders issued under the Quarantine Act.

Emergency Measures Act: Several Canadian premiers have advised the Liberal government not to invoke the Emergency Measures Act at this late date. The provinces already have their own emergency powers acts and public health regulations in place that are needed to deal with the coronavirus epidemic. The provinces are no doubt right. The time for the federal government to have invoked the Emergency Measures Act to provide leadership, direction, and a unified national approach to the blocking the importation of the Coronavirus, and its containment once present in Canada, is long past.

As to Prime Minister Trudeau, he has never had any intention of invoking the Emergency Measures Act. He has gone on record several times in stating that he regards the Emergency Measures Act as "a last resort" which he "hopes will never be needed". One could ask, if the Emergency Measures Act was not needed -- in the judgement of Prime Minister, Justin Trudeau -- to combat the devastating impact of the coronavirus epidemic on Canadians, when will it ever be used for its intended purpose by a Liberal government? Could it be that Justin Trudeau associates the Emergency Measures Act with the former War Measures Act that was invoked by his father, the late Pierre Trudeau, in deploying the Canadian Army on the streets of Montreal and Quebec City during the FLQ crisis of October 1970, in an episode that constitutes a black mark in the history of civil rights in Canada, and on history of the Liberal Party.

Coronavirus Cases: Canada has upwards of 28,000 coronavirus cases to date, with 1,000 deaths. However, the increases in new infections in Ontario, Quebec and British Columbia have been concentrated in long-care home facilities for the elderly where to date over the majority of the deaths have occurred. In Canada, over 94 percent of the coronavirus deaths are among persons over 60 years of age, and the elderly living in close quarters in long-care home facilities are particularly vulnerable to the spread of the virus once it appears. In response, the Ontario provincial government has announced that it is forming 'hospital teams' of doctors, nurses, and support staff to rush to long care homes on the onset of an outbreak to screen, test, isolate and treat the sick. Moreover, now that face masks and test kits are becoming more readily available, Ontario plans to provide all long- care home residents and workers with face masks, to undertake a screening and testing of both residents and caregivers, and an aggressive tracking of all contacts of the infected. As of today, Ontario is currently administering upwards of 9,000 tests per day on those most vulnerable to the virus. Moreover, care workers have been banned from working at more than one long-care home to prevent the transfer of infections.

In Quebec, there are currently well over 15,000 confirmed virus cases and some 600 deaths; the virus is sweeping through long-care homes for the elderly; and 1200 public support workers have contracted the virus. The provincial government has appealed to doctors and nurses to volunteer to work in the long care homes and had requested that the federal government authorize the Army to help as well. It was announced today that 125 military medical personnel have been dispatched to Quebec long-care homes.

Several provinces had reported no new cases for a day or two, raising hopes that the rate of new infections is beginning to fall, except for Ontario and Quebec. Across Canada, the number of confirmed cases of coronavirus is now upwards of 29,000 and the number of deaths at

1,200 persons. Worldwide, the number of coronavirus cases has reached 1,420,000, with 510, 480 recoveries, and 137,000 deaths. As of today, the epicentres of the pandemic are in Europe – Spain, Italy, France, and Britain – as well as the United States, with New York City and Seattle being particularly hard hit.

Thursday, April 16, 2020

Leadership Failings: Both Justin Trudeau and Conservative opposition leader Andrew Scheer returned to Ottawa after Trudeau spent the Easter weekend with his family at the Harrington Lake 'cottage' in Quebec, and Scheer flew back to Ottawa from Regina with his entire family – his wife and five kids – on a small nine-passenger Challenger Jet after spending the Easter Weekend at his home in Saskatchewan. Both leaders are being roundly criticized for their hypocrisy, after admonishing Canadians to 'stay at home' during the Easter weekend and to avoid going to the cottage. Scheer should have known better, but for young Trudeau, it is just another indication that he does not regard rules and regulations as applying to him.

Vacation Conflict of Interest: One needs only to recall that in December 2016, Trudeau and his family, and the President of the Liberal Party of Canada, accepted an invitation from the Aga Khan to spend the Christmas vacation on his private island in the Caribbean. They flew out to the island on the Aga Khan's private helicopter, stayed for the Christmas holidays, and Trudeau and the Aga Khan exchanged gifts. Upon returning to Canada, Trudeau was roundly criticized for what appeared to be a clear violation of the conflict of interest rules for public office holders. The Aga Khan Foundation – of which the Aga Khan was the head – was in receipt of grants totalling anywhere from $15 to $25 million per annum from Canada, in support of the work of his foundation in improving the lives of marginalized peoples worldwide.

Trudeau denied that the Aga Khan was trying to curry favour with his government and maintained that they had been personal friends for years. Subsequently, it was revealed that there had been no personal contact between the Aga Khan and Justin Trudeau for over thirty years since his father, the late Pierre Trudeau, had been a friend of the Aga Khan. After an investigation, the Ethics Commissioner, Mary Dawson, ruled that Justin Trudeau had violated Canada's Conflict of Interest Act, but no penalties were applied. The caucus of the then-majority Liberal government took no action to displace Trudeau as 'first minister', and no steps were taken by the Liberal Party hierarchy to remove Justin Trudeau from the leadership of the party. Trudeau emerged unscathed from a scandal that would have ended the career of most MPs or Public Servants, with no sign of contrition on his part.

Other than an outright vote by party members in the House to withdraw their support from a sitting Prime Minister of their party – an unheard of event in Canada -- there is only one way for party members in parliament to removed their leader, which is under the provisions of the Reform Act (2015). It was introduced by a Conservative MP, Michael Chong, to give members of parliament a greater role in parliament. Among its provisions is a clause (49.2) that specifies if 20 percent of the entire caucus request a review of whether a party member should continue to sit in caucus, a secret ballot will be held with only a majority vote required to expel the member from the caucus. However, the caucus expulsion clause is not mandatory. An amendment was made to the original bill in the House of Commons. The Act states that the expulsion clause does not apply to a caucus unless the caucus votes after an election to have the clause apply to their caucus. The Liberal Party caucus has never voted to accept the caucus expulsion clause. Apparently, the Liberal Party hierarchy does not want Liberal backbenchers in parliament to have the power to remove their anointed leader from the headship of the Party. In contrast, the Conservative Party caucus has adopted the caucus expulsion clause after each subsequent election. As long as the Liberal Party caucus lacks the courage to vote openly to adopt clause 49.2 of the Reform Act, the caucus has no control over its leader, and only the leader of the Liberal Party in Parliament can expel a party member from caucus.

Criticism of WHO: In parliament on Wednesday, April 15th (and again, on Thursday, April 16th), Andrew Scheer, the leader of the Conservative Party Opposition, expressed a concern about the close relationship apparent between the World Health Organization (WHO) and the Chinese government, and the poor track record of WHO in giving misleading, and often conflicting, public health advice during the coronavirus pandemic. He expressed a serious concern about the accuracy of the information being provided by WHO on the nature of the coronavirus threat, and declared that it was incumbent upon the Liberal government to explain why it was basing its public health decisions strictly on the advice from WHO. Scheer pointed to the initial claim by WHO that the coronavirus did not spread easily between people, and its early advice against countries closing their borders to U.N. members states, such as China.

More generally, the Liberal government is being criticized for adhering to the position taken by WHO on the controversial question of the wearing of face masks. The WHO has advised against the wearing of face masks by the general population and has maintained that face masks are only necessary for medical personnel and frontline workers in direct contact with infected persons. The Chief Public Health Officer for Canada, Dr. Therea Tam, who has served on WHO committees, was quite outspoken in discouraging the wearing of face masks during the early stages of the coronavirus spread in Canada.

Another criticism made against the Liberal government was that, based on WHO guidelines, the federal government refused demands from various Canadian health authorities and provincial governments, to close the border to foreign nationals when coronavirus cases began appearing in Canada. However, the Liberal government did not do so until March 18th, when it could no longer plausibly be denied that such an action was absolutely necessary to stop any further importation of the coronavirus from abroad. (On its part, the WHO did not declare the COVID-19 a global pandemic until a week earlier, on March 11th, when it was evident to all and sundry that the virus was already spreading rapidly in Europe and in the United States.)

In concluding his speech in parliament, Andrew Scheer claimed that the "autocratic, human rights abusing government" of China had had an inordinate influence on the WHO; that the WHO had suppressed information concerning the potential devasting impact of the coronavirus; and that the Liberal government must be held accountable for its decisions "if it's decisions are based on the advice of the World Health Organization".

Among members of parliament, there was a similar concern. The Health Committee of the House of Commons -- which comprises representatives of all parties in the House of Commons -- had unanimously issued a summons calling for Dr. Bruce Aylward, one of the Assistant Directors-General of the WHO, to appear before the Committee for questioning. Initially, he had agreed to do so, but then abruptly cancelled at the last minute. Clearly Liberal members of the House of Commons are concerned about their governing Liberal Party leadership following the advice of the WHO, and want the situation investigated, as do the members of the parties of the Opposition.

The criticism levelled by Andrew Scheer echoed criticisms made of WHO several day earlier by the Trump administration in the United States, and an announcement by President Trump -- on Tuesday, April 14th -- that the United States was going to suspend its $400 million per annum contribution to the WHO, which accounts for 15 percent of the funding on which WHO relies. Moreover, on the Wednesday, the Associated Press accused the Chinese government of suppressing evidence of the rapid rate of transmission of the virus for six days in early January before informing the WHO of the scale of the outbreak in Wuhan.

When questioned by the media about the charges levelled by the Trump administration against the WHO – and by Andrew Scheer in parliament -- and the American threat to withdraw its funding contribution, Patty Hajdu, the Minister of Health, maintained the Canadian government still placed its confidence in the WHO. She asserted that: "Canada values the work of the World Health Organization, and we continue to commit to contribute toward the work of the organization".

Prime Minister Trudeau deflected the criticism of WHO. He maintained that now is the time to focus on what needs to be done to protect Canadians from the coronavirus, and that Canada would continue to work with "the United Nations affiliate agency [the WHO] because the virus demands a global coordinated response". We "lean on experts in international institutions and in partner countries around the world who are making recommendations alongside our domestic experts on what we need to do now". Moreover, he added: there would be months and years in future to reflect upon the various institutions and systems, domestically and internationally, to learn from our responses, and how "we could have done better in this process". In sum, Prime Minister Trudeau is saying that: we are going to ignore the mistakes of my government; we are going to leave any investigation of the conduct of my government to sometime in the future; and my government will continue to rely on the World Health Organization for direction. When asked how much financial support Canada provides to the WHO, Trudeau replied that he did not know.

Economic Situation: With Canada's GDP falling a record nine percent in March, from February levels, and several provincial governments strapped for liquidity and unable to borrow monies in the global market, the Bank of Canada announced that it will commence buying up to $50 billion worth of provincial debt, as well as $10 billion of investment-grade corporate bonds. The stated intent is to maintain liquidity, prevent major structural damage to the economy, and, hopefully, lay the basis for "a relatively fast recovery".

Although there has been some speculation as to when the provincial lockdowns can be removed, Prime Minister Trudeau warned that it "would be absolutely disastrous for us to open up too early or too quickly and have another wave hit us that could be just as bad as this one and find ourselves in a situation of having to go back to quarantines".

Friday, April 17, 2020

Farmers & Seasonal Workers: Farmers are reportedly worried about losing their crops, and the millions of dollars invested, if a recurrence in the spread of the coronavirus should strike the farming sector during harvest time. They are asking for some type of crop insurance program to be offered by the federal government. At present the federal government has provided a $2 billion loan program for farmers, but the farmers maintain that they cannot afford to take on more debt. The federal government also has financed a $50 million program to pay farmers $1,500 for each seasonal migrant worker that they employ to cover the wages of the worker, and the cost of room and board, during the 14-day compulsory isolation period for seasonal workers upon their arrival. Travel restrictions have been lifted through classifying foreign seasonal workers as essential workers in the farming sector.

To ensure that famers will comply with the 14-day isolation period for seasonal workers upon their arrival, the federal government has prescribed heavy fines that might be imposed on farmers and farm organizations who fail to isolate the seasonal workers. The fines range from $1,000 to $100,00 per violation, up to a maximum of $1 million for a major violation. However, the federal government has no system of inspection. It is relying on local health units and provincial labour ministries to enforce the regulations on behalf of Services Canada. Advocates for seasonal migrant workers are demanding that the federal government provides a dedicated office to enforce the 14-day isolation requirement, to inform migrant workers of their rights in their own language, and to provide support for workers who lodge complaints. In contrast, the agricultural industry is worried that the huge financial penalties that might be levied against farmers who inadvertently contravene some requirement, or are judged to have done so, will discourage them from seeking seasonal migrant workers with a resultant loss of major crops, and of an employment income for the prospective migrant workers.

The critical problem is how to keep seasonal migrant workers isolated for 14-days in practicing social distancing. On a large fruit or vegetable farm, up to forty seasonal workers might be employed, and accommodated in five or six dormitories where they eat in a common area. Isolating the seasonal migrant workers individually upon arrival on a farm, and maintaining a social distancing, will be impossible for all practical purposes. The only alternative would be to place each seasonal migrant worker in a hotel room. However, in doing so the farmers will incur a heavy expense, whereas the federal financial subsidy covers only the added wage cost and a basic room and board costs for a migrant worker while remaining idle in isolation for 14-days.

A much better approach would have been for the federal government to quarantine seasonal migrant workers at the border for 14 days after their arrival, and then to test them to ensure that they are free of the virus before proceeding to the farms where they will be employed for the summer. In that case, the federal government would not have to pay a wage subsidy to farmers to compensate them for the payment of two weeks of wages, and room and board, while the seasonal workers are in isolation on the farm. The worst thing for a farmer is to have a seasonal migrant worker become sick with the coronavirus soon after arrival. It would introduce the virus on the farm, and it would put at risk the local community which most likely is not equipped to deal with a coronavirus patient or patients. The response of the federal government to the seasonal migrant workers problem is typical of the approach of the Trudeau Liberal government to any problem. A large sum of public money is thrown at a problem without the government taking any action on its part or making any effort to look for a practical solution to the problem.

Although seasonal migrant workers have been classified as essential workers and are admissible to Canada, a general ban on foreign travellers is in force in most countries. During the current coronavirus pandemic, there are almost insuperable problems for farmers to overcome to secure seasonal migrant workers. Employment and Social Development Canada is projecting a shortage of 20,000 farm labourers this year. One solution proposed by a member of parliament is that the government allow unemployed Canadians, who are receiving the $2,000 monthly CERB payment, to be permitted to work on farms and in processing plants without losing their payment benefit. However, the hours of work in the fields are long; the work is often exhausting for those who are not accustomed to hard physical labour; and the basic skills involved are not easily grasped by novices, and the work in processing plants is onerous. Hence, the engaging of unemployed company and retail store employees in farm work is a non-starter.

Statistics Canada has reported that Canada lost a million jobs in March.

Canada and the United States announced that they have renewed their ban on non-essential travel across their joint border for another 30-days until June 21st. The cross-border travel ban was introduced in March, with the intention of renewing it on a month by month basis, if required.

Financial Aid Programs: Prime Minister Trudeau announced that $962 million will be provided to help rural businesses, $500 million for the arts, sports, and cultural sectors, and a further $250 million to support start-up companies working on innovative technologies.

Oil Industry: In his announcement, Prime Minister Trudeau stated that the federal government would spend $1.7 billion for the remediation of abandoned oil wells, and $750 million to reduce methane gas emissions. These initiatives will create upwards of 10,000 jobs in total and were hailed by environmentalists. However, Canadian oil company executives are calling for the federal government to do more in providing lines of credit or making repayable loans available to the oil industry. They are not seeking handouts. Nonetheless, a rumour that the federal government was preparing a $15 billion aid package for the oil industry, drew an immediate protest from a well-organized consortium of 84 environmental groups from around the world. Why these environmental zealots are crucifying the Canadian oil industry when two of the real culprits in global warming – China and India – escape their wrath, is puzzling until you realize that it is the Trudeau government alone that heeds their alarmist rhetoric. Before the Canadian oil industry was crippled with the twin blow of the oil price collapse and the COVID-19 lockdown, Canadian carbon emissions contributed less than 1.6 percent to global warming, and probably close to a zero impact when taking into account the carbon sink of Canada's boreal forest, tundra, wet lands, and agricultural lands.

Criticism of WHO: In threatening to withdraw American funding from the WHO, President Trump criticized the WHO for placing all other nations in jeopardy by uncritically relaying misleading coronavirus information from China during the early stages of the COVID-19 outbreak. However, Prime Minister Trudeau has refused, as of mid-April, to respond to a demand by the Conservative opposition that a parliamentary inquiry be launched into what transpired with respect to the misleading WHO reports, and has deflected repeated demands from the Press for comment. To date, the Prime Minister has stated only that: "it is really important that we stay coordinated as we move through this". The stance of the Liberal government -- as expressed by Christya Freeland, the Deputy Prime Minister -- is that all countries need to cooperate during the pandemic in "working actively with WHO".

On April 17th, it was reported that two retired Canadian diplomats -- a former ambassador to China, and a former envoy to China – have criticized the federal Liberal government for its complaisant attitude towards China, and its glossing over of China's deliberate misleading of other countries as to the threat posed by the coronavirus. Health Minister, Patty Hajdu has characterized such criticisms of China as being dishonest, and as 'conspiracy theories originating on the Internet'. Dr. Tam, the Chief Minister of Health, is more circumspect and diplomatic. She took the stance that Canada is involved in "a learning exercise" and is dependent on cooperation with other countries more than ever.

What is evident beyond dispute is the extent to which the Liberal government has been submissively following the recommendations of the World Health Organization and has resisted calls from Canadians that airports and borders to be closed to travellers from China. The lack of action by the Trudeau government was based on a mistaken belief in the honest and integrity of the government of China that the virus threat was modest, a faith in the competence and integrity of the WHO, and political correctness -- a desire not to offend the sensibilities of the Chinese people and their government by immediately banning Chinese travellers from entering Canada.

What is equally disturbing is a report that the WHO, as of mid-April, still considers the wearing of face masks by non-infected persons as being unnecessary. Still another startling revelation was made by a former Chief of Staff (2010-2015) in the Ministry of Public Safety and Emergency Preparedness (now Public Safety Canada). He claims that a "quietly Malthusian" belief existed among his colleagues in that department, and that it consisted of a general acceptance that in any virus outbreak "the strong will live, and the weak will perish". There was also a lack of any belief in the doctrine of containment and the closing of borders. The mindset of the Canadian public health authorities was to rely solely on health care services to treat those who succumbed to a virus infection. Sadly, it is these same officials – the cited former colleagues -- who are now advising the Canadian government during the present coronavirus epidemic. Enough said!

Indigenous Financial Aid: Prime Minister Trudeau announced that $306 million will be provided by the federal government in aid of small and medium-sized Indigenous businesses suffering from the effects of the COVID-19 lockdown. The financial aid program will be administered through the existing Aboriginal Capital Corporation Association which offers financing and business support services to First Nations, Inuit, and Métis businesses. The financial aid will take the form of short-term, interest free loans, and non-repayable grants. Prime Minister Trudeau stressed that the money would enable thousands of aboriginal businesses, many owned and operated by women, to survive the economic downturn during the COVID-19 lockdown.

Indigenous Services Minister, Marc Miller, stated that many Indigenous businesses are in rural or remote locations, and lack a ready access to capital. It is expected that 6,000 Indigenous-owned businesses are in danger of closing. They are experiencing a dramatic drop in business, and in revenue, during the COVID-19 epidemic. In announcing the new Indigenous business financial aid package, Prime Minister declared that more help would be coming soon.

City of Ottawa: In Ottawa, the nation's capital – population 934,000 -- the total number of coronavirus cases has reached 728, with 21 deaths, and a daily rate of new infections as high as fifty cases. In Ottawa, as well as in Ontario and Quebec more generally, the new cases are largely in long-term care homes for the elderly. However, in Ottawa, the four city-owned and managed long-care homes -- a total of 717 beds, with 1,100 staff -- have not experience a single COVID-19 infection to date. The protection of the elderly residents from infection was due to actions of the Director of the facilities, Dean Lett, who upon becoming aware of the virus threat, implemented simple precautions to secure his facilities. Visitors were banned; staff and contract service personnel entering the facilities were required to wear personal protective equipment – face masks, gloves and gowns -- which the facilities had in stock; residents were screened twice daily for any symptoms of the disease; staff were banned from working at more than one facility, long before the Ontario government issued that regulation; new arrivals and residents returning to a facility were isolated in a room for 14-days; a liberal use was made of disinfectants, and social activities at the homes were altered to maintain a safe social distancing.

The prevention of the spread of COVID-19 is not rocket science. It requires only simple precautions to be instituted before the virus is present to preclude it from being imported and spread locally if it should become present. Unfortunately, these precautions were not taken by the federal government. Canada took no action, at an early date, to keep the coronavirus out of the country, and to keep it from spreading into the local population wherever and whenever it might have been imported.

Medical Services: Emergency departments at hospitals, doctors and medical clinics are reporting a dramatic drop off in their normal numbers of patients. People with milder forms of sickness, with infections, injuries, sprains, and chronic health problems are staying at home out of a fear of contacting the COVID-19 virus in waiting rooms. In Ontario, a survey by the Ontario Medical Association (OMA) has revealed that doctors are experiencing anywhere from a 20 to 90 percent drop in income. Faced with paying office rent, staff, for diagnostic equipment, and other overhead expenses, with a drastically reduced income, doctors are laying off their support staff, and a significant number have temporarily closed their private practices. Provincial governments are responding to the plight of doctors and medical clinics in various ways. In Ontario, the government has provided doctors with billing codes to bill the Ontario Hospital Insurance Plan (OHIP) for telephone consultations with patients. In Saskatchewan, the government has introduced an income stabilization program for doctors. In Newfoundland-Labrador, doctors are being paid 80 percent of their average billings to the provincial health plan on condition that they keep their practice open and assist when needed to deal with a COVID-19 outbreak.

Sports Leagues: The major North American sports leagues, and minor leagues, are facing an uncertain future as to when sports can be played again. Both the National Basketball Association (NBA) and the National Hockey League (NHL) want to complete their 2019-2020 season; Major League Baseball and Major League Soccer want to get their playing season underway, and the Canadian Football League (CFL), and the National Football League (NFL) are anxious to set a date for the commencement of their 2020 season.

At present both the NBA and NHL are investigating the possibility having their 2019-2020 season re-commence – once the lockdown and travel restrictions policies are lifted -- with games held at several neutral sites. The idea is to gather the players to live together temporarily in a 'bubble' at a designated neutral site or sites, where they can be tested regularly for the coronavirus, and play their games before TV cameras without any fans in attendance. Eventually, the hope is to admit a limited number of fans spaced out in the seating areas, and then eventually to return to their home arenas under normal conditions. However, there are numerous problems. Both the NBA and the NHL have teams in both Canada and the United States that will have to cross the border, which has just been closed for another 30-days; there are different self-isolating restrictions in force in the different cities, states and provinces of North America; and both leagues have a significantly large number of international players from countries where regulations governing travel will be maintained for different lengths of time depending on the severity and duration of the outbreak in each country. The logistics appear to present a nightmare.

Starting up a season to play games after players have been in a long period of enforced idleness --in being literally quarantined at home without being able to workout regularly -- will be disastrous in terms of potential physical injuries, not to mention tiredness and sloppy play that can lead to even more injuries. One of the most asinine proposals is for the NHL to complete the final dozen games of its season and to enter into a full playoff schedule, over the summer and through the fall. The intent is to have the players of each division of teams to be isolated in hotels at several neutral sites to play in arenas empty of fans for the first few months before transferring to their home arenas and playing before their home fans. Apparently, no thought has been given to the health and well-being of the players with the extended season running into the start of yet another full season of hockey, or whether players are willing to be separated from their families for a potential two months or more during the aftermath of a virus epidemic.

[Somewhat later, the NHL brass realized that the smaller cities proposed for hosting the early neutral site games – three in the United States and

Saskatoon in Canada – were not really suited for that purpose. In the smaller cities, there was a lack of the hotel accommodation near or adjacent to the arenas where the teams would need to house the players in isolation, and the arenas were not equipped with TV broadcasting facilities. Hence, attention shifted to having games played in several NHL arenas, which would be designated as neutral sites, where there are hotel accommodations adjacent to the arenas.]

If the NHL and NBA are to re-commence play this year, it would be better to write off the remaining regular-season games, hold a brief round-robin tournament for the teams within five points of a playoff spot, and then have a shortened playoff of five-game series. It would enable the delayed playoffs to be wound up in time to give the players an off season break before starting the regular 2020-2021 season of play. Otherwise, both the NHL and the NBA might better just end their 2020-2021 seasons, declare the team in first place in the standings as the champion -- with an asterisk in the record books -- and vote the individual awards based on the play of the players during the truncated season.

For the baseball, soccer, and football leagues the situation appears to be far less complex. They can simply delay the start of their season until quarantine and travelling restrictions are lifted, start playing before empty stadiums for TV coverage, gradually let a restricted number of fans attend the games with social spacing in the stands, and then evolve into removing all restrictions on fan attendance at various stadiums depending on how the virus threat has dissipated in the different cities concerned.

Saturday, April 18, 2020

Personal Care Workers: Prime Minister Trudeau has announced that the federal government would provide financial assistance to personal care workers earning less than $2,500 per month, and that the federal government was in negotiations with the provinces who are responsible for long-care homes. To that end, the Minister of Seniors, Deborah Schulte, announced that the federal government will increase federal health transfers to the provinces to enable them to 'top up' the wages of personal care workers in long-term care homes for the elderly. The intention is to encourage the personal care workers, who are receiving the minimum wage, to stay on the job in the face of the current rapid spread of the coronavirus through long-care homes in many areas of Canada, and particularly in Quebec and Ontario. Moreover, many part time personal care workers have suffered a loss of income in being forbidden by the provinces from working in more than one institution.

Quebec has announced that it will pay personal care workers an additional $4.00 per hour which is to compensate the workers for the enhance danger that they face of contacting the COVID-19 virus. With outbreaks raging thought long-care homes in Quebec, many personal care workers are staying home and applying for the $2,000 per month federal CERB payment. Technically, they are not entitled to the receive the CERB payment as they have not lost their job due to the coronavirus epidemic. However, no one is reviewing the applications to determine whether payments are being issued to personal care workers, who are refusing to report to work, are sorely need, and have numerous employment opportunities.

In addition, a temporary pay increase of eight percent has been introduced by the Province of Quebec for frontline medical personnel in direct contact with virus cases, and a four percent pay increase for medical personnel in supporting roles. The two new initiatives will cost the province a total cost of $287 million. The provincial police have been ordered to crack down on people ignoring the self-isolation order and on non-essential businesses that have remained open, with the imposition of major fines. The Province of Quebec is currently the epicentre of the coronavirus epidemic in Canada with 5,518 cases recorded to date, and 36 deaths.

Ontario has announced that it will wait to see what the federal government plans to contribute before deciding on what monies to contribute to increase the wages of personal care workers in private long-care homes. In both Ontario and Quebec, the coronavirus is reportedly spreading like 'wildfire' among the elderly residents of a small number of long-care homes. More generally, it is elderly resident who already have serious health problems who are accounting for most of the virus-related deaths. In Ontario, the number of admissions to hospital has slowed appreciably, the number of COVID-19 patients in Intensive Care Units has remained constant at 247 for the past two weeks, inclusive of 193 patients on ventilators. The surge in coronavirus cases that it was feared would occur in the month of April, has not materialized.

(Subsequently, the Ontario government announced that front-line health care workers in long-care homes and retirement residences, will receive a $4 per hour pay increase, which will also apply to hospital personnel directly involved in providing health care to COVID-19 patients. In hospitals, the pay increase covers nurses, personal support workers, developmental services workers, mental health and addiction workers, respiratory technicians, and auxiliary workers. It excludes positions where workers are not directly involved in the care and treatment of COVID-19 patients, such as maintenance staff, lab workers, clerical staff, and dieticians.)

South Korea: Articles are beginning to appear in the press and on the Internet that provides insights into the recovery process in South Korea from which lessons can be drawn. In that country, citizens were encouraged to self-isolate if feeling ill, but there was no general lockdown of businesses. Three weeks ago -- after only a four-week period of some restrictions on public gatherings and self-isolation for those who were experiencing coronavirus symptoms – South Koreans resumed their normal social and work activities. Citizens during the recovery stage are wearing a face mask and following a government directive regarding washing their hands and maintaining at least a one-metre social distancing in so far as possible. Since the lifting of the self-isolation, new coronavirus infections have been few and far between. The feared second wave of virus infection has not materialized.

In South Korea, schools were closed during the pandemic, and people were advised to wash their hands, and to maintain a physical distance from others, and large gatherings were banned. One advantage that South Korea had in combatting the spread of the coronavirus is that 90 percent of the urban population wore face masks during the epidemic. Stores and business remained open; although they suffered economically during the self-isolation period through a lack of customers and clients, with some bankruptcies occurring.

With the return to normal activities, some types of businesses are experiencing a slow recovery as people are reportedly afraid to travel, to go to restaurants, clinics, movie theatres, and sports centres, or to use public transportation, which are all situations where a physical spacing cannot be observed. However, on Wednesday, April 15th, South Koreans managed to hold a national election. Voters wore masks and gloves, stayed one metre apart at the polling stations, where they had their temperature taken and their hands disinfected before receiving their voting slip and entry to the polling booth. In mid-April, South Korean had the coronavirus well contained with only 100 new cases a day, while coronavirus cases were soaring by the thousands in the European countries and the United States. Why?

Like Taiwan, South Korea took immediate action to limit the importation of the coronavirus by closing its borders to foreign travellers at an early date, and to contain the spread of the virus by employing modern technologies in a tracking and testing program. The first virus infection was recorded in South Korea on January 21st, and by February 4th a testing kit for the virus was developed by Kogene Biotech of Seoul, and rapidly approved by the health authorities. As early as February 10th, testing commenced on an initial group of 2,776 individuals of whom 27 tested positive and were quarantined. By February 27th, two other South Korean biotech companies had developed testing kits, and testing stations were established in urban areas, inclusive of drive-thru testing centres, to serve the public. Additional laboratories were also set up to conduct a PCR analysis of the swabs.

On its part, the health authorities focussed on containment with an effort made to identify and locate any contacts made, and the areas visited, by infected individuals over the previous 48 hours. The purpose was to locate and test all contacts who were potentially exposed to the virus, to quarantine anyone who tested positive, and do disinfect the contact areas. In tracking the contacts made by the infected individual, the health authorities used electronic transactions data (credit card purchases) and mobile phone location logs, as well as police surveillance cameras once a specific area of contact was identified for disinfecting. The mobile phone tracking system was highly efficient, and efficient in tracking contacts and enabling the coronavirus to be contained, because 95 percent of South Koreans possess a smart phone.

South Korea had another advantage in that it learned from its experience in dealing with the Middle East Respiratory Syndrome epidemic of 2015 which struck the country harder than any other nation outside of the Middle East. In response, the South Korean government secured the passage of the Infectious Diseases Control and Prevention Act which gave health authorities the authority to access GPS tracing data from credit card transactions, smartphones, and cars that would be needed to track a virus infection threat, and the health authorities had not hesitated to use that authority.

All technically advanced western countries have the technology readily available that the South Korean government employed to efficiently, and effectively, contain the spread of the coronavirus. The key difference is that the South Korea government had the will and determination to implement an emergency measures act to take control and direction at a national level of the effort to combat the virus, with a willingness to provide the citizens with full disclosure of what the government was doing and why. That commitment to take command and provide leadership has been totally lacking in Canada under the Liberal government of Prime Minister Justin Trudeau. The federal Liberal government under young Trudeau has refused to invoke the Emergency Measures Act, has responded in an ad hoc manner to the coronavirus threat, and has left it up to the provinces and provincial and municipal health authorities to take whatever actions might be required to combat the coronavirus threat and contain the virus spread.

The difference in the response of the South Korean government and the federal Liberal government of Canada can be seen later in the differences in the impact of the coronavirus pandemic on society. As of April 30th, South Korea, with a population of 51.2 million has had a total of 10,728 coronavirus cases, 247 deaths, and 9,059 recoveries from the virus infection, and is well advanced in its social and economic recovery. Canada, with a population of 37.6 million, has had a total of 53,013 cases, 3,180 deaths, and 21,187 recoveries from the infection, and only as of the end of April are the Canadian provinces tentatively approaching a partial lifting of their lockdowns and a gradual re-starting of the economy. Moreover, that difference fails to account for the heavy economic cost Canadians are paying, and will pay, for the lockdown of the Canadian economy, which South Korean businesses and industries did not have to endure.

Drugs from India: Mary Ng, Minister of Small Business, Export Promotion, and International Trade, has reportedly intervened directly with her counterpart in India to secure the release of a shipment of five million capsules of hydroxychloroquine that was ordered by Canada several months earlier for the treatment of auto-immune diseases, such as lupus and multiple sclerosis, as well as for the treatment of malaria and rheumatoid arthritis. With the coronavirus ravaging India, in March the export of the drug was banned along with over twenty other drugs produced in India. Today, some countries are using hydroxychloroquine as an experimental drug in the treatment of patients infected with the COVID-19 virus, although there is no clinical evidence of its effectiveness. In Canada, Dr. Theresa Tam, Chief Public Health Officer, revealed that Canada is now studying the hydroxychloroquine drug which is "definitely one on the list" of possible treatment drugs for patients suffering from the coronavirus disease.

What is particularly disturbing is the revelation that India produces and exports to Canada anywhere from seventy to ninety percent of the drugs that Canadians need when they fall ill; and that, in our current global economy, there is no secure Canadian source for needed drugs. This is yet another argument for a government policy of national self-sufficiency in all areas pertaining to the basic needs of Canadians, and not just for self-sufficiency in food and energy. Government cooperation at all levels is necessary to ensure that henceforth generic drugs are produced in Canada by Canadian companies or a Crown corporation, and that private manufacturers of patent drugs establish branch plants to manufacture the drugs in Canada.

Such a policy can be implemented by the Provinces through announcing that within a period of five years, they will no longer pay for drugs produced in a foreign country. If that requires the abrogation of international free trade agreements, so be it! With health care cost soaring, and the payment for prescription drugs taking up a larger and larger proportion of provincial health budgets, it is imperative as well that the monies expended by government on drug purchases stay in Canada to provide employment for Canadians and Canadian tax revenues, rather than going abroad for the profit of international drug corporations and cartels. In the existing system, the federal government – and Canadian taxpayers – are locked into ever increasing, massively large health transfer payments to the provinces to cover drug purchase costs for an aging population.

If need be, a federal Tory conservative government might well consider the establishing of a Crown corporation to produce generic drugs, on a cost-plus basis, to reduce drugs costs and the necessity for increasingly large federal health transfer payments to the provinces to pay for the exorbitantly priced drugs being produced and marketed by international pharmaceutical corporations.

Chapter Four

Sunday, April 19, 2020

Recall of Parliament: When Parliament recessed on March 13th, with the coronavirus threatening Canada, MPs supported a motion for Parliament to reconvene on Monday, April 20th. Subsequently, emergency sessions were held on March 24th and April 11th, with a reduced House of 32 MPs embodying a proportional representation of all parties based on the number of seats held after the October 2019 election. On each date, a debate was held with respect to a financial aid package intended to provide support for Canadian workers and Canadian companies who were suffering a severe financial blow because of the lockdowns initiated by the provincial governments to contain the spread of the coronavirus. Both financial packages received a swift passage through the cooperation of all parties. In a one-day sitting, on both March 24th and April 11th, parliament passed – with the unanimous vote of all parties – two separate major financial aid packages for unemployed Canadian workers, businesses and companies devastated by the coronavirus lockdown legislation. Now the political parties are negotiating as to how a recalled parliament will operate.

Liberal Virtual Parliament Proposal: The Liberal government favours having a small number of MPs – representative of all the parties – to return to the House of Commons for one day a week until a system of virtual representation can be set up which will enable all 338 MPs to participate in the business of the House from their own homes, with Parliament no longer in session. The Prime Minister, Justin Trudeau, has proclaimed that the position of the Liberal Party is "a way to keep the important work of our democracy going while at the same time respecting public health". To date, no one has questioned the authority, and legality, of members of parliament passing legislation outside of parliament through a virtual connection with parliament no longer in session. Sovereignty resides within parliament, not in the hands of individual MPs sitting in their own homes across the country. As a former Liberal Prime Minister, Pierre Trudeau – the father of Justin -- not so subtly once put it: 'MPs are nobodies outside of the House of Common".

Conservative Reduced Representation Proposal: The Conservative Party -- as set forth in an "Open Letter to Canadians" (April 18th) from the Conservative leader, Andrew Scheer – is proposing that parliament sit for three days per week for a full parliamentary session, with the reduced representation of 32 MPs as adopted earlier. (A quorum of twenty parliamentarians is required to conduct the business of the House of Commons.) Where the virtual parliament idea is concerned, the Conservative Party is willing to accept a proposal before the Standing Committee on Procedure and House Affairs, which is already being studied: viz. the feasibility of having all 388 MPs hold a meeting in a virtual sitting, once a week, to keep all MPs abreast of what has transpired during three-day parliamentary sittings, and to give the wider body of MPS an opportunity to express their views. However, the virtual meeting would be only a one-day supplement to a regular three-day per week reduced parliament.

The Conservative Party position is that parliament must remain in session; and that it is a question of defending the rights, prerogatives, and powers of parliament. When parliament is in session, the MPs of all parties have two hours each day to question the Prime Minister, and his ministers, on government policies and expenditures; MPs are able to debate and vote on essential legislation; and parliament is able to exercise its customary oversight over expenditures and to expose government actions to public view and to hold the government accountable to the Canadian people. Moreover, the Conservative contention is that parliamentary debate, discussions, and tough questions lead to an improvement in government programs and policies. With a reduced number of MPs practicing social spacing in the House of Commons, and a reduced support staff equipped with face masks and gloves, there is little appreciable danger of a virus outbreak in the House of Commons chamber.

With parliament able to follow its normal procedures during a three-day sittings each week, it would facilitate parliamentary committees in being able to investigate government actions and expenditures through calling witnesses, passing motions, and forcing the government to produce documents for perusal. During the first emergency session of parliament on March 24th, the Health Committee had demanded, and secured, documents relating to the Cabinet's initial response to the coronavirus threat. At present, there are parliamentary committees that have been meeting virtually online, but the Trudeau government has denied them the exercise of their regular powers outside of parliament.

When in session earlier, parliament tasked the Auditor General with reviewing the unprecedently high levels of government expenditures being made during the coronavirus epidemic, to ensure that the monies are not being misspent. However, that task is complicated in that there is currently an interim Auditor General in office. Hence, the Conservative Party is calling on the Prime Minister to appoint a permanent Auditor General so that the review -- ordered by parliament -- can be got underway.

In this dispute, the Conservative Party has taken the position that the functioning of parliament is an essential service; and that the Conservative Party is proposing 'a common sense' arrangement to enable parliament to continue to perform its function. Andrew Scheer has pointed out that the parliaments of other democratic representative governments have continued to meet during the coronavirus pandemic: viz. the European Parliament, and parliament in Japan, Italy, France, Germany, Greece, Sweden and Finland, not to mention the U.S. Congress. Why not the Canadian parliament in regular sittings, for three days per week with a reduced representation? (The one exception is Great Britain, where a parliament of reduced members passed a package of emergency powers to enable the government to combat the coronavirus epidemic, after which parliament was immediately prorogued for a month – March 25th to April 21st – for an extended, but customary, Easter break. On April 21st, the British Parliament will be recalled for its regular sittings, presumably with a reduced representation, present in the House of Commons.)

Only the Trudeau government in Canada has tried to totally dispense with parliament during the coronavirus crisis. It appears that the Liberal government is trying to avoid facing a parliamentary scrutiny of its expenditures and of its blind following of misleading and incorrect advice from the World Health Organization in dealing with the coronavirus threat.

Virtual Parliament Proposal: With parliament due to be recalled on Monday, Prime Minister Trudeau has made a last-minute announcement that a tentative agreement has been reached with the NDP and the Bloc Quebecois to a Liberal proposal for establishing a virtual parliament. When the skeleton parliament resumes sitting on Monday, the intention is to put the Liberal government proposal to a vote. The proposal is to hold two 90-minute virtual sessions per week (on Tuesday and Thursday) with all MPs to participate via video conferencing, and a Wednesday sitting of the House of Common with the reduced representation of MPs based on a proportional representation of the political parties according to their numbers in the House.

How having 338 MPs tuned into a virtual session will function without the application of House of Commons rules through the Speaker formally recognize speakers and controlling the time allotted the various opposition parties, remains unanswered, as does the question of how will the parliamentary committees fulfill their functions in that proposed hybrid system. However, having a one-day session each week, as opposed to the original Liberal government proposal of a totally virtual parliament, will permit legislation to be debated and legally enacted by Parliament, but it will be done in a rushed one day period.

Otherwise a one-day sitting each week will permit little more than routine government business to be transacted, and for financial packages to be voted on without much discussion. There will be little time, if any, for penetrating questions to be posed and answered by government ministers, or for parliamentary House committees to table demands for government documents to review. One presumes the proposed virtual sessions will be little more than the Prime Minister and government ministers expounding on what a great job the government is doing in combatting the spread of the coronavirus -- for TV consumption -- with opposition members struggling to express a coherent critique in whatever brief time is allotted them on screen. Moreover, in the House of Commons MPs are free to speak their minds without any fear of being sued for libel or slander, but that would not be the case in a speech made by MPs from their own home via a virtual connection.

Prime Minister Trudeau has continued to insist on a one-day sitting each week of the House and two virtual days of virtual sittings per week, as negotiated by Liberal party with the NDP and Bloc Quebecois. At one point, Trudeau commented that the Conservative were not "taking a responsible approach" because if an agreement were not reached all 338 members of parliament would have to reconvene in the midst of a coronavirus epidemic, along with the Parliament Hill clerks, interpreters, security and cleaners. One might ask: who is the dishonest, misleading, and irresponsible person in this political dispute?

It appears that the Conservative Party will be outvoted by the Liberal Party minority in combination with the members of the NDP and Parti Quebecois, and the Conservative members of parliament will have to abandon their efforts to maintain the function of parliament in holding government accountable for its actions and expenditures. The Liberal Party has positioned itself to paint the Conservatives as 'the bad guys' who are holding up what is being presented as a reasonable way – virtual sessions -- to involve all MPs in House business without exposing them to the danger of contacting a coronavirus infection if they gathered in Ottawa for the recall of parliament. What is being ignored is that under the Conservative Party counter proposal, parliament would continue to fulfill its proper constitutional function with three days of sittings per week with a reduced proportional representation of MPs, and one virtual session per week to keep all MPs abreast of parliamentary business and able to voice any particular concerns. Otherwise parliament would continue to function, with all of its powers, rights and prerogatives intact, but with a reduced representation.

The Liberal plan to dispense with parliamentary sitting, except for a one-day session to pass necessary legislation, is a political manoeuvre to escape parliamentary scrutiny, and House committee investigations in a situation where the minority Liberal Party government has a minority representation on the committees and cannot control their agendas. The Liberal plan has escaped condemnation by reporters of our Liberal Press who are ignorant of the true function of parliament, and unaware of how essential the workings of parliament are to the preservation of the rights and freedoms of Canadians in holding government accountable for its actions and expenditures. Not only is the holding of virtual sessions outside of parliament of a questionable legality, it will effectively emasculate parliament. It is yet another example of the deception practiced by the Justin Trudeau Liberal government in pontificating to Canadians about the Liberal Party beliefs in democracy, transparency, and parliamentary government, while consistently seeking to govern without any parliamentary scrutiny in ignoring the elected representatives of the people.

Monday, April 20, 2020

Virtual Parliament Adopted: The House of Commons met today, with a reduced proportional representation of the political parties, and the MPs representing the Liberal Party, the NDP, and the Bloc Quebecois, outvoted the Conservative Party representatives, to adopt the Liberal Party proposal of a one-day sitting of parliament (each Wednesday), supplemented by two days of a virtual parliament (each Tuesday and Thursday). A motion was passed that gave the House administration the authority to limit the number of MPs attending the Wednesday parliamentary sitting, which will leave it up to the Party Whips to work out.

The next day, the Speaker of the House, Anthony Rota – the Liberal Party MP for Nipissing-Timiskaming – addressed MPs on the House Affairs Committee -- which had been meeting to discuss how the virtual parliament concept will work. He admitted that the lack of regular sittings of parliament will present "a major barrier to the functioning of parliament"; that the virtual meetings of parliament 'present challenges to all members to fully participate in the exercise of their roles'; and that the thirty standing committees that usually meet to examine issues and legislation cannot function. Furthermore, the Speaker called on all MPs to "recognize that not everything is possible during a pandemic". It was also explained that the one day – Wednesday -- sittings of parliament, with the reduced representation, will be reserved for questioning the Prime Minister and Ministers on the government response to the COVID-19 impact.

(In effect, the House of Commons is being constituted as a COVID-19 Committee. Apparently, there are no other issues that the Liberal Party government deems important enough to be raised in parliament.)

With respect to the video-conferencing technology, the Speaker informed the House Affairs Committee that there were security and connectivity issues to be addressed, as well as procedural issues. A glimpse of what is to come was revealed in the sitting of the House of Commons on Monday that adopted the Liberal virtual parliament proposal. The Liberal Party members continually spoke of the dangers to the public health of having all 338 members assemble in regular four-day sittings of parliament – a non-issue. The Liberal Party failed in its earlier attempt to establish an absolutist government with an unlimited power to tax, borrow and spend without the consent of parliament, but it has succeeded, through the introduction of its virtual parliament concept, in emasculating parliament and freeing itself of any effective parliamentary oversight on government spending and borrowing.

Canadians ought to be asking themselves: Why can all other parliamentary governments worldwide continue to function, with a reduced representation of members, during the COVID-19 pandemic, when the Canadian parliament supposedly cannot. The ease with which the Liberal Party has duped the NDP, the Bloc Quebecois, and the Canadian media into accepting a dispensing with the workings of parliament, makes one wonder if Canadians are worthy of the gift of the parliamentary system of government bestowed on them by their forefathers.

Oil Industry: The commitment of Saudi Arabia and its OPEC allies to reduce oil production by 10 million barrels per day, and by the G20 energy nations to reduce their production by 3.7 million barrels per day, has had no appreciable impact in raising oil prices, despite the hopes of the promoters of the oil production cuts. With the lockdowns, travel restrictions, and factory closures, the world demand for oil has fallen by 30 million barrels a day which continues to drive down global oil prices.

Tuesday, April 21, 2020

Economic Recovery: Ontario and Quebec are still seeing large increases in coronavirus cases – up to as many as nineteen a day in Quebec, primarily among the elderly in long-care homes – and Nova Scotia is reporting a dozen or more new cases daily, with thankfully only ten virus-related deaths in that province. However, there has been a significant flattening of the curve of new cases in British Columbia, and in Newfoundland-Labrador, Saskatchewan, Manitoba, Alberta, and Prince Edward Island, the daily number of new cases has decreased to five or less. New Brunswick has reported no new cases during the last two days. Several provinces are contemplating ending the lockdown in May, to permit some businesses and schools to re-open. Both Deputy Prime Minister Freeland, and Dr. Theresa Tam, the Chief of Public Health Canada have warned the provinces to be 'thoughtful about taking that next step' to avoid the risk of "slipping backwards". To date, the number of confirmed coronavirus cases in Canada has reached 36,823, with 99 virus-related deaths.

Foreign Takeovers: The federal government announced that it is taking steps, similar to what several other countries have done, to tighten the rules governing foreign takeovers. The intention is to protect Canadian companies during the recovery transition period when companies that are short of capital and struggling to recover in the market share, will be easy prey to foreign takeovers. A singular scrutiny is reportedly to be paid to foreign corporations and state-owned entities seeking to invest in, or take over, Canadian companies in the public health field and in the provision of critical goods and services. If the objective is to strengthen and enhance the self-sufficiency of Canada to supply its own needs in the fields of health care, basic foods, and energy; that is a national policy that Tory conservatives can heartedly support.

United States: The number of coronavirus cases in the United States has reached 775,000 with 42,000 virus-related deaths, which far exceeds that of any other country. The next worst afflicted country, Spain has but 200,000 cases. Italy has the highest death rate, currently at 24,000 deaths, followed by Spain with 21,000 deaths. (These rankings depend on the reliability of Chinese government statistics, which indicate a lower number of coronavirus cases and virus-related deaths in China, which many have questioned.) President Trump has announced that he will temporarily ban -- by an executive order – any further immigration to the United States during the duration of the coronavirus epidemic to prevent potential new importations of the virus. At present, roughly 460,000 immigration vias are issued annually by the American government, and 580,000 green cards to foreigners applying for permanent residency. Seasonal agricultural labourers have been classified as 'essential workers'. To date, there is no immediate prospect of the United States beginning to re-open the economy with the coronavirus still spreading in many areas of the country.

Economic Recovery: Germany is the first European country to commence its economic recovery program. When the coronavirus first appeared in Germany, and was raging in neighbouring countries, the German government acted quickly to impose a nation-wide lockdown, social spacing, and the introduction of testing with an aggressive policy of tracing the chain of contacts of infected persons. Through good planning, Germany was sufficiently supplied with testing kits and medical care supplies. It did not experience any shortage of personal protective equipment for medical personnel and personal support workers, and did not have to compete in the costly struggle for medical supplies in the global market. A widespread testing program was rendered efficient through the existence of a network of laboratories to carry out the swab analyses, which enabled infected persons to be relatively quickly identified and quarantined. Overall, Germany had 139,897 confirmed cases of COVID-19 and 4,294 deaths out of a population of 83 million during the coronavirus pandemic, but as of April 20th, the coronavirus threat was deemed to be under control. Some German states are reporting no new cases. The City of Jena saw a decided flatlining of virus cases following the introduction of the compulsory wearing of face masks.

In Germany, small shops, bookstores, and car dealerships have been authorized to re-open, and schools will be opened as of May 4th in most areas. To be followed by beauty salons and some cultural venues and restaurants with social spacing rules remaining in place. Moreover,

Germany is distributing 50 million respiratory masks, which Germans are "strongly advised" to wear in public, and the wearing of a respiratory mask will be compulsory on some state transport systems. Large stores and industries remain closed for the moment, and large public venues – sports stadia – will remain closed to the public until August 31st. Individuals who have developed antibodies to the disease will immediately be issued "immunity cards" and permitted to move freely in working, travelling domestically, and socializing. During the coronavirus epidemic, Germany provided an $800 billion financial package to ensure that firms retained their liquidity during the lockdown. The financial aid was distributed through massive state loans to businesses and funds for companies to pay laid off workers, and through deferring billions of euros in tax payments.

Personal Protective Equipment: If the COVID-19 pandemic has provided any lessons, it is that non-medical cotton face masks, social spacing, and attention to washing one's hands and disinfecting common objects being touched by the public, are the keys to preventing the acquiring of a virus infection, and that widespread testing, the quarantining of infected persons, and the tracking of the chain of contacts of infected persons, and the quarantining of those who test positive, are critical to containing the virus once it is present in a local area. There is every prospect that the German recovery will proceed as planned so long as face masks are worn in public, the requisite social spacing is maintained whenever practicable, and the prescribed basic hygiene is practiced.

Tuesday, April 21, 2020

Personal Protective Equipment: In Canada, the shortage of the N-95 respiratory masks, and personal protective equipment for medical personnel and public support workers in long-care homes, continues. Prime Minister Trudeau revealed today that two million N-95 respiratory masks, and thousand of pairs of medical gloves were destroyed in 2019 because they were past their due date for use; and he pledged that federal stockpiles of such equipment would be used in future, and not destroyed. It was also revealed that a cargo plane – chartered by the federal government – had returned empty from China on Monday without the medical protective equipment that had been ordered. Canada is now dependent on the respiratory masks, plastic surgical face shields, surgical gowns, and gloves that Canadian companies are beginning to manufacture. The delay by the federal government in failing to act quickly to purchase that equipment early on, and a concurrent failure to turn immediately to Canadian manufacturers to gear up to produce personal protective equipment and ventilators, once the critical need was identified, is inexcusable. Now, the Minister of Public Health, Patty Hajdu, has finally admitted that the federal government stockpile of personal protective equipment is totally inadequate to meet provincial needs.

When Bell Canada (BCE Telecommunications) saw the need weeks ago to secure N-95 respiratory masks to protect thousands of Bell technicians from infection who were doing essential work across Canada, the company acted immediately to secure the masks, gloves and coveralls in bulk from foreign suppliers. Now, having supplied its own workers, Bell has a surplus of 1.5 million N-95 respiratory masks and K-95 respiratory masks (a similar Chinese design) which it is donating for distribution to frontline health care providers, first responders, and various health agencies across Canada. Similarly, Canopy Growth Corp, which purchased personal protective equipment early on, in bulk, to protect is employees working in cannabis sheds, is donating 25,000 N-95 respiratory masks and 40,000 plastic shield surgical masks to the Province of Ontario for distribution.

Charities: Prime Minister Trudeau announced that $350 million will be provide to Canadian charities and public service organizations – United Appeal, the Red Cross, etc. -- to enable those organizations to continue to provide a sorely needed social assistance and social functions to the communities dependent on them. The organizations that depend on support from the public have suffered a severe drop in donations during the coronavirus epidemic and have not been able to stage their traditional fundraising events.

Wednesday, April 22, 2020

Personal Care Workers: This is unbelievable. An association that provides personal care workers to Ontario long-care homes has just announced that it has managed to procure a supply of personal protective equipment – face masks, gloves, gowns. – for its employees. In effect, for over a month during the height of the coronavirus epidemic in Ontario, personal care workers have been entering long-care homes, and the homes of patients in private care, without any personal protection equipment. Indeed, there was apparently a provincial directive – given the scarcity of personal protective equipment, and the priority need to protect medical personnel in constant contact with the virus – that personal care workers in long-care homes were to wear whatever personal protective equipment they had only is situations where a patient exhibited COVID-19 symptoms, or if a patient has flu-like symptoms, or had travelled outside the country.

One company that supplies personal care workers to long-care homes has had two employees test positive for the COVID-19 virus, and there may be more now that a broader testing is underway. My God! No wonder the virus is currently raging among the elderly residents of the long-care homes in Ontario. One Ottawa woman, with a bed-ridden husband requiring home care services, took the initiative and paid $500 to have face masks, gloves and gowns specially made locally for the personal care workers to put on before entering her home. The personal care workers had been arriving at her home without any personal protective equipment. The simple wearing of a face mask is one of the most simple and effective way for asymptomatic individuals to prevent the spread the virus when in contact with others. Why have the companies that employ personal care workers, not taken the initiative to have face masks made locally for their employees to wear? Any type of face mask is better than none!

Recovery Strategies: A newspaper columnist has reported that Catherine McKenna, the Minister of Infrastructure and Communities, is 'reading up' on how President Franklin Delano Roosevelt sought to overcome the severe economic impact of the Great Depression of the 1930s through the policies introduced in his "New Deal" legislation. Roosevelt promised "bold, persistent experimentation" to get the American economy going again, and introduced a number of government programs and initiatives to create jobs.

Clearly, the Trudeau government is searching for ways to jump start the economy once the coronavirus epidemic is under control and the number of new infections begin to trend strongly downwards. Among the Roosevelt "New Deal" achievements were two major construction projects: the Tennessee Valley Authority (1933 to present) hydro-electric dam building on the Tennessee River that provided thousand of jobs, flood control, and low-price electricity to the population of six states; and the Hoover Dam (1931-1936) construction project on the Colorado River that employed thousands of workers, created the largest water reservoir in the United States, and provided flood control, irrigation water, and hydro-electric power to the western states.

It is highly unlikely that our present Liberal government with its poor record of infrastructure development, and its inability to get things done, is capable of planning a major infrastructure project. Of course, there are several energy development projects – oil sands development projects, several major pipeline projects, and two major LNG projects, for which the planning is already in place, which have achieved the support of the Aboriginal peoples through whose lands the pipelines will pass, which will created tens of thousands of good-paying jobs, and which will attract billions in foreign investment monies. However, such major national projects are hamstrung by a Liberal federal government that is derelict in its duty to maintain the rule of law in arresting protester engaged in illegal activities, and that adheres to a economy destroying global emissions reductions targets that three-quarters of our competitors in the global market are ignoring.

Tourism & Real Estate: Concerns are being expressed about the economic collapse of the tourism industry, and the real estate market. Across Canada, the ban on travel and the lockdown has devastated hotels and the tourism industry. Hotels across Canada have less than a five percent occupancy rate, have laid off over 250,000 employees, and have experienced a revenue decline of 90 percent. Moreover, they are worrying about losing their summer season. The hotel owners are asking the federal government to make loans available of up to $6.25 million per business -- on a per property basis, rather then by owner – with a loan guarantee to enable hotels to retain some liquidity during the lockdown period.

The $102 billion tourism industry, which employs about 1.8 million Canadians, has already shed a million jobs through a complete loss of business during the lockdown. The tourism industry, which is unable to qualify for loans with no revenue flow, and with concerns about when tourism will revive and to what extent, is asking the federal government for financial assistance. The criteria for accessing the existing financial support programs – the wage subsidy for workers, the payroll wage subsidy for companies, and the rent relief program – do not fit the tourism industry in which the major revenue stream is during the summer tourism season. Melanie Joly, the Economic Development Minister, has declared that the government is investigating ways to help the tourism industry.

Wednesday, April 22, 2020 (continued)

Vaccines: Great news from Germany. A COVID-19 vaccine, that was developed jointly by a German biotechnology company and the American pharmaceutical company, Pfizer, has been approved for testing on humans. Two hundred volunteers will participate in a clinical trial of the vaccine. In the United States, 2,000 volunteers have been recruited to test the Pfizer vaccine.

Long-Care Homes: In Ontario, the provincial government has requested that the federal government send military medical personnel to private long-care homes in the province to free up personal care workers to focus on the non-medical care of the elderly residents. Initially, the intention is to deploy the military medical personnel in five long-care homes where the coronavirus disease is sweeping through the residents. At one of the worst hit homes in Ottawa, 38 residents in the 240-bed institution, and five personal care workers, are sick with the virus – an almost a sixteen percent infection rate among the residents – and one resident has died. At another hard hit long-care home of 303 beds in Ottawa, 51 residents and 28 staff -- full time and part time -- are sick with the virus, and there have been eleven virus-related deaths. One the worst hit long-care homes is a 60-bed facility where 51 of the residents and 24 staff members – full and part time – with five residents having died, a death rate of almost ten percent. Six days later, the Ontario government reported that out of 892 coronavirus deaths in Ontario, 671 virus-related deaths were among long-term care and retirement residents.

(Three days later, on April 25th, some light was cast on why some private long-care home in Ontario are currently hotbeds of virus infections, while other long-care homes in the province have only a handful of cases and very few, if any, deaths. Personal care workers at one of the hardest hit homes have revealed what transpired.

At this one particular long-care home, staff were not provided with medical protective equipment, had to make do with ill-fitting, flimsy dust masks, and had to reuse the disposal probes that cover thermometers. There was no enforcement of social spacing, residents continued to eat in a communal dining room, a patient who was visibly sick with the virus continued to use the elevator to visit another floor of the home, and part-time staff continued to work at more than one home in ignoring the provincial ban against that practice. As a result, some staff refused to work at that particular long-care home out of a fear of contacting the virus.

The personal care workers who remained healthy, and on the job, were greatly overworked and were unable to properly care for the health and hygiene of the residents, or to control the movement of the residents within the facility. What we have here is a dismal failure on the part of those in authority – the owner and manager responsible for operating the private long-care home -- to realize the seriousness of the coronavirus threat, and to introduce even elementary protective measures to minimize exposure by the residents and staff to the virus. One suspects that is a similar case with respect to the other half dozen long-care homes in Ontario where the coronavirus is raging like a wild-fire among the residents.)

In Quebec, Premier Francois Legault has requested that a thousand Canadian Army soldiers be send to Quebec to provide non-medical personal care support in the long-term care homes that are being ravaged by coronavirus infections. At present, there are 125 military medical personnel – doctors and nurses – deployed in Quebec at long-term care facilities. However, Quebec is facing a particularly severe health care crisis. Over 1200 personal care workers have become infected by the COVID-19 virus, in a situation where there is a shortage of personal protection equipment. As of Wednesday, the number of personal care workers absent from work -- across the province -- had reached 9,500, inclusive of those who are sick. In Quebec, many personal care workers are staying home inbeing unwilling to risk their lives by going to work.

The staff absentee problem is particularly acute at the long-care homes where there is a dire need for their personal care support services. Hence, the request made to the federal government by Premier Legault for military personnel to be deployed to provide basic personal care for the long-care home residents, while doctors and nurses attend to the sick.

Canada Emergency Student Benefit (CESB): Today, April 22nd, Prime Minister Trudeau announced a new Canada Emergency Student Benefit (CESB) program to provide financial aid to students who are unable to secure a summer job because of the COVID-19 provincial lockdowns. If approved by parliament, the new CESB program with provide Canadian and permanent resident students who are graduating secondary school or graduate school with a payment of $1,250 per month from May to August. The CESB program is expected to cost $9 billion. Students with disabilities, or who care for others, will receive a higher stipend of $1,750 per month. The program is to fill in a benefits gap in that only workers who have lost their job are eligible to receive a $2,000 per month payment under the Canada Emergency Response Benefit (CERB) program established earlier.

Moreover, student who return to school when things are back to normal, and who are eligible for a government grant under the existing Canada Student Grants program, will receive double the former grant level: up to $6,000 for a full-time student; and $3,600 for a part-time student.

The existing financial program for First Nations, Inuit, and Metis Nation students pursuing a post-secondary education will be increased by $75.2 million.

In addition, under the new Canada Emergency Student Benefit (CESB) program, students who volunteer to participate in COVID-19 response efforts – unspecified activities – will be granted a bursary of up to $5,000 towards the furthering of their education. Prime Minister Trudeau also declared that the federal government plans to create 76,000 new jobs for students this summer, which will be in addition to the jobs provided through the regular Summer Jobs program of the federal government. However, no information has been provided as to how the 76,000 new jobs will be created, what the students will be doing, or how the work creation system will be organized and the students equipped to do whatever work is required, was not explained.

When questioned about the statement that 76,000 summer jobs would be created for students, the Employment Minister, Carla Qualtrough, was not that positive. She replied that the federal government was consulting with the provinces about opportunities for student employment, but the reality was that the lockdown has derailed any real prospect of undertaking major job-creation initiatives. What she offered was a forlorn hope that "students will find ways to keep themselves occupied to contribute to upskill and just not stay sitting around for the whole entire summer". In other words, the Trudeau government has no idea how to create 76,000 summer jobs, or any jobs for that matter, during the current coronavirus epidemic.

In the Liberal La La Land approach to student employment, there was one positive development. The federal government is asking for student volunteers to help with COVID-19 data collection, case tracking, and contract tracing, and several universities are encouraging their students to participate.

(Much later – on July 17th, during an investigation by the House of Commons Standing Committee on Finance -- it was discovered that a major Canadian international charity, the WE Charity, had just submitted, as of April 22nd, a proposal to the Prime Minister's Office (PMO) and several department heads for a massive new employment scheme for student volunteer workers to be employed for the summer in working for charities and not-for-profit organizations. In the April 22nd announcement of the new Canada Emergency Student Benefit (CESB), Prime Minister Trudeau did not mention any proposed new summer employment program for student volunteer workers; yet the claim that 76,000 new summer jobs would be created for students indicates that the Prime Minister must have had the WE scheme in mind. It is clear, that Employment Minister, Carla Qualtrough, was not aware of the WE student employment scheme at that time.)

Ad Hoc Government: Following the April 22nd announcements by Prime Minister Trudeau, he was questioned by the Press as to why the Liberal government has not created a single universal benefit to cover all Canadians who have lost their jobs, or are suffering a major loss of revenue through the impact of the coronavirus epidemic. Prime Minister Trudeau replied that the government's approach is "to target emergency financial assistance in stages to those who clearly need it, rather than a universal system wherein assistance might go to some who do not need it". The leader of the NDP, Jagmeet Singh, called on the government to simply make the existing Canadian Emergency Response (CERB) a universal benefit to allow any Canadian experiencing financial distress due to COVID-19 lockdown, to apply for the benefit under broader criteria.

Clearly, the Trudeau Liberal government is continuing its ad hoc, spur of the moment, approach to governing, with massive financial aid packages being thrown together as yet another community makes it known that its members are suffering economic distress due to the coronavirus lockdown or, in the case of students, are expected to be impacted with the loss of an expected income. The patchwork approach of creating more and more financial aid programs involving the expenditure of billions of dollars, each of which targets different types of worker and businesses, with different qualification criteria, and different payment amounts for different periods of time, is creating a veritable nightmare for government administrators. The soaring costs and payments being made under various programs, are far outstripping any effort to keep track of where the monies are going.

What is striking about the daily TV announcements of the new financial aid packages by Prime Minister Trudeau, is how closely the aid packages follow upon news stories -- on the Internet and in the print media -- of economic problems being experienced by a particular industry, or economic sector, or community within Canada, or simply demands being made by an interest group. One wonders whether the Prime Minister is spending his time in confinement at home in the 'Rideau Cottage' in scrolling the Internet new stories, and ordering his ministers to come up with yet another financial aid package for him to announce at his daily TV presentation. If so, it explains the ad hoc, spur of the moment, response of the federal Liberal government to the impact of the coronavirus. On its part, the Trudeau government has proclaimed that it is 'working with provincial and territorial partners, industry, Indigenous communities, and stakeholders to identify negative impacts from the evolving COVID-19 situation'.

Rather than the government developing a measured proactive program response to the impact of the coronavirus, and relying on members of its own caucus and members of the opposition in parliament, to raise serious concerns that need to be addressed, the Prime Minister appears to be relying on the Press to fulfil that role. What we have here -- with parliament having been emasculated -- is an exercise in direct democracy filtered through the national press with an elected dictator – a benevolent despot -- deciding upon whom the favours of government will be showered. This is not to deny that the financial aid packages are sorely needed in many instances. The problem is that Canada is being governed by one man. It is Prime Minister Justin Trudeau who is deciding to whom billions of dollars in public money will be given, and to whom it will be denied – viz. the oil and gas industry – without any questioning or any oversight by parliament which has been reduced to a rushed rubber stamping – in a one day a week sitting -- of financial aid packages already presented and promised to the public by Prime Minister Trudeau in his daily 'morning show' TV appearances.

Thursday, April 23, 2020

Student Work Placement Program: What has remained unacknowledged in the announcing of the new Canada Emergency Student Benefit (CESB), and the hint of a new student employment scheme to provide summer jobs for 76,000 students, is that the federal government already has an existing, long-established program for employing students: the Student Work Placement Program (SWPP). That existing program has a mandate to facilitate the securing of employment for Canadian and international post-secondary students, either part-time work through the year and/or summer employment.

Under the SWPP, Employment and Social Services Canada work with companies – "employer delivery parties" – to place students in work positions, with the employer eligible to receive a wage subsidy of $5,000 for every student employed under the program, and $7,00 for every first year student and student employed from under-represented groups, inclusive of women in Science, Technology, Engineering, and

Mathematics (STEM studies), persons with disabilities, newcomers, and Indigenous students.

One might ask why the existing student job placement program -- which is already in place -- could not have been simply expanded, with a broadening of the eligibility criteria for students, the provision of additional funding, and a slight change in the program mandate – to facilitate students to find summer work, and pay students the stipend to be provided by the new CESB program. Why is the Liberal government rolling out the new Canada Emergency Student Benefit (CESB program) that overlaps many of the responsibilities of the existing Student Work Placement Program, when the establishment of any new government program invariably involves delays in establishing a new administration and administrative system, and in getting the system up and running?

(One might ask also why Canadian taxpayers are providing a wage subsidy to employers -- under the existing Student Work Placement Program -- to provide employment for 'international students' entering Canada under a student work visa? Jobs for students are scarce for Canadian students. They should not have to compete with international students entering Canada on a student work visa for the available jobs. Canadian citizenship should have its privileges, and partially so when it is the families of Canadian students, through paying taxes, that are providing the funding for government wage subsidies to employers who hire students.)

Long-Care Homes: The Ontario government has ordered public health units across the province to test every resident and staff member in long-care homes, inclusive of the few homes where there have been no outbreaks. The testing will be quite broad to include anyone who has come in direct contact with a COVID-19 patient at a home. The intention is to identify those who have contacted the virus, including asymptomatic residents and staff, so that the individuals can be isolated to better manage the current outbreaks. Concerns were expressed by municipal health units regarding how to secure enough personnel to administer the tests, whether the needed testing kits were readily available, and whether laboratories would be swamped in analyzing the nasal swabs. In Ottawa, recreational staff -- who are currently laid-off with the closing down of municipal recreational facilities -- are going to be retrained to administer the required coronavirus detection tests, and perhaps to provide support in the feeding of residents in the long-care homes that the municipality operates.

Ventilators and Face Shields: In the United States, the 3M company and other medical supplies companies have partnered with car manufacturers – Ford, General Motors, Toyota, and others – who have geared up and are producing plastic face shields, surgical masks, and ventilators. Furloughed auto workers have responded to appeals to volunteer to return to work to produce the medical personal protection equipment even though they had been receiving their pay while at home during the coronavirus epidemic.

Municipalities: The Federation of Canadian Municipalities has asked the government to provide $10 billion in financial aid to Canadian municipalities in the form of $7.6 billion distributed on a per capita basis and $2.4 billion distributed to cities that have major transportation systems. Canadian cities are caught in a situation where their tax revenues, user fees, and revenues from public transit have plummeted and their costs in providing public services – garbage pickup, policing, social assistance and social housing, road repairs, water and sewage, city payrolls, and administration expenses – are fixed. In the City of Ottawa, tax payments have been deferred to October for hardship cases, inclusive of low-income seniors and the disabled, which has further reduced City tax revenues in the short term. Moreover, the city transit system – OC Transpo – has experienced a 90 percent drop in ridership during the coronavirus lockdown, with a heavy loss in revenue from a system that normally brings in $50 million per quarter. Overall, Ottawa is paying out $1 million per day in fixed costs. More than 4,000 part-time employees – in recreational and cultural programs -- have been laid off, but that only saves $2.7 million a month, as the City deficit has continued to climb.

The Federation of Canadian Municipalities has calculated, based on the current rate of municipal indebtedness, that if the lockdown lasts for six months longer, the City of Ottawa would have a municipal debt of $187 million for this fiscal year, Montreal of $538.5 million, and Calgary at $400 million, and Edmonton at $216.7 million. Toronto would have a municipal debt of $1.7 billion, which is equivalent to fifteen percent of the total city budget. With the lockdown, the Toronto Transit Authority is currently suffering a $90 million per month revenue loss.

Municipalities need emergency funding to keep essential services going. They are in a financial bind because in Canada, municipalities are not allowed to borrow money to meet day-to-day expenses; whereas the federal and provincial governments are able to do so to meet their emergency needs during the COVID-19 crisis. In Canada, municipalities can only borrow money for major infrastructure projects.

Provincial Finances: Several Canadian provinces are seeking federal government financial aid and are asking the government to create an emergency credit agency to lower provincial borrowing costs. Newfoundland-Labrador is in a financial crisis situation. In that province an existing heavy provincial debt and a drastic drop in oil revenues, have resulted in a poor credit rating. Alberta is suffering a severe economic hit with the plummeting of oil prices, and a severe drop in provincial government revenues during the lockdown. The situation will be helped by the Bank of Canada, which has announced that it plans to purchase a total of $50 billion in provincial debt to help the provinces maintain their liquidity. All provinces are experiencing a drastic decline in revenues during the coronavirus lockdown.

Economic Recovery: Andrew Scheer, the Conservative Party leader, has called on the Trudeau government to establish a national plan for coordinating the restarting and re-opening of the economy to avoid a patchwork approach with each province proceeding differently. In response, Prime Minister Trudeau confirmed that restrictions will be eased across the country on a province by province basis, with the each provincial government deciding on its own approach based on its own particular situation with respect to the virus containment in the province. The federal government will eventually 'attempt to pull together all the different experiences to establish a set of guidelines and principles'.

Farmers & Ranchers: Ranchers and farmers are suffering substantial financial loses from the closure of major slaughterhouses, meatpacking and pork processing plants while infection controls are being carried out in the plants where there have been outbreaks of the coronavirus among the workers. In High River, Alberta, the Cargill meat packing plant closed on April 21st, when 759 employees who are either sick or have tested positive for the COVID-19 virus,, and over 300 virus cases have been reported in the local Filipino workers' community and the adjacent Stoney-Nakoda First Nations reserves. The plant which processed 4,500 head of cattle per day, and produces 36 percent of Canada's beef, is expected to be shut for two weeks while employees self-isolate and the plant is disinfected. To date, the Cargill plant is the epicentre of the COVID-19 cases in Alberta.

The next day, April 22nd, the JBS meatpacking plant in Brooks, Alberta, had 67 employees either sick or testing positive for the Coronavirus, and one employee – an older woman – died from the virus infection. JBS is staying open, but the plant is operating at a reduced capacity with only one shift on which the healthy workers – who tested negative – have been placed, with the requisite personal protection equipment. Meatpacking is an essential food supply industry. However, given the nature of the work in close quarters, it is difficult to enforce social spacing. Together, Cargill and JBS provide 70 to 75 percent of Canada's processed beef. No shortage of beef is expected, but prices may rise.

During the closure of the Cargill plant, many ranchers are incurring extra costs in feeding their stock which cannot be sold and moved to the meatpacking plant. Moreover, the international market is closed off. Canada exports upwards of 45 percent of its beef and cattle-on-the-hoof annually to fifty-six different countries, with the United States accounting for 74 percent of beef exports. If the export market remains closed until the end of June, Cattle ranchers/cattle farmers expect to lose $500 million.

Marie-Claude Bibeau, the Minister of Agriculture and Agri-Food Canada, has expressed a concern about the health and safety of the packing plant employees, and announced that the federal government has set up a working group to establish a national approach on meat and poultry issues. The federal government has already committed $20 million to the Canadian Food Inspection Agency for the hiring of additional staff to work with the provincial inspectors of the processing plants.

A similar situation exists in the hog processing industry under the impact of the coronavirus, with several major abattoirs having been closed owing to workers getting sick or testing positive for the virus infection. One of the largest pork packing plants in eastern Canada, the Olymel plant in Quebec – north of Montreal – closed on March 29th when nine employees became sick with the COVID-19 virus and 100 employees tested positive. The modern, highly automated, plant, normally employs about 1,000 workers on two shifts, and processes 28,000 hogs per week from local Quebec farms and from eastern Ontario farms. The finished product is shipped – in refrigerated transport – to urban markets in Quebec and to over fifty different countries.

On the outbreak of the coronavirus sickness, the employees were sent home to self-isolate for 14-days while the plant was disinfected. The intention was to re-open the plant on April 14th, but that was delayed until April 23rd, while masks and glasses were secured for employees and panels constructed to increase the safe distancing on the production line. With the gradual resumption of production, a local doctor is being employed to constantly monitor the health of the workers entering the plant. With similar processing plant closures elsewhere in Canada, hog farmers are losing money in the delays being experienced in being able to deliver their animals to be processed. Hog producers are claiming that the delays are costing them anywhere from $30 to $50 per animal. They are asking for an emergency payment from the federal government of $20 per hog to partially compensate them and to provide a sorely needed revenue source.

Another serious financial loss is being incurred by farmers who raise piglets for sale within Canada and in the American market. It cost $40 to raise a piglet ready for market, and other farmers are not buying "feeder pigs" as they cannot sell their mature pigs owing to abattoirs being closed because of coronavirus infections. American farmers, who account for twenty percent of the market for Canadian piglets, are refusing to purchase piglets for the same reason. Three of the largest pork processing plants and several others, have been forced to close in the United States. In most years, the U.S. market absorbs six million Canadian piglets, which accounts for 20 percent of the market for Canadian farmers. Now, the farmers are being saddled with extra feed and care costs for unwanted animals that they cannot sell.

It was announced further that the Minister of Agriculture and Agri-Food, Marie-Claude Bibeau, is currently consulting with the provinces to provide some level of support to farmers and ranchers while investigating how their respective processing bottlenecks can be rectified.

Friday, April 24, 2020

Immunization: A controversy has erected over a proposal by a leading biochemist at the Advanced Centre for Detection of Cancer in Toronto that special hospitals programs be established in which volunteers could be deliberately infected with a mild dose of the COVID-19 virus to build up a natural immunity. The context is that many medical personnel are convinced that the only way the economy can become fully operation again without triggering a second wave of infections -- in the absence of a vaccine -- is when a large segment of the population has built up a natural immunity through having been infected, and having recovered, from a COVID-19 virus attack. At present, there are only 16,438 individuals who have recovered from the coronavirus disease in Canada, which is a quite small, almost insignificant, 'background immunity' pool in a Canadian population of 36.5 million people. Hence, the proposal to establish a program of variolation with a mild dose of the coronavirus to produce a natural immunity. At present, the federal government is encouraging everyone to 'stay at home' to avoid becoming infected with the virus. However, people cannot remain at home forever, and by staying at home the population is not building up a natural immunity to the coronavirus. No 'herd immunity' can be achieved.

Several Canadian bioethicists have condemned the proposal for medical practitioners to deliberate infect volunteers with a mild dose of the COVID-19 virus, as constituting a direct violation of the Hippocratic Oath taken by new physicians 'to do no harm'. Presumably they are thinking that, given the unknown character of the coronavirus, the injecting of even a mild dose might cause a full scale infection with the risk of death. The bioethicists argue that a herd immunity ought to be achieved only through vaccination with a COVID-19 vaccine, and not with a program of variolation with the injection of a mild dose of the virus itself. However, that stance ignores the fact that there is, as yet, no proven vaccine readily available to vaccinate a large segment of the population, and that governments are faced with an immediate need to prevent a total economic collapse by opening up economic activity, and of doing so without creating a second wave of infections.

To date, it is not known to what extent the natural antibodies, which are developed by the immune system of an infected COVID-19 patient, will give any long-lasting immunity against a future re-infection.

Political Correctness: The Liberal Press is all in an uproar over a critique that a candidate for the leadership of the Conservative Party, Conservative MP Derek Sloan, sent to members of the Party. In the critique, Sloan claimed that the World Health Organization (WHO) has been "a puppet of the People's Republic of China for over a decade"; that Canada's Chief Public Health Officer, Dr. Theresa Tam, has "continually cited the WHO as an authority" on how to respond to the coronavirus threat; and that in accepting the pronouncements of WHO at face value, without questioning them, Dr. Tam had consistently misled Canadians about the serious threat posed by the coronavirus outbreak in China. In particular, Sloan cited several statements made to Canadians by Dr. Tam early on: that "the virus doesn't spread from person to person'; that "face masks don't work"; and that "closing borders to travellers from virus hotspots wouldn't work". More generally, Derek Sloan claimed that Dr. Tam appeared to be concerned more with 'saving face' for China than protecting Canadians in her downplaying the seriousness of what was happening on the ground in China during the early stages of the virus impact in that country.

Up to that point, everything that Derek Sloan complained about in his critique respecting the deficiencies of Dr. Tam in exercising her responsibilities as the Chief Public Health Officer of Canada, was, and is, utterly true. However, he crossed the line as to what constitutes an acceptable criticism in his closing remarks, which disparaged the personal integrity and loyalty of Dr. Tam. After mentioning that Dr. Tam was formerly involved with WHO – through her membership on a number of WHO committees – Sloan declared that Dr. Tam should "either resign or be fired"; and that "Canada's Chief Public Health Officer needs to work for Canada. Not for the WHO or any other foreign country".

Other than the utterly uncalled for, and disparaging personal remark in his closing statement, which questioned Dr. Tam's loyalty to Canada, there is nothing in the critique of the work of Dr. Tam that is not merited. Moreover, the Sloan comments are not the least bit racist. Dr. Tam is of Chinese descent, but her race was never mentioned in the critique circulated by Derek Sloan. For the Conservative Party, the critique is an embarrassment not for its criticism of the performance of Dr. Tam in her capacity as the Chief Public Health Officer for Canada, but for the concluding statement that questioned her loyalty to Canada. For that disparaging personal remark, Derek Sloan owes an apology to Dr. Tam, personally.

However, for the politically-correct Modern liberals, and the Liberal Press, that concluding statement was a trigger point for a diatribe of denunciations of Derek Sloan for being supposedly 'a racist', 'an xenophobe', and someone of whom 'white nationalists would approve'. How all that was read into Derek Sloan's closing statement is beyond belief. A National Post columnist, John Ivison, even managed to work in a swipe at the Conservative Party in exclaiming that "the coded Canada-first language was a thinly disguised appeal for support from the intolerant fringe of the Conservative Party" with Ivison pointing out that Dr. Tam was born in Hong Kong. To that point, the birthplace of Dr. Tam and her race had not been mentioned by anyone. Her birthplace was left unspoken by Derek Sloan in questioning her loyalty, but granted it was viewed by many as an underlying factor in the questioning of her loyalty by Derek Sloan. However, it is not necessary to be born in a foreign country to be 'disloyal' to your country. Moreover, there were equally good grounds for objecting to the characterization of a supposed 'fringe of the Conservative Party' as being 'intolerant'. Is it because they do not share the Modern liberal values of John Ivison?

In his article, Ivison takes a swipe at the current leader of the Conservative Party, Andrew Scheer, who is denounced for his failure to 'decry the intolerance' of a member of the Conservative Party, Derek Sloan. Scheer is condemned as well for his deficiencies in failing "to articulate a contemporary conservatism that recognizes the modern Canadian mosaic". To top it off, Mr. Ivison throws in a general comment that: "In a multi-ethnic country where visible minorities make up a quarter of the population, no party tainted with racism can win power". Who is that comment aimed at? None of the political parties in Canada are racist, or tolerant of racists.

Derek Sloan responded that he has no intention of apologizing to Dr. Tam, which is highly regrettable. An apology is definitely in order, not for his criticism of the failings of Dr. Tam as Chief Medical Officer of Canada, but for his questioning of her loyalty to Canada. However, the story had taken on another dimension. An article posted on an Internet news site the next day – April 25th – accuses Derek Sloan of being "a racist", and a "misogynist" -- for making the comments that he did concerning the failings of Dr. Tam in responding to the coronavirus threat -- and calls for Andrew Scheer to expel Derek Sloan from the Conservative Party.

One can see the mentality behind the demands for the ouster of Derek Sloan, and what it bodes for Canadians and political discourse in this country. In future, any Conservative who speaks out about preserving Canada's heritage, national culture, and the sovereignty of the nation, against the threat posed by globalism – 'open borders', and 'the free movement of peoples, goods, services and capital' -- is going to be branded by the Liberal Press as using a 'coded Canada-first language'. That is apparently a Liberal code phrase implying that the person so described is a closet 'racist' and 'xenophobic.

It is not easy being a conservative in a country that is dominated by a Liberal Press that is committed to propagating Modern liberal values, that is bent on disparaging and denigrating conservative values, and that quickly brands anyone who voices any disagreement with, or criticism of, Modern liberal globalist values as being a 'racist' and a 'reactionary'. It is an unfair, unmerited, and highly biased negative treatment that the Liberal Press reserves for prominent conservatives. It was a treatment that Stephen Harper experienced some years ago, when he was continually condemned in the Liberal Press for supposedly having "a hidden agenda" to destroy the Canadian social benefits system. Yet, history will attest that Stephen Harper (Prime Minister, 2006-2015) governed well in protecting and promoting the well-being and common good of Canadians and the national interests of Canada.

What we have in play, with the personal attacks on Derek Sloan, is a rather absurd situation. In his newspaper column, John Ivison implies that Derek Sloan is a closet racist for his critique of Dr. Tam; yet, in the same column, Ivison sets forth a long list of the faults and failings of Dr. Tam in her capacity as Chief Public Health Officer of Canada. The Iveson list agrees with, and even exceeds, the criticisms made by Derek Sloan. Apparently, it is acceptable for a Liberal to criticize the failings of a Liberal party appointee to office -- the Chief Public Health Officer – but if a Conservative does so, it is unacceptable because of the assumption by Liberals that there must be some darker and deeper racist and/or misogynist motivation in the conservative psyche. My god! Has political correctness progressed in Canada to the point where a male Conservative member of parliament cannot critique the performance of a female and visible minority office holder without being accused of being a misogynist and a racist?

If we are going to have gender equality with females occupying many prominent public positions and half of the political leadership positions and offices of government, then they must accept the public scrutiny and the criticism that goes with it when they make major mistakes in judgement. The same goes for members of a visible minority when they occupy prominent public positions. To the credit of Dr. Tam, she has not complained about being criticized. Her position is that mistakes have been made by all government agencies and authorities everywhere, but that "we're all in this together, learning as we go".

Following the publication of the Ivison article, Prime Minster, Justin Trudeau weighed in on the Derek Sloan controversy obliquely with a truism -- "Intolerance and racism have no place in our country", and a political opinion: "Canada has succeeded because of our diversity". Andrew Scheer took a responsible position on the issue in stating that Derek Sloan was wrong to question the loyalty of Dr. Tam to Canada: "I believe it is not appropriate to question someone's loyalty to their country. I believe that it is a very serious accusation that you have to have some very substantial evidence to make". The Ontario caucus of the Conservative Party called on Derek Sloan to apologize to Dr. Tam, or retract his comment questioning her loyalty. Many Conservative MPs have voiced a similar view in maintaining that the comment "went too far".

Subsequently, Sloan declared that he was not questioning Dr. Tam's loyalty, that he had "never mentioned Dr. Tam's race or sex", and that he did not doubt her intentions. "However, she is responsible for relying on the flawed data of both the WHO and the Chinese government for her decision making. This has literally cost lives". (Derek Sloan is a social conservative candidate for the leadership of the Conservative Party who has been seeking support among Chinese social conservatives and anti-communist Canadians who are strongly opposed to the communist People's Republic of China. Ironically, Sloan is the only candidate with a Chinese language section on his website.)

The coronavirus epidemic is revealing to Canadians the strong biases of Modern liberals, the self-righteous mentality of the Liberal elite, and the inadequacies of the Liberal government of Prime Minister Justin Trudeau.

Chapter Five

Friday, April 24, 2020

Recovery Proposal: Government everywhere in the world are struggling with how to re-start and re-open their economies without triggering a second wave of infection by the coronavirus. One approach is to gradually ease restrictions on some businesses, starting with small businesses on a local basis, in areas where the number of new cases has flatlined or rapidly declined. It is at best, a 'hope for the best strategy', which if it works will lead to the lifting of restrictions on more and more different types of work and recreational activities over time. The problem with this gradualist approach is that even if it works, and a second wave of infections is avoided, it is a slow process that can stretch over months in an ongoing disruption and distortion of a struggling economy striving to recover from an almost total lockdown.

In Canada, the federal Liberal government has announced that it is taking a 'hands-off approach' to the short-term opening of the economy. It is the provinces, who have taken the lead in combatting the spread of the coronavirus, who will now make the decisions as to what businesses will be permitted to open and when, based on their local rates of infection. Once the different provincial programs are in place, then the federal government intends to produce guidelines on best practices and principles, which will be based on observations of the successes and setbacks being experienced under the different provincial approaches.

(The next day, the Trudeau government reversed its stance. After a face-time conference with the provincial premiers, it was announced that the federal government and the provinces have agreed "to work together to develop a joint set of national guidelines" on how best to re-open the economy while avoiding a second wave of coronavirus infections. The objective is to establish a national standard 'way of doing things', while incorporating some provincial flexibility. It sounds good, but whether there be any real follow-up in providing a set of national guidelines for Canadians, remains to be seen.)

Where the long-term recovery is concerned, the Trudeau government has announced that it will commit over $1 billion to COVID-19 research to better understand the nature of the virus, to develop a vaccine, and to formulate a long-term recovery strategy for the country. It is rather late in the day to begin to work on a vaccine and a recovery strategy, but the initiative is praiseworthy. The projected funding breaks down into $40 million for viral sequencing to track the different strains of the virus; $23 million for vaccine research; $600 million for private-sector trials of drug treatments and vaccines, and $114 million to the Canadian Institutes of Health research to investigate measures that can reduce the spread of the virus.

Some Canadian public health officials are arguing that the provincial governments can only fully lift the lockdowns when a 'herd immunity' has been developed within the population of Canada. That those who have recovered from the disease and have a natural immunity will need to be reinforced by a widespread program of vaccination – once a vaccine has been developed – to attain a 'herd immunity' among the general population. The problem, where vaccination is concerned, is that as soon a vaccine is developed, it may take anywhere from twelve to eighteen months to test and secure an approval for its use in humans. Moreover, even more time will be required to get a vaccine into a large-scale production, and to vaccinate upwards of sixty percent of the population to develop a 'herd immunity'.

Herd Immunity Approach: In Canada, Dr. Theresa Tam, the Chief of the Public Health Agency, has cautioned that there is "not enough evidence" to back 'herd immunity' based on a natural immunity as an approach to re-opening society in the absence of a vaccine. On its part, the WHO has issued a brief that there is "no [scientific] evidence" that people who have recovered from COVID-19 have antibodies in their blood sufficient to protected them from a second infection; although several days subsequently, the WHO issued a second brief statement that most of those who recovered from a coronavirus infection would have "some level of protection".

It is preposterous that public health professionals are spending their time in discussing the concept of a natural 'herd immunity', and its potential contribution to renewed economic activity in Canada, when its patently impossible to attain a 'herd immunity level in Canada without a major program of vaccination over a period of months with an as yet to be developed vaccine. At present, there are only 16,438 individuals who have recovered from the coronavirus disease in Canada, which is a quite small, almost insignificant, 'background immunity' pool in a Canadian population of 36.5 million people. The scientific approach of counting on the development of a vaccine promises a long-term solution to eradicating the coronavirus threat, but a more immediate pragmatic and practical approach is needed to prevent the spread of the coronavirus.

Despite the dismissal by its Chief -- Dr. Tam – of the concept of building up a natural 'herd immunity', the Public Health Agency of the federal government is setting up an Immunity Task Force to establish a tracking program to determine the number of people who have recovered from being infected with the virus, and who now are 'believed to be immune' to the virus. The hope is that if there are a lot of people with this 'background immunity' in some geographical regions, it will be less risky to lift the lockdown in those regions at an early date. In effect, such regions will have a small pool of people that have acquired an immunity. What is Immunity Task Force envisages is the establishing of a program of widespread testing across Canada for the presence of the coronavirus among Canadians, together with a serology test (blood test) of infected persons who have recovered from the disease to determine the level of antibodies in their bloodstream. It is expected that it will take months to complete the immunity testing, in conjunction with a continued testing of those who are getting sick. Apparently, the intention is not only to trace the spread of the virus to facilitate its containment, but to allow those with a 'natural immunity' to resume their jobs and social activities, while retaining in isolation those who test positive for the virus.

What is unreal about the whole concept of a nation-wide immunity testing of a very large segment of the Canadian population is that several critics familiar with the testing procedure -- within the bio-technology field in universities and the private industry -- are pointing out that a nation-wide immunity testing program is an impractical exercise of questionable value where the proposed establishment of a 'herd immunity' is concerned. The existing testing system of taking nasal-throat swabs/laboratory analysis cannot be simply upscaled to administer the 100,000 to 500,000 tests that will be required daily to cover every Canadian showing the coronavirus symptoms, as well as the general population to identify the asymptomatic carriers. Nor does Canada currently have a sufficient quantity of personal protective equipment to protect the army of health care workers who would be administering the tests in the field.

Undertaking such a national immunity testing program presents a number of practical problems: the securing and supporting of the personnel required to administer the testing, and the number of testing kits required, as well as the swabs need for taking the test sample and the enzyme needed in the laboratory analysis, which are already in short supply in struggling to meet the existing testing demand. Moreover, false negative can be reportedly as high as 30 percent, which is caused where the amount of virus matter in the secretions picked up by the nasal swab is insufficient to indicate the present of the COVID-19 virus, or the infected person is in the first few days of an infection and does not test as infected. Thus, pre-symptomatic persons who test negative, would feel free to circulate in public and could inadvertently spread the virus. What we have here is yet another impractical public health approach to combat the coronavirus from our Public Health Agency of Canada. God save us from these public health bureaucrats, so- called 'experts', who have no real idea of how to eradicate the novel coronavirus threat!

It appears that the portable testing kit developed by Spartan Bioscience of Ottawa, with its hand-held DNA "Cube' analyzer -- which is reputedly 100 percent accurate with the capability to produce a test result on-the-spot in less than an hour – will address most of the testing problems with the older nasal swab/laboratory testing process in identifying whether a person is positive or negative for the virus infection. However, severe practical problems will still remain in upscaling to take the number of tests required across Canada to identify and isolate infected persons – both symptomatic and asymptomatic carriers. Moreover, recovered patients will have to undergo a blood test to determine the level of immunity antibodies in their bloodstream to determine if they have developed an immunity.

Several countries – notably Germany – are considering issuing an 'immunity passport' that would enable those who have established their immunity through undergoing serology test to confirm that they have developed antibodies that provide immunity to the COVID-19 virus. Immunity passport holders would then be free to return to work, to socialize, and to travel without fear of becoming re-infected. However, one potential problem is how will the immunity pass system be enforced in public to distinguish those who have been tested, and deemed to have an immunity to the virus, and those who have no such immunity but do not respect government regulations. There are always irresponsible individuals who would not hesitate to carry a fake immunity card to gain employment and/or their social freedom.

Serology Testing: In the United States, the Federal Drug Administration (FDA) has already approved a coronavirus antibody test, and a Canadian company, Roche Canada, has developed a antibody test that will be available by late May or early June. A Halifax company, MedMira Inc. has developed a rapid antibody test that can be performed in three minutes using a drop of blood.

In serology testing, an anti-body test is performed on a blood sample – usually taken from a finger prick -- to look for the antibodies that are produced by the immune system for a defence against a particular virus, in this case the coronavirus. The antibodies attach themselves to an invasive virus, and are capable of neutralizing, destroying, and removing the attacking virus from the body. It is known that one type of antibody (IgM antibodies) appears in the blood within a week after a body becomes infected by the coronavirus, and a more durable antibody (IgG) is detectable after two weeks. The problem with serology, or blood antibody, testing is that the level of immunity protection afforded to recovered patients is not known with respect to the duration of the immunity, and what level of antibodies is necessary to convey an actual immunity to a second infection.

Recovery Strategies: One thing that is most striking about the various proposals of the federal government concerning how to approach the re-opening of the national economy, is the emphasis on investigating the disease pathogen, on a widespread immunity testing over several months to get a clear picture of the spread of the virus and the background immunity levels, and on the development of a vaccine. Granted, the investigating of the disease pathogen and the development of a vaccine are critical undertakings, but they are long-term priorities. However, Canada is dealing with an immediate need to get the economy functioning again, while avoiding a second wave of infections. Hence, there is a crucial need for a more immediate and practical approach. What is being ignored is how effective the wearing of a face mask can be -- if widely adopted -- in limiting the spread of the virus, and in preventing asymptomatic individuals from spreading the coronavirus.

Face Masks: One needs only to look at the experience of South Korea and Japan, where face masks have been widely worn among the populace. Based on the experience of those two countries, and of Hong Kong, it is obvious that the wearing of plain cotton masks, by the general public, is surprisingly effective in preventing the spread of infections by infected persons and asymptomatic individuals, thereby eliminating or greatly reducing the occurrence of new infections. However, the World Health Organization continues to maintain that the wearing of face masks in public is not necessary, and Dr. Theresa Tam, the Chief Medical Officer for Public Health Canada is still maintaining that face masks are only necessary for frontline medical personnel dealing directly with infested persons.

What determines the view of both the WHO and Dr. Tam is that there are currently no 'scientific studies' proving that face masks are a significant factor is limiting the spread of the COVID-19 virus. Hence, the use of face masks is not being recommended. God save us from these academic science types with a mind bounded by their professional medical journals, who are incapable of independent thought and action based on practical experience, observation, and pragmatic considerations. They do not have the independence of mind and discernment that distinguishes great leaders in a time of crisis. Why the Trudeau government continues to adhere to the recommendations of the WHO and the Public Health Agency of Canada, is beyond belief given their recent history of providing misleading, and often plainly wrong, public health advice concerning the coronavirus threat. Where the re-opening of the economy is concerned, Prime Minister Trudeau has declared that Canada will 'follow the science', although he added that efforts to contain the spread of the coronavirus will focuss on physical distancing and personal protective equipment, which includes the wearing of face masks.

Recovery Strategies: On April 24th, the present diarist forward to Dr. Vera Etches, the Chief Medical Health Officer for the City of Ottawa, Ontario. 'a recovery plan' that is based on a low cost and practical approach to protecting Canadians from a second wave of coronavirus infections while re-opening the economy. The letter is self-explanatory.

Dr. Vera Etches
Medical Health Officer
Ottawa

After reading intently the coverage of the COVID-19 virus pandemic, and the various proposals for re-opening the economy, the one thing that has been overlooked is the effectiveness of the N-95 respiratory mask in preventing infections. Hence, what is needed is a recovery plan that takes advantage of the capabilities of the N-95 respiratory mask which, when made compulsory for wearing in one city in Europe – Jena, Germany – caused infections to flatline.

A Recovery Plan

1) Focus testing on persons who had contact with an infected person, and on those who have apparently recovered from an attack of the COVID-19 virus to determine whether they are virus free or need to be placed in or retained in quarantine;

2) Place the N-95 respiratory masks -- millions of which are now being purchased by government -- on Amazon.ca for purchase at a nominal price to cover shipping and handling costs and to prevent hoarding;

3) Make it compulsory to wear a respiratory face mask when going out in public;

4) Let all businesses, companies, transportation systems, and public activities recommence that can function with staff, workers, customers, clients, and participants wearing a respiratory mask; and

5) Keep those who are sick, or have been sick, quarantined until they test free of the virus.

The wearing of respiratory masks by the public, in conjunction with a continued emphasis on the washing of hands, the use of hand sanitizers, and the disinfecting of public contact surfaces, will keep virus infections flatlined during the initial stages of re-opening the economy.

Yours sincerely,

Robert W. Passfield
Ottawa, ON

Thereafter, the diarist forwarded the 'recovery plan letter' to the Ministry of Heath for Ontario, with the following addendum:

"The N-95 respiratory masks ought to be manufactured in three different sizes – small, medium and large – to better fit the contours of the face of Canadian of all ages and head sizes. One complaint about the current N-95 respiratory mask, is that some users have found that in fitting the mask to get a complete seal against the contours of the face, they need to tighten the mask to the point where it leaves deep marks in their face after hours of wear.

Where the N-95 respiratory cannot be readily obtained for immediate use, a resort can be had to hand-made cotton gauze masks – washable and re-usable – that have proven to be effective in preventing virus infections during previous pandemics. In the United States, the Center for Disease Control of the U.S. Food and Drug Administration, has recommended that cloth face masks be worn by the general public for the duration of the coronavirus pandemic; yet that recommendation has yet to be publicized. At present, governments are thinking in terms of grandiose undertakings, at an horrendous expense over a long period of time, to get their national economy open, while avoiding a second wave of coronavirus infections.

The safest way to re-open the economy at a minimal cost and delay is simply for the government to make the wearing of face masks compulsory in public with a continued commitment to the washing of hands, the use of hand sanitizers, the constant disinfecting of common surfaces touched by the public, and the maintenance of social distancing whenever practicable. Government must supply the N-95 respiratory mask to the fullest extent possible, given our current domestic manufacturing capacity, while supplementing that effort by encouraging Canadian companies to manufacture a cotton gauze mask, and by publishing instructions on how to make a cotton mask or different types of cotton masks so that Canadians can make a mask for themselves."

Respiratory Masks: It has just been announced that GM Canada has started up an assembly line capable of producing a million respiratory masks per month at its Oshawa, Ontario, plant, and will supply the masks to government at cost. Currently, the company has 50 employees working two shifts per day. In Michigan, GM is not manufacturing the N-95 respiratory mask; it is producing a different type of respiratory mask in its Ontario plant. No explanation was provided.

Saturday, April 25, 2020

Spanish Flu: A recent study of the impact of the Spanish flu pandemic on the United States, in 1918-1919, has concluded that the early introduction of an aggressive policy of physical distancing measures – inclusive of the wearing of face masks – was effective in containing the virus spread with a 50 percent lower peak death rate in 1918 than the cities that took no such precautions. (Presumably, the death rate would have been even lower in the cities practicing social distancing and the wearing of face masks if everyone had obeyed the city ordinances.) However, where restrictions on social distancing and the wearing of face masks were lifted after a six-week period, the cities that had escaped the initial wave of infections were struck severely in the second wave of virus infections. Only the cities that maintained their various physical distancing practices and the wearing of face masks far beyond the initial six-week period, were spared the second wave of infections and the high death rate associated with the Spanish flu virus in other cities.

In Canada, the Spanish flu was introduced in September 1918 by invalided soldiers returning home from the Great War (World War I), and, subsequently, it spread quickly through the towns, villages and farms of the country when well over 500,000 Canadian soldiers were demobilized and returned home following the Armistice of November 11th. In total during 1918 and a resurgence of the virus in 1919, over 50,000 Canadians died from the Spanish flu, out of a population of 8 million Canadians. Worldwide, well over 20 million people died from the Spanish flu.

It was a virus that struck rapidly among the young and the healthy. Symptoms were fatigue, coughing, muscle and joint pain, loss of appetite, and a mucous build-up in the lungs that blocked the respiratory system. The virus was highly contagious, and a significant number of the sick died anywhere from one day to several days after the initial infection. At the time, doctors were not familiar with the virus, or viruses more generally, but public authorities took a common-sense approach from the onset of the appearance of the disease in their community.

People were advised to avoid crowds and anyone who was coughing and sneezing, to avoid using common drinking cups, to cover their mouth when coughing or sneezing, to stay a home if suffering from cold symptoms, and to wear a cotton gauze face mask when in a sick room or in a crowded area. Instructions were published on how to make a four- layer cotton gauze mask, and on its use: change every two hours, and either burn a used mask or boil it in water for four to five minutes before drying and re-using. In addition, people were advised to wash their hands before eating, to use 'destructible dishes, or dishes that were sterilized in boiling water.

In the larger cities, churches, schools, movie theatres, billiard halls, dance halls, and public bathhouses were closed, and large public gatherings were banned. Limits were put on the number of persons allowed on a streetcar and in grocery stores. Many businesses were closed by the authorities, and in some provinces the wearing of face masks in public was made mandatory. The sick were quarantined either at home, in a hospital, or in temporary facilities. Although doctors were not familiar with the virus, they recognized the danger of an influenza attack, and advised that these elementary precautions be taken immediately. However, during the onset of the coronavirus in Canada in February 2020, public health officials were slow to advise and adopt such elementary measure for the protection of Canadians.

Testing: Dr Theresa Tam has stated that the national target for testing should be about 60,000 tests per day, and that the testing should include nasal swab/laboratory tests for the virus infection, as well as serological tests to screen the blood for virus antibodies, with the testing to proceed in conjunction with contact tracing and the continuance of social spacing. To date, testing has been restricted for the most part to those who are ill, or in immediate contact with an infected person. The shortage of testing kits, and particularly of the swabs used in testing, has prevented any general testing among the population at large. Hence, there is no clear idea as to how extensive the spread of the corona virus is among Canada's population, and epidemiologists are being frustrated in their efforts to build a model of the spread of the virus.

In eastern Ontario, the Ontario Regional Microbiology Laboratory, which serves sixteen hospitals, is now conducting 1,132 tests per day – about half of the tests in the greater Ottawa urban area – but the testing is limited due to a shortage of the speciality swabs used to collect nasal secretions for testing. The swabs are imported primarily from Italy, and there is a high demand in the global market as other countries are likewise experiencing a shortage. As a result, the regional lab is running at only 50 to 60 percent of its capacity.

Spartan Bioscience Cube: The Spartan Bioscience 'aluminum cube' DNA-analyzer, which enables an on-the-spot testing, one-hour, testing for the COVID-19 virus, is in high demand. During the past two weeks since its approval by Health Canada, the Ottawa company has received a total of two million orders for the COVID-19 test kit cartridge from Ontario, Quebec, Alberta, and the federal governments. In response, Spartan Bioscience had entered an arrangement with a Toronto manufacturer which will increase production to several hundred thousand test kits per week by July. The company expects no problem with securing swabs for collecting the DNA samples. The swabs used with the mobile 'cube' testing kit are manufactured locally.

(Subsequently, on May 4th, the effort to test Canadians for the coronavirus suffered a serious setback when the National Microbiology Laboratory in Winnipeg found that the swabs being used with the revolutionary Spartan Bioscience testing cube were unreliable in collecting a sufficient quantity of the virus DNA to ensure accurate readings by the Cube. There is no problem with the reliability of the cube analysis. The problem is strictly with the capability of the new swab to consistently collect a sufficiently representative sample of secretions to ensure that the test is 100 percent reliable, or a close approximation thereto. This is a major setback to the achievement of a viable testing program for the general Canadian population.)

Canada Emergency Commercial Rent Assistance: Prime Minister Justin Trudeau announced a new rent relief program to aid small business tenants who have been forced to close or have suffered a drastic decline in revenues during the coronavirus epidemic. The Canada Emergency Commercial Rent Assistance (CECRA) program will be funded jointly – within each province -- by the federal government and the province concerned, and will provide emergency loans as a temporary financial relief to landlords who agree to reduce the rent of their small business tenants. The emergency loans to 'commercial property owners' will cover fifty percent of the rent payments that they would normally receive from a commercial tenant for April, May, and June, if the landlord agrees to reduce the rent of his small business tenants to 25 percent of the normal rent for the said three months, and promises not to evict the tenant.

In effect, the new Canada Emergency Commercial Rent Assistance program is intended to help small business owners, who are commercial tenants. It will help the retail store tenants to survive a severe drop in revenues during the coronavirus epidemic by reducing their rent payment to their landlord to just 25 percent of the normal rent, while protecting landlords -- with commercial retail store tenants -- from suffering a severe loss or total loss of rental income.

The emergency loans to landlords with commercial tenants are forgivable as of December 31, 2020, if the landlord recipient complies with the regulations governing the CECRA program, and refrains from seeking to recover the rent abatement granted the commercial tenant – the 25 percent of the rent dispensed with under the CECRA agreement.

To qualify for the emergency forgivable loan, a landlord must have small business tenants who pay less than $50,000 a month in rent and who have suffered a revenue decline of at least 70 percent from the pre- COVID-19 levels, or small business tenants who have been forced to close their business because of pandemic restrictions. Landlords who have non-profit and charitable organizations as tenants are also eligible. The Minister of Finance, Bill Morneau, has estimated that the new program will cost $2 billion, and will be fully operational by mid-May, when loan requests will be back dated to cover the month of April.

Real Estate Market: Companies owning retail real estate have been particularly hard hit by the coronavirus lockdowns. Mall owners are reporting – with malls totally shut down -- that retail tenants have paid as little as 40 percent of the rent owed for April and, what is totally surprising, two major brand companies, with retail outlets in a large number of malls across Canada, have failed to pay any rent in April. In response, mall owners have begun approving rent deferrals for some of their retail tenants but are worried that rental deferral requests might reach as high as forty to sixty percent for May. In contrast, the real estate companies have reported that upwards of 96 percent of their residential tenants have paid their April rent. One suspects that small retail business tenants -- who fear that they may be forced into bankruptcy -- are hanging on to whatever liquidity they possess, rather than paying their mall rent while their business remains closed. In contrast, residential renters want to maintain possession of their rental units, and do not want to be evicted once provincial controls on evictions are lifted. In the Greater Toronto Area, residential real estate listings are down 67 percent below last year.

Canadian Seafood Stabilization Fund: In Ottawa, Bernadette Jordan, the Minister of Fisheries, Oceans, and the Canadian Coast Guard, announced another new financial aid program: the Canadians Seafood Stabilization Fund (CSSF), which will provide $62.5 million in financial aid to the fish and seafood processing sector. The program is intended to address the financial strain and instability that the fish and seafood processing industry is facing both long term and during the economic dislocations being experience during the coronavirus lockdown. It is also intended to provide a long-term employment for the women and men working in the industry.

The financial aid program will enable the industry to access short-term federal government financing to pay for maintenance and inventory costs; to add cold storage capacity for unsold product; to comply with new health and safety measures for workers; to support the introduction of new manufacturing/automated technologies to improved the productivity and quality of the finished seafood products, and to enable the industry to adopt their products in response to changing market demands.

The new Canadian Seafood Stabilization Fund program will be delivered on the east coast by the Atlantic Canada Opportunities Agency, and in Quebec by the Canada Economic Development for Quebec Regions, and on the west coast by Western Economic Diversification Canada. Strictly speaking, this financial aid program is not a direct response to the economic impact of the coronavirus lockdown. It is a financial aid program designed to address long term economic problems and dislocations in the fish and seafood processing industry that the industry does not have the financial capacity to address for itself, and particularly so during a coronavirus lockdown.

Sunday, April 26, 2020

Virus Statistics: To date, in Canada, there are a total of 45,354 confirmed cases of coronavirus infection, a total of 2,465 deaths, and 16,438 resolved cases. Quebec and Ontario are the epicentres of the virus infections in Canada. The Province of Quebec has 23,267 confirmed cases, 1,446 deaths, and 5,507 resolved cases; while Ontario has 13,995 confirmed cases, 73 deaths, and 7,509 resolved cases.

Recovery Plans: The United States and the European Union are currently engaged in working out viable approaches to gradually lifting their lockdowns – or in the words of British Prime Minister Boris Johnson, 'to modify the lockdown' – while remaining highly conscious of a need to avoid triggering a second wave of virus infections. In Canada, several provinces have begun to partially lift their lockdown restrictions. Both Ontario and Quebec – the two hardest hit provinces by the coronavirus – have announced that they will reveal, next week, their plans for commencing the re-opening of the economy in their respective provinces.

The devastating economic impact of the coronavirus has caused many free-trade globalists to re-think their commitment to a laissez-faire economic policy on the part of government. In the United States, as part of its groping towards a recovery plan, the Trump administration is proposing to purchase equity stakes in oil and gas companies to aid that sector to recover from the devastation it has experienced from a double blow: the coronavirus lockdown, which has drastically reducing demand, and the plummeting of world oil prices owing to Saudi Arabia flooding the market with oil in its price dispute with Russia.

Monday, April 27, 2020

Tracking of Contacts: One of the critical steps in any recovery plan, by way of containing any new onslaught of virus attacks, is the identifying and isolating of infected persons, the tracking of their immediate contacts for testing, and the quarantining of those who test positive and the self-isolation of the other contacts. The tracking of contacts is a labour- intensive work on the ground in tracking the movements of the infected person and identifying and notifying those individuals who were in an immediate contact. The contacts of an infected person are traced back over a 48-hour period from the first evidence of symptoms in the infected individual.

The City of Ottawa public health unit has responded by adding 350 people to its staff – retired nurses, medical students, and re-assigned City staff, and is seeking further volunteers. To greatly facilitate the tracking of contacts of an infected person, and the establishing of contact with the individuals who have been exposed to the virus, the City is looking into using smartphone tracking. The intention is to acquire an existing app for downloading by the public. Singapore has successfully used a smartphone app, working through the Bluetooth system, to trace contacts and to contain the spread of the coronavirus. Moreover, contact-tracking apps are under development in several countries, and Google and Apple are jointly developed an app for tracking contacts that will be available shortly.

As of early April, if not earlier, several prominent Canadian government officials and medical officers have speculated that government might need to introduce smartphone tracking surveillance to ensure that mandatory quarantine orders are being obeyed by infected persons. Taiwan has used smartphone surveillance quite effectively, as has South Korea, and Singapore which launched the initial program on March 20th. In those countries, the spread of the coronavirus was contained through an aggressive quarantining of infected persons, the identifying and testing of contact persons, the mandatory quarantining of those who tested positive and self-isolation if they tested negative. Moreover, all three of these countries imposed strict border closures at a very early date to prevent foreign travellers importing the virus. With these aggressive coronavirus control policies in place, major lockdowns of the populations were not required.

Canadian public health authorities are convinced that the most effective way stop the spread of the coronavirus is to track down the persons who had contact with an infected person to warn them of threat, and to encourage the contact persons to self-isolate until they can be tested. Both Alberta and Ontario have adopted an aggressive tracking strategy, and perhaps other province as well, with the assembly of tracking teams. However, the task has proven to be overwhelming, and the manual tracking of contacts is too slow in tracing where an infected person has been and in tracking down and notifying the individuals with whom the infected person had contact during the time when he or she was contagious.

Among medical authorities, smartphone tracking is becoming widely recognized as being a highly effective and efficient system for identifying individuals who ignore their quarantine restriction, and in identifying and tracking the individuals who came in contact with the infected person so that they can be notified of their exposure, be tested, and self-isolated while monitoring their health. The system works through tracing smartphone interactions. Moreover, a smartphone tracking system can be used to compile aggregate data to identify where people are congregating in defiance of the social distancing advisory. The tracking system can also be used for locating people at risk through identifying the patterns of virus movement to enable an intervention to be made to quarantine effected areas, and to encourage self-isolation in the areas under threat. In Europe, smartphone tracking is now being widely adopted.

In Canada, it was reported (April 9th) that Daniel Leung of LivNao, a Vancouver software start-up, has developed a ready-to-use smartphone app that can automatically identify persons who have come in contact with an infected person, and that can automatically notify any individual coming into contact with the infected person so that they can isolate themselves. However, to date contacts with provincial and federal health departments have reportedly produced little interest in the LivNao cell-tracking technology, and a spokesperson for the Canadian Civil Liberties Association has objected that the new smartphone tracking system, if applied by government, constitutes a threat to privacy and might be used to discriminate against infected persons. (No explanation has been offered as to how a government smartphone tracking system would 'discriminate against infected persons' – by government acting to prevent them from circulating socially?)

Various newspaper accounts have made it clear that contact tracking is a common response to containing epidemics around the world, and more recently is credited with breaking the chain of transmission of the Ebola epidemic in West Africa (2013-2016). What smartphone tracking offers is a more efficient and critically faster method of identifying individuals exposed to the coronavirus so that they can be tested, quarantined if they test positive, and provided with immediate medical care if they become sick.

In a volunteer tracking system, members of the public will be asked to download the app, and when individuals show symptoms of the disease, they are expected to notify the individuals whom the tracking app has identified as contacts. In a mandatory system, the app is downloaded by government on all smartphones, and the public health authorities track and notify the contacts of an infected person directly. Nonetheless, some concerns have been expressed about the implementation of a smartphone tracking system.

One concern that has been expressed is that the system of smartphone app tracking, to identify infected persons and map the virus spread, might lead to 'the stigmatization of communities, groups, or places as high risk'. Hopefully, the view being expressed is merely the recognition of a potentially regrettable secondary effect of contact tracking, rather than a distorted politically correct view that the avoidance of offending the sensibilities of particular individuals and ethnic groups is more important than the health and lives of their fellow citizens. Whatever the case, if there are individuals or particular groups who do not practice social distancing, who do not self-isolate, and who are not practicing proper hygiene in washing their hands, then they are a threat to the health, well-being, and even lives of their fellow citizens, and society has a right to know. Hopefully, once the transgressing individuals or groups are identified, they will change their habits, conform to the public health regulations, and cease to be a danger to others. Individuals and groups need to be held accountable for their actions, or inaction, in a national crisis. That is likewise the case, with the identification of high-risk places, so that they can be avoided by most people to protect their health and lives.

For a Tory conservative, there is no privacy issue involved in a temporary smartphone tracking surveillance when public health, and the well-being and lives of Canadians are under threat during a deadly virus outbreak.

Indeed, the forced quarantining of infected persons to protect the health and lives of Canadians is fully acceptable in law, and consistent with common sense, with the protection of the public health, and with public morality. A surveillance of the public activities of Canadian citizens, as distinct from their private activities and private business, during a deadly virus epidemic is not a privacy, civil liberties, or human rights issue. The right to privacy relates to one's private life, not to one's public activities which, by definition, are public.

More generally, whether it is a case of smartphone tracking of the public movements of individuals, or cameras mounted in high crime areas or installed for traffic monitoring, where the motive is the protection of the public from harm or the threat of death, privacy is not an issue. To the Tory mind, people who complain that any monitoring of public activities is an invasion of privacy, are either are up to no good, are not accomplishing anything worthwhile, or are engaging in criminal activities. Those who obey the law, and always do what is right, fair, and just, have nothing to fear from a public surveillance system. Indeed, public surveillance systems enhance the personal security of law-abiding citizens.

What is particularly surprising about the slowness to adopt smartphone tracking surveillance is the failure of Ontario to do so. Premier Ford is a populist, but he has revealed staunch Tory elements in his mindset in stepping up to take command in combatting the coronavirus threat, in his moral outrage in taking steps against companies engaging in price-gouging, and his concern for the health and well-being of all Ontarians. Why his government has not acted quickly to adopt a smartphone tracking surveillance system at a time when he is encouraging his provincial health authorities to aggressively engage in contact tracking, remains puzzling.

Food Security: Articles are beginning to appear in the Canadian press, as of mid-April, that are calling on the Canadian government to take positive steps to re-establish a domestic food processing industry. In the decades after the implementation of NAFTA (1993), the fruits and vegetable food processing and canning industries migrated to the United States where the growing season is longer, and canning plants can stay in operation longer. What is alarming is that Canadian grocery stores have canned vegetables on their shelves from as far afield as China, with oddly enough even canned vegetables from Peru, of all places.

During the coronavirus pandemic, Canadians have experienced no shortage of food, but at least ten countries since mid-March have introduced bans on the export of grain or rice. Moreover, transport bottlenecks caused by lockdowns in many countries, have caused shortages of food in some countries and have posed a serious threat to food security. This has let to several countries setting up a national task force to examine the food supply chain vulnerabilities. There is a new emphasis on local food production to attain a national self-sufficiency in basic foods.

Both the Canadian, Ontario and Quebec governments are expressing a need to produce more fruits and vegetables domestically, as well as medical supplies. Of course, the United Nations is maintaining the states must work together to avoid 'beggar-thy-neighbour policies'. How growing more of one's own food and attaining a national self-sufficiency in basic foot stuffs is begging thy neighbour, remains unexplained. A national self-sufficiency policy leaves other countries free to grow whatever crops they need to feed their own people. Without major export sales of their crops to western nations, the developing nations may well experience a slower growth rate, but it might well benefit them in having less social unrest and a better food supply in becoming more self-reliant. It is western countries who are hurting themselves in relying on basic foods sourced from less-developed countries. In being dependent on a global market for basic foods, the western nations are vulnerable to prices surges when social, political, and economic instability strikes the primary producers of food.

Not only does the existing global multilateral food supply chain fail to provide security of supply, but it represents a loss of domestic employment, the tax revenues that would be yielded by domestic growers and industries, a lack of quality control, manufacturing standards, and health inspections over the crop grown, the animals raised, and canning/packing of food products, as well as a lack of control over additives. That is equally the case with production of drugs in other countries. Moreover, the manufactured goods and food products purchased overseas are transported in ships that are using bunker fuel for their diesel engines that make a significant contribution to carbon emissions, and pollute our waters through dumping their bilge waters in our harbours. With the dislocations suffered by the global supply chain during the coronavirus, and the continued the depreciation of the Canadian dollar against the U.S. dollar – a 72 to 74 cent Canadian dollar, it is predictable that prices of food imports to Canada, which are already high, will increase between ten and fifteen percent as is being predicted at present.

What is encouraging are reports -- as of mid-April -- that federal and provincial departments of agriculture are concerned about the security of Canada's food supply, and that investigations are underway concerning the potential for increasing Canada's greenhouse growing capabilities. At present, Canada imports $15 billion (Can) worth of worth of fruits, nuts, and vegetables per annum, and Canadian greenhouses produce $1.3 billion worth of food, mainly tomatoes, cucumbers and peppers on a mass scale, with lesser crops of lettuce, green beans, eggplants, and some herbs and microgreens. Oddly enough, 65 percent of the greenhouse tomatoes, cucumbers and peppers are exported, primarily to the United States. At present, Canada has a surplus of underutilized greenhouse capacity – built to accommodate the growth of cannabis in an industry which has failed to take off.

The advantages of greenhouses over outdoor farms in growing vegetables is that they provide a year-round growing season in Canada, are not subject to the vagaries of weather that plagues outdoor farming, and the temperature and watering can be controlled – with no waste of water -- which is a plus with Canada facing the impact of global warming and potential future droughts. Investigations are reportedly underway to determine the variety of crops that can be readily adopted to greenhouse growth on a commercial scale. The Canadian and provincial agricultural sectors ought to be investigating drought resistant crops as well.

What the supply-chain problems indicate is a need for Canada to de-couple from the globalized economy, which is dominated by a China hub, and to develop a national self-sufficiency in the products and produce needed by Canadians that will not be available in times of international crises. What is needed is a new national economic strategy policy that aims at maintaining a domestic research and production base to secure for Canada a domestic source of medical supplies and equipment, generic drugs, critical manufactures goods, and basic food products, with the development of a highly-skilled and knowledgeable work force, and a domestic capacity to gear up to meet Canadian needs during pandemics, natural disasters, and war.

Tuesday, April 28, 2020

Closing Borders: In an interview with CBC News – posted on the Internet yesterday -- Dr. Theresa Tam, Chief of the Public Health Agency of Canada, was asked: Why did Canada not close its borders at an earlier date than March 18th for foreign travellers and March 21st for American visitors, to keep the coronavirus out of the country?; and, why has a health screening program not been established in international airports and at border entry ports? Her answers are astounding.

First, Dr. Tam claimed that closing the border to travellers from China and 'other COVID-19 hotspots' might not have made much difference as it would not have stopped the virus coming in from other countries. Although the WHO was reporting in January that the coronavirus was highly contagious in human to human transmission, Dr. Tam maintained that there were "very, very few cases globally" and only ten cases in Canada that could be traced back to travel from China; and that the coronavirus "had already travelled somewhere else", including Iran and some European countries. Hence, the closure of the Canadian border to Chinese travellers would not have been effective in preventing the entry of the coronavirus into Canada.

(This is a totally absurd argument. What Dr. Tam is arguing is that travellers from China, including from Hubei Province, were allowed to continue to enter Canada during January, February and early March, because the coronavirus disease had spread to other countries already, and closing the border to Chinese travellers would not have prevented the entry of the coronavirus to Canada as there was already a small number of coronavirus cases in Canada. What this argument ignores is that Canadians were demanding the closure of the border to all foreign travellers, not just Chinese travellers. Moreover, this is an unbelievably passive, and fatalistic, attitude on the part of a public health official: viz.

'the coronavirus will enter Canada from somewhere, somehow, so why close the border to any one country, or group of countries'.

This in mind boggling! Apparently, no thought was given to trying to prevent potential virus carriers from other countries from entering Canada and adding to the spread of the coronavirus. It was only the action of President Trump in banning European travellers from entering the United States on March 13th, and a growing public pressure from Canadians, that forced the Trudeau Liberal government to finally close Canada's border to foreign travellers in mid-March.)

Secondly, Dr. Tam stated -- during the CBC interview -- that the closing of Canada's borders was not "in the playbook" of most health experts during the early days of the coronavirus outbreaks. 'They never envisaged the world shutting down'. Moreover, the closure of the U.S. border was not part of the pandemic preparedness plan: the "North American Pandemic Avian Influenza Plan" (2007). She also defended the current system of informing new arrivals in Canada of the symptoms of the coronavirus disease, advising them to self-isolate for 14 days, and informing them of the public health agencies to contact in the event of illness. Dr. Tam added that screening measures at international airports and border crossings 'likely would have failed because many carriers don't display symptoms', and that it is "highly unlikely" that screening will "be picking up people with symptoms as they are crossing the international borders".

 (My god! These comments are bizarre coming from a supposed public health authority. Since screening systems are not 100 percent accurate, Dr. Tom sees no need to introduce a screening system in Canada's international airports and at border entry points.)

The public health preparedness plan that she refers to, does provide for the closure of Canada's borders to non-North American countries in the event of a threatening influenza outbreak in other countries, and does call for the imposition of a strict screening process at airports and ports of entry. The "North American Plan for Animal and Pandemic Influenza" (2009 update) provides for a collaborative approach among Canada, the United States, and Mexico to correlated their activities in combatting and slowing the entry of an avian and human influenzas into North America, and commits each government to: the detection of novel human strains of influenza, the minimizing of illness and deaths, and the maintaining of the economy and functioning of society. Chapter 5, "Border Monitoring and Control Measures Associated with Pandemic Influenzas", states that the three countries will prevent infected individuals from entry to their respective countries, and will institute "strong disease surveillance systems coupled with appropriate screening at all North American airports, seaports, and regional perimeters" to further delay "the entry of a novel strain of human influenza" into North America.

Hence, there is no excuse for the laxity of the federal Liberal government – in acting on the advice of Dr. Tam and her Public Health Agency – in refusing to close the Canadian border to citizens from countries with a high rate of coronavirus infections during the month of February and the first two weeks of March. Nor is there any excuse for why returning Canadians, permanent residents, and those exempted from the ban on international travellers entering Canada, are not undergoing a strict health screening, and testing ever today upon entering Canada.

(One suspects that President Trump tired of the insistence of the Trudeau Liberal government that border controls and a strict screening of foreign travellers were not necessary. The recalcitrance of the Canadian Liberal government in refusing to impose border controls banning foreign travellers (non-North Americans), probably accounts – at least in part -- for the United States unilaterally imposing border closures first on foreign travellers who had visited China (January 31st), and subsequently on travellers from Europe (March 13th). [Iran is another country with a high rate of coronavirus infections, but Iranians are already banned from the United States under an earlier political travel ban imposed by the American government because the Iranian government is supporting terrorist activities abroad.]

During the CBC interview, Dr. Tam admitted that some of Canada's pandemic control actions 'could have been taken sooner', and that the response of the federal government was 'not perfect'. (Others might say that the slow response of the federal Liberal government to closing the Canadian border to foreign travellers, and its continuing failure to institute a strict screening and testing at Canada's international airports and border entry points, constitutes a case of gross negligence. Dr. Tam and her senior advisors at the Public Health Agency ought to be eased into retirement for any good that they are doing.)

Returning to Work: In Ottawa, public servants have been expressing their concern that social distancing cannot be maintained once they return to work in their office towers. Workers take crowded public transit vehicles to work, enter a common door, take elevators with a common push-button pad, will share washrooms, lunchrooms, meeting rooms, and office equipment. Moreover, the federal government offices have been introducing the asinine 'activity-based workplaces' system whereby desks are used in rotation by different individuals depending on their work activity; and individuals do not have an assigned office space. A temporary solution would be to extend the home-based work system -- currently in place for many public servants during the coronavirus epidemic -- for a longer period during the recovery phase. However, that is not a viable long-term solution, even during later stages of a recovery phase. The obvious solution is to make it mandatory for public servants to wear face masks and gloves at work, and for the government to insist that everyone leaving their home must wear a face mask. Within government offices, there should be a recommitment to each public servant having their own office cubicle, computer, printer, filing cabinet, and phone.

Payroll Wage Subsidy Program: This program, officially the Canadian Emergency Wage Subsidy (CEWS) program, is intended to ease the costs of small business by paying 75 percent of their payroll costs – up to a maximum of $847 per worker per week -- in return for the company recalling their laid off workers or committing to maintain workers on staff rather than laying them off. To date, the program has received almost 10,000 submissions from businesses for the payroll wage subsidy, which is only a small fraction of the astonishing seven million applications received from laid off workers applying for the workers' wage subsidy, the Canada Emergency Response Benefit (CERB), and which opened for applications much earlier on April 6th. The Canadian Federation of Independent Business does not see small businesses taking advantage of the payroll wage subsidy to recall laid off workers. Small businesses lack cash flow, during the lockdown and cannot afford to pay even the 25% of their normal payroll wages that the CEWS program requires them to do. Only the larger companies have the reserves of liquidity required to take advantage of the program, which will pay 75% of the payroll wages for the period March 15th to June 6th, for the workers rehired in anticipation of the re-starting of business activity on the lifting of the lockdown.

The Canadian Manufacturers and Exporters association does expect some of its member companies to take advantage of the CEWS payroll wages subsidy program to rehired workers to fulfill orders that were pending before the lockdown. However, the recovery of the manufacturing and export trade sector will depend, for the most part, on the pace of the recovery in the United. States.

Social Inequities: A University of Ottawa professor in the School of Social Innovation has complained in the press that the worker wage subsidy program – Canadian Emergency Response Benefit (CERB) – exacerbates social inequalities in failing to cover migrant workers and international students when their work permits expire and they lose their jobs. What this complaint ignores is that when foreigners are granted a work permit by the Canadian government to enter Canada and to work while in the country – a Visa code W-1 – the work permit covers a specific period of time in Canada with the understanding that the individual will return to their country of origin when the work permit expires. Why should the Canadian government pay a wage subsidy to foreigners who are unemployed and remaining in Canada illegally? One wonders what social innovations they are teaching at the University of Ottawa.

Secondly, the professor has complained that the Canada Pension Disability Plan provides a maximum payment of $1,387.66 per month for individuals no longer able to work because of a "severe and prolonged" disability, and that the disability pension payment is often lower depending on how much the individual contributed to the CPP while working. The inequity complained of is that under the CERB workers, who have lost their job during the coronavirus lockdown, will receive a subsidy of $2,000 per month, which is much greater than the monthly disability pension payment under the federal Canada Pension Disability Plan. What is being lost sight of here is that the CERB payments are a temporary benefit of four months duration – a total of $8,000 – for workers who have been laid off due to the coronavirus; whereas the disability pension is of an unlimited duration, and individuals with a disability have access to provincial financial aid programs for the disabled, as well as superior health care benefits and income tax benefits. If one were to total the financial and health care benefits received by a disabled worker each year – from the federal Canada Pension Disability Plan and provincial support programs -- it would greatly exceed the temporary $8,000 total payment received by a furloughed worker under the CERB.

Airport Taxi Drivers: Taxi drivers serving the Toronto Pearson Airport have complained about their vulnerability to the coronavirus as the airport continues to serve Canadians returning home from abroad. Their major concern is that individuals who show signs of illness in their screening at the airport are being directed to take a taxi to a hospital or testing station to be tested for the coronavirus infection. To date, fourteen taxi drivers have tested positive, and four have died. Taxi drivers are demanding that protective shields be installed in their taxis to separate them from the passengers, and that personal protective equipment – face masks and gloves – be issued to them. The Greater Toronto Airport Authority has agreed "to source personal protective equipment" for the taxi drivers.

Wednesday, April 29, 2020

Airports & Airlines: Canadian airlines have lost 90 percent of their business; and Air Canada alone has furloughed 16,500 employees – 15,200 unionized staff, and 1,300 managers. Senior managers who remain on staff are taking 15 to 50 percent pay cuts. Canadian airports collectively are expecting to lose $1.8 to $2.2 billion in revenue this fiscal year, and it is expected that international air travel will not re-open until Christmas. In the interim, planes worth hundreds of millions of dollars are parked, earning no revenue, but draining the airlines of money in insurance costs, leasing payments on the planes, and maintenance.

More generally, it is estimated that 250,000 jobs -- in Canada and the United States -- are dependent on the air transport industry. What is worse, the industry expects the economic impact to continue for the remainder of the year and well into 2021, regardless of when the airport shutdowns are lifted. Another factor of concern is whether the public will feel safe from the risk of a coronavirus infection within the close confines of an aircraft. Will the public quickly re-embrace air travel?

At present, laid off Canadian airline personnel are eligible to apply for the worker wage subsidy (CERB), and airlines can apply for the CEWS payroll wage subsidy. To be eligible to receive the payroll wage subsidy, which pays 75 percent of the wages of furloughed workers recalled to work -- with a maximum payment of $847 per worker per week for each recalled worker -- an airline would have to have a annual payroll of less than $1 million. Clearly, the major airlines do not qualify for CEWS payroll wage subsidy which is intended to provide support for small and medium sized businesses. Hence, Airlines are seeking a separate financial support package from the federal government.

In the United States, the airlines industry has suffered the severest drop in revenues of any industry. At present, the U.S. government has set aside $29 billion for loans to airlines, re-payable at a reasonable interest rate; and Congress has designated $50 billion in direct financial support for U.S. airlines. Airlines that apply must agree not to cut pay or lay off employees, to accept limits on executive compensations, and cannot buyback stock or pay dividends until September 2021. Moreover, the Trump administration, at one point, was considering –rather surprisingly -- the possibility of the government taking an equity share in the airlines as part of the bailout plan being developed.

Clearly, the U.S. government has learned its lesson about unconditional financial bailouts of the major banks and investment houses during the mortgage default crisis of 2008. At that time, the U.S. government established a $700 billion emergency fund to buy up 'toxic' mortgage-backed securities to stabilize the market, while the major banks and investment houses -- who were being saved from bankruptcy -- continued to pay large compensation packages, stock options, and bonuses, to their investment managers and executives who have caused the mortgage crisis.

While Canadian airlines have suffered greatly from the impact of the coronavirus lockdown, whether the Trudeau government will abandon its penchant for dispensing unconditional financial grants remains to be seen. The Canadian Transportation Agency has already suspended the new passenger protection regulations that had required airlines to compensate passengers for cancelled flights with a refund, rather than a voucher for a future flight. Currently, Air Canada is reimbursing ticket holders for cancelled flights with a voucher for the equivalent value of any future flight. However, the voucher must be used within 24 months.

At present, the Canadian pilots and flight attendants who are employed on the planes that remain in service in transporting Canadians home to four major airports – Montreal, Toronto, Calgary and Vancouver -- are wearing face masks, glasses, gloves and gowns. Planes are well-equipped with hand-sanitizers; there is no food or drink service; and passengers on entering the plane are given a snack box and a bottle of water. Transport Canada has ruled that all passengers boarding a plane must wear face masks. At least one airline, WestJet on its remaining domestic and international flights has instituted a spacing policy of leaving the middle row of seats empty on its Boeing 737 and 787 passenger jets, as well as a policy of disinfection the cabins after a flight. The Airline Pilots Association Canada is asking for the federal government to institute a better screening of passengers to identify coronavirus carriers before the plane is boarded, as well as an expedited testing process for aircrews.

More generally, airports worldwide are enforcing a two-metre distancing, except for family members, and are encouraging travellers to thoroughly wash their hands before and after passing through a screening process. In Hong Kong, travellers must enter a disinfectant booth where they are sprayed with a disinfectant – a 40 second process – that kills bacteria and viruses on skin and clothing. In addition, the Hong Kong airport is employing automated cleaning robots that kill microbes by zapping them with ultraviolet light and has set up check-in kiosks for travellers to obtain their boarding pass without interacting with airline personnel. Moreover, in most Asian airports, thermal detection screening is in place to detect travellers with a high temperature, which is indicative of a coronavirus infection, although thermal detection screening does not detect asymptomatic virus carriers.

On international airlines, flight attendants are wearing face masks and gloves, and planes are being sanitized and cleaned after each flight. South Korea, which is determined to eliminate the COVID-19 virus, rather than just contain it, has the Korean Air cabin crews wearing surgical gowns, gloves, eyeglasses, and face masks. In addition to WestJet, various airlines worldwide -- including Air Canada – have adopted the middle row empty spacing policy on their planes. However, according to the latest reports, most airlines are now abandoning that policy owing to the high cost of flying with one-third of the seats empty.

Fearful of losing their tourist season, some countries in Europe have opened 'tourist corridors' along which tourists from certain countries -- individuals who have tested negative for the virus – are permitted to fly to the tourist summer holiday meccas.

Vaccine Research: The University of Oxford in England has developed a potential coronavirus vaccine, which is undergoing clinical trials in healthy young British volunteers. One dose appears sufficient to generate a strong immune response. If the vaccine is proven, and approved, it is hoped to produce a million doses by September for initial use in the United Kingdom. Elsewhere, upwards of eighty research institutes worldwide, at universities and private pharmaceutical companies, are working on the develop of alternative coronavirus vaccines to find the most effective vaccine for combatting the virus.

In Ottawa, the Thistledown Foundation established by the founder of Shopify – Tobias Lütke and his wife Fiona McKean – has contributed $5 million in support of research grants to researchers working on developing a coronavirus vaccine. The Foundation is currently providing funding for 23 Canadian researchers. Among the grant recipients is a leading immunotherapy research scientist at the Ottawa Hospital, Dr. John Bell, the Senior Scientist, Cancer Therapeutic Program, Ottawa Hospital Research Institute, and Professor of Medicine and Biochemistry, Microbiology & Immunology, University of Ottawa.

The previous work of Dr. Bell has focused on the identification and characterization of novel cancer killing therapeutic viruses that selectively infect and kill cancer cells, while leaving healthy cells and tissues unharmed. Dr. Bell has received a $250,000 grant to pursue research to develop a COVID-19 vaccine. He will be working with University of Ottawa researchers, and Dr. Carolina Ilkow – a professor working in the areas of virology, tumour biology, and biotherapeutics -- to combine a bit of genetically engineered DNA material from the

COVID-19 virus with a cancer-fighting virus by way of working towards the development of a COVID-19 vaccine.

Earlier, in February 2020, Chinese researchers managed to map the complete sequence of the DNA genetic material in the coronavirus genome and published their results in a scientific journal. It was found that the coronavirus – subsequently named the COVID-19 virus -- is part of the COV family of viruses, which includes the SARS-CoV and the Middle East Respiratory Syndrome (MERS-CoV). Seventy percent of the COVID-19 genome sequence is about 79 percent similar to the SARS-CoV, and about 87 percent similar to the MERS-CoV. Moreover, the findings clearly indicate that the COV-19 virus originated with bats.

Health of Children: With the closure of medical clinics and doctors' offices during the lockdown, a concern has been expressed that babies and toddlers are missing their first series of immunizations. Locally, here in Ottawa, the Children's Hospital for Eastern Ontario (CHEO), local pediatricians, Ottawa Public Health, and CANImmunize, have responded to that critical need by establishing a children's immunization clinic. The fear is that young infants and children will be particularly vulnerable to a variety of potentially deadly diseases once social distancing ends. The initial aim is to inoculate children under the age of two with the primary series of vaccines, as well as the children and adolescents of immigrants who did not receive the primary series of vaccines in infancy.

The primary series of vaccinations includes: the five-in-one vaccine (diphtheria-pertussis-tetanus-olio-Hemophilus influenzae type B), pneumococcal conjugate vaccine, rotavirus vaccine, meningococcal conjugate type C, measles-mumps-rubella vaccine, and the chickenpox vaccine. Canadians have much to be thankful for in benefiting from the scientific achievements of western civilization.

In response to a 50 percent drop in admissions in the emergency department during the COVID-19 lockdown, CHEO has opened a virtual emergency department online for children requiring medical attention. A secure online self-tirage form has been posted for a parent to fill out to provide details of the child's health or injury problem, after which the parent is contacted, within a half hour, by a CHEO registration clerk to book an virtual appointment with a physician. In a virtual viewing and assessing of 'the patient', the physician can provide advice on a treatment or recommend a visit to the emergency department for tests and/or treatment. CHEO is thinking of maintaining the virtual emergency department online after the COVID-19 crisis ends. It will address the overcrowding and long wait times normally encountered in visits to the emergency department.

Easing the Lockdown: With New Brunswick and Saskatchewan, and surprisingly Quebec, starting to ease the lockdowns in their respective provinces, the Ontario government has announced its recovery plan framework. It will proceed in three stages, over a period of two to four weeks. The transition to each successive re-opening phase will be governed by the rate of new coronavirus cases being recorded in the various public health regions of the province. The aim is to guard against the danger of incurring a surge in infections as the lockdown is being lifted, and to ensure that any outbreak can be quickly identified and contained. Each phase has a distinct focus for re-opening the economy.

Phase One: Selected workplaces will be permitted to re-open if they can modify their operations to meet physical spacing requirements, some parks will be re-opened, and a greater number of people will be permitted to gather for funerals, church services, etc. Hospitals will start to re-schedule elective surgeries and other medical services. The key to entering the first phase is a two-to-four-week period with decreasing number of COVID-19 cases and an appreciable decrease in the number of coronavirus patients to hospitals.

Phase Two: Most workplaces will be permitted to re-open, including service industries, retail, and offices, as well as outdoor spaces and larger public gatherings will be permitted. This will depend on the hospital system possessing enough personal protective equipment and critical care beds to handle any surge in coronavirus cases.

Phase Three: All workplaces will re-open, and restrictions on public gatherings will be relaxed still further. Large gatherings such as concerts and sporting events will remain restricted "for the foreseeable future". The third phase will focus on having enough public health officials to effectively track the contacts of new cases – the ability to reach contacts within a day – to test and quarantine any contact that tests positive. The intent is to have a capacity to quickly detect new outbreaks, and to maintain high testing rates.

No timeline has been assigned for the inauguration of the various stages. Premier Ford has referred to the framework as a map, not a calendar.

Thursday, April 30, 2020

Canada Emergency Student Benefit (CESB): During the Wednesday sitting of parliament, the government put forth its proposed emergency financial package of support for students who are unable to secure a summer job because of the coronavirus lockdown. The financial package bill provides $9 billion in emergency support for students, of which $5.2 billion is intended for post-secondary students. In the initial bill, students, who cannot find summer work because of the coronavirus lockdown, were to receive $1,200 per month, from May to August, and students with dependants and students with disabilities were to receive $1,750 per month for the same period. However, the bill was amended by the minority Liberal government to take account of the views of the opposition parties.

In response to a demand from the NDP, the projected monthly payment for students with dependants and students with disabilities was increased to $2,000 per month to match the CERB payments. Furthermore, to meet Conservative concerns the bill was amended. As revised, the bill requires student applicants to attest that they have been searching for work but were unable to find a job, requires Service Canada to continually inform students, who are in receipt of student benefit grant, of jobs available through government job postings, and enables students to earn up to $1,000 – before taxes – during the benefit period, without losing their emergency student benefit financial aid.

The amendments were made in response to objections by Conservative Party members that the government should not be just giving the students a financial each month for doing nothing, with no recognition or commitment on the part of the student to seek a job. For Conservatives the hope is that the new legislation will make students aware that they are expected to try to find a summer job and will encourage them to take jobs that are available, rather than sitting home doing nothing. A reliance is being placed on the work ethic of the individual students, their sense of what is the right thing to do, and, hopefully, their desire to earn a greater income through working. Subsequently, the program was named the Canada Student Emergency Benefit (CESB).

It had been reported that some businesses upon re-opening in Manitoba are finding that workers receiving the Canada Emergency Response Benefit (CERB) payment are preferring to stay home rather than work. Hence, Conservatives MPs are concerned that the projected student emergency payment benefit might also serve as a disinclination for students to seek a summer job. Hence, the provision in the new student benefit legislation enabling students to benefit further, financially, from working part-time – at whatever jobs might become available -- while receiving the CESB payment. For Conservatives, it was, and is, a moral issue. Government grants ought not to undermine the work ethic by promising to pay students as much, or more than they might make in working at a summer job.

The new Canada Emergency Student Benefit (CESB) also introduced modification in the existing student grant programs of the federal government. The eligibility for existing student loans was broadened, the total number of non-repayable student grants available to students was doubled, and a new grant of up to $5,000 was introduced for post-secondary students who volunteer to work in support of community initiatives aimed at combatting the spread of the coronavirus. (This new grant was subsequently established, and funded, as a separate student volunteer summer work project, the Canada Student Service Grant.)

Coronavirus Impact: Over the first quarter of the year, 40 percent of Canadian businesses have laid off staff, with massive layoffs concentrated in the travel accommodation, tourism, retail, and food services sectors where almost three-quarters of businesses have reported laying of 80 percent or more of their workforce. To date, 7.26 million Canadians have applied for the Canadian Emergency Response Benefit (CERB) wages subsidy for having lost their job owing to the coronavirus lockdown, and that single program alone, which was launched just over a week ago – with payments backdated to March 15th – has already cost the federal government $25 billion. More generally, fifty percent of

Canadian businesses have experienced a decrease in revenue of over 20 percent compared to the same quarter last year. Yet, some sixty percent of businesses are confident that they can return quickly to 'normal operations' if all lockdown and physical distancing regulations are removed. Whether their customers and clients can so quickly shed their social distancing cautions and fears of activities and gatherings that might lead to a revival of the coronavirus, remains to be seen.

Canine COLVID-19 Detection: In the United States, researchers at the University of Pennsylvania have found that viruses give off specific odours. Hence, they have eight Labrador retriever dogs who are being trained to detect the coronavirus odour. Once trained, the dogs will be tested for their suitability for use in screening for the virus, and, if the tests are successful, they will be used to help identify asymptomatic coronavirus carriers. In England, a similar experiment is underway. The London School of Hygiene & Tropical Medicine has joined with a charity, Medical Detection Dogs, to train six dogs to detect the coronavirus. If successful, the intention is to deploy the coronavirus detection dogs at U.K. Airports.

Province of Quebec: Despite soaring virus infection cases in long-care homes and senior residents in Quebec, Premier Legault announced that the provincial government has a timetable for lifting lockdown restrictions across the province. Quebec intends to move quickly to re-start its economy, while Ontario is following a much more cautious phase by phase approach. In Quebec, most stores will be allowed to re-open May 4th, construction and manufacturing will re-open on May 11th along with elementary schools and daycares, and the removable of most travel restrictions. As early as May 4th, access to cottage country north of Montreal will be allowed, but out-of-province visitors and cottagers from Ontario will continue to be turned back at the provincial border. The intention of the government is that social spacing will continue in force to the fullest extent practicable, and with a monitoring of the health of the workers to enable any retail store, school, manufacturing plant, or construction site, and the surrounding area, to be quickly locked down if struck by COVID-19 outbreak. Lockdown restrictions are continuing in force in the greater Montreal area, which is the coronavirus epicentre in the province.

At present, 1.2 million Quebecers have lost their jobs during the provincial lockdown, and it is hoped that the plan for a partial re-opening of the economy will restore 450,000 jobs. One of the largest employers in the province, Bombardier Inc., declared that it will phase in the recall of its 11,000 workers over a two-week period, and will introduce temperature checks, tool disinfection stations, and Plexiglas shields to separate workers as much as possible.

Given that public health authorities do not know what to expect, and the fact that the feared second wave of infections has not materialized in countries that have begun to lift their lockdown, one can admire the Quebec government for saying 'enough is enough' in starting to lift the lockdown. The intention to monitor the situation, and quickly re-impose self-quarantining and a lockdown in any area where there might be a virus outbreak, is quite sensible. C'est un bon risqué! Yet another worthwhile precaution would be for the provincial government to insist that everyone wear a face mask when in contact with others in public, and at work or school where a physical or social spacing is not possible.

Personal Protective Equipment: A team of eighty medical students at the University of Toronto have taken the initiative to produce thousands of medical plastic face shields using 3D printers. Almost ten thousand plastic face shields have been produced and, to date, a total 8,000 have been delivered to hospitals, clinics, first responders, and long-care homes in the Greater Toronto Area. Medical students at several other universities across Canada have taken up the idea and are producing medical plastic face shields on 3-D Printers.

With millions of N-95 respiratory masks now being manufactured by Canadian companies, and tens of thousands of medical plastic face shields, surgical face masks, surgical gowns and gloves being produced domestically, where are they being distributed? What services have received the Canadian-manufactured personal protection equipment? Where are the reports in the media of the distribution of personal protective equipment to hospitals, to first responders and to long-care homes? Has the shortage of personal protective equipment been fully addressed for hospital staff, first responders, and personal care workers? If so, how can Canadian citizens acquire the N-95 respiratory face mask, face masks, and surgical gloves to enable them to go out in public, and return to work in stores, factories, and businesses, without running a high risk of becoming infected with the coronavirus?

Thursday, April 30, 2020 (continued)

Investigating the WHO: The House of Commons has been informed that Dr. Bruce Aylward, a Canadian Medical doctor-epidemiologist, and one of the Assistant Directors-General of the World Health Organization, has refused to testify – via a virtual conference hook up from Switzerland -- before the parliamentary Health Committee in response to a summons. Earlier, the Committee had voted unanimously to investigate the directives issued by the World Health Organization on which the Canadian government had relied in its response to the coronavirus threat.

Dr. Aylward led a WHO delegation to Wuhan in February 2020 to examine the coronavirus situation on the ground. In his initial report, Aylward praised the effectiveness of China's efforts and methods in slowing the spread of the virus, and asserted that during his time in China, that there 'was a steep decrease in new cases', that fewer people were showing up at clinics for assessment, and that treatment beds were opening up. These assurances were utterly false; yet western countries relied on the assurances of the WHO that the coronavirus outbreak was under control in China, and not an immediate threat to themselves.

On Thursday, April 30th, the parliamentary Health Committee unanimously voted to issue a mandatory summons to force Dr. Aylward to appear to testify. However, the mandatory summons can only be enforced on Canadian soil should he return to Canada.

(A week later, on May 6th, a dossier prepared by the "Five Eyes " intelligence organization – U.S., U.K., Australia, New Zealand, and Canada – would be leaked to the press. It confirmed that China has refused to admit until January 20th that the coronavirus could be transmitted human-to-human, and that China had deliberately downplayed the infection threat posed by the virus. Despite Hong Kong and South Korea expressing alarm in late December, the WHO had slavishly repeated the information provided by China as late as February 2020.)

The final report, issued by Dr. Aylward on behalf of the WHO – which appeared sometime in March -- states that COVID-19 is "a new pathogen that is highly contagious, can spread quickly, and must be considered capable of causing enormous health, economic and social impacts". It is an accurate assessment, produced after-the-fact, and it constitutes a complete contradiction of what Dr. Aylward and the WHO were asserting in their communiques and directives as late as early March 2020. What is the point of the WHO preparing an after-the-fact report on the nature of the coronavirus threat, when the contagious nature and magnitude of danger posed by the virus threat, is now obvious to everyone worldwide? Moreover, there is no statement regret, of apology or of contrition, for producing the totally false and misleading initial report of February 2020.

(Statistics Canada would report later -- on June 15th -- that Canadian manufacturing sales fell by 28.5 percent in April during the coronavirus lockdown. Motor vehicle sales (trucks and cars) plunging 97.5 percent, the auto parts industry sales dropped 88.1 percent, and the fossil fuels industry sales declined by 46.4 percent. Food sales, despite grocery stores remaining open as an essential service, fell 12.8 percent in April.)

Chapter Six

Friday, May 1, 2020

Lockdown Policy: Finally, someone has publicly questioned the need for a complete lockdown of a country to combat the spread of the coronavirus. Such a discussion is pertinent to current discussions over how soon, and how completely, to re-open the economy of Canada. To date, the discussion has been dominated by top level national health officials who are risk adverse in an unknown situation, and by political leaders and pundits who are in salaried positions unaffected economically to any great degree by the lockdown. They are not suffering the economic consequences of unemployed Canadians who have no income, who cannot pay their rent or mortgage, and/or who are trying to contact Social Services to apply for the Employment

Insurance (EI) benefit. (Reports are that it is a totally frustrating experience in getting a constant busy signal from offices that are working only regular hours in a normal five-day week, while being called upon to field potentially tens of thousands of calls per week during a period of massive layoffs.)

Top government officials, including Prime Minister Trudeau, can talk blithely about continuing the lockdown into July, with public health authorities speculating that some form of lockdown might need to be continued into September. Public health officials in Canada are calling for a slow return to normality, with the pace to be determined by the capacity to conduct widespread tests for the virus and to trace contacts for testing so that workers can be safe on the job. Prime Minister Trudeau stated earlier in the week that: "Restarting our economy will be gradual and careful and will be guided by science". Why not be guided by common sense and the experience of other countries that have already advanced into the recovery stage.

There are medical professionals worldwide who are questioning whether total lockdowns are needed but, unfortunately, they are not attracting much attention from the public health care agencies and health departments that are advising western governments. The medical personnel are citing the experience of several countries where practical measures were adopted to successfully prevent the spread of the coronavirus, and its recurrence, without a resort to a complete national lockdown, or even the need for a partial lockdown.

Stuart Thomson, a *National Post* columnist has argued "The Case Against Lockdowns", based on the views of medical personnel familiar with the experiences of Hong Kong, Taiwan, and South Korea where the coronavirus has been contained and strictly limited without a resort to a lockdown. Their common experience provides good evidence that a massive lockdown is not necessary to prevent the spread of the coronavirus. The lessons to be learned from the countries cited, the citizens of a country can be protected from a coronavirus infection without a general lockdown by immediately taking six practical initiatives: viz.

1) the practice of social distancing, avoiding crowds and a frequent washing of hands. These practices were followed by the people in the countries and territory mentioned out of a fear of contacting the virus infection, even before it was recommended by government. There was no lockdown, and social life and business life continued under these precautions. Even restaurants remained open with a requisite physical distancing between tables.

2) the wearing of face masks in going outdoors and in public places. In Asia, the wearing of face masks in crowded cities is customary on the outbreak of a cold virus or flu virus, and that practice was followed during the coronavirus threat. In Hong Kong, 99 percent of the population wore face masks in public during the height of the coronavirus threat with many continuing to do so thereafter.

3) the immediate closure of schools. Children do not respect social distancing, or cannot do so in a school environment, and children are believed to be major spreaders of virus.

4) the early imposition of travel bans on foreign travellers entering the country. As soon as the outbreak of a contagious virus in China became known, travellers from China were banned by the three Asian governments, and when outbreaks occurred in other countries, all foreign travellers were banned from entry.

5) the immediate testing of citizens returning home from abroad, and the mandatory quarantining of those who test positive. The sick and asymptomatic carriers of the virus were provided with medical staff outfitted with respiratory masks, surgical gowns, and gloves.

6) the introduction of a broad testing program within the country to test for the virus presence, with any individuals testing positive to be quarantined, in conjunction with the use of a smartphone technology tracking system to trace, identify, and test contacts who were potentially exposed to the virus, and the quarantining of those who test positive. The identification of contact persons to be coupled with a spaying of disinfectants in the immediate areas of cities where a cluster of infections were found.

In following an aggressive policy in taking immediate action to implement the six practical actions, Hong Kong, Taiwan and South Korean, managed to greatly limit the introduction of the coronavirus into their respective countries, to contain the spread of the virus when it appeared within their local communities, and to keep the number of coronavirus cases and the death rate surprisingly low. They did it successfully without the closing down of all social and economic activity through the imposing of a costly lockdown. In contrast, the governments of Canada and the western European countries (except for Sweden) followed the guidelines of the WHO in imposing a complete lockdown on their countries, which was based on the apparent success of the lockdown of Wuhan in China. However, what was ignored was that China had also resorted to several of the practical actions utilized by Hong Kong, Taiwan, and South Korea, to contain the spread of the coronavirus.

During the lockdowns in western countries, people have been ordered to stay at home, except for essential trips to get food or prescriptions, and all non-essential businesses, stores, businesses, factories, and cultural and recreational facilities have been closed. One needs only to compare the coronavirus statistics of the western countries that focused on a national lockdown strategy to combat the spread of the coronavirus – countries such as Canada, the United Kingdom, Spain and France, with the coronavirus statistics of Hong Kong, Taiwan and South Korea, to see the fallacy of relying on a nation-wide lockdown to prevent the spread of the COVID-19 virus.

The fallacy of the nation-wide lockdown approach is further illustrated by what Canada has experienced with the severe outbreaks in its long-care homes. Once you let the coronavirus into the local community of long-care home residents, it takes only one personal care worker -- who is an essential worker not subject to the lockdown -- to infect a whole population of elderly residents. As of May 1st, with recovery programs being introduced in the European countries, the coronavirus statistics are:

Hong Kong: population 7.4 million, 1,044 coronavirus cases, four deaths, and 859 recovered.

Taiwan: population 23.8 million, 429 coronavirus cases, six deaths, and 324 recovered.

South Korea: population 51.2 million, 10,774 coronavirus cases, 248 deaths, and 9,072 recovered.

Canada: population 37.68 million, 53,670 coronavirus cases, 3,224 deaths, and 22,095 recovered.

Britain: population, 67.8 million, 177,454 coronavirus cases, 27,510 deaths, and 1,918 recovered.

Spain: population 46.7 million, 242,988 coronavirus cases, 24,824 deaths, and 114, 678 recovered.

France: population 65.25 million, 130,185 coronavirus cases, 24,594 deaths, and 50212 recovered.

The coronavirus has had a severe impact on Italy as well, but Italy did not impose a national lockdown until the number of coronavirus cases was soaring in the northern provinces. (Italy: population 60.47 million, 207,428 coronavirus cases, 28,236 deaths, and 78,249 recovered.) One oddity is that Italy, with the oldest population in Europe, has an average age of 81 among those who have died from the coronavirus disease. The United States presents a complex situation as the American government has not imposed a uniform national lockdown. Each state has responded in different ways to outbreaks of the coronavirus, with the individual states imposing different levels of lockdown at different times. New York City and Seattle are the current epicentres of the American epidemic. (United States: population 333.5 million, 1,130,494 cases, 65,605 deaths, and 141,706 recovered.)

CERB Fraud: Reports are surfacing that in the rush to get money to Canadians in need, the $2,000 monthly wage subsidy payment – the Canada Emergency Response Benefit (CERB) -- is being issued to applicants who are not qualified to receive it. A Canada Revenue Agency (CRA) employee has confided that she has knowledge of a case where a senior applied for, and is receiving, CERB payments for herself and two adult disabled children – a total of $6,000 per month -- to a household already receiving government pensions and ineligible for the CERB.

Another incident cited was that of three prisoners in a Quebec jail who applied for and received CERB cheques, which fortunately were intercepted by correctional authorities.

Carla Qualtrough, the Minister of Employment, Workforce Development and Disability Inclusion, has taken the position that Canadians are basically honest, that the government is counting on their honesty, and that the monies will be recovered when Income Tax returns are processed. However, the fallacy of that approach is that the CERB monies will already have been spent, and how can monies be recovered from individuals on an old age or disability pension, or who are receiving welfare or EI payments, or are serving a prison sentence. What is needed is for the government departments responsible for administering the various federal financial aid programs to establish a dedicated unit to run random checks of applicants against government pension and other financial aid program lists, and to immediately investigate any submissions that departmental employees suspect may be fraudulent. Kevin Page, a former parliamentary budget officer, has pointed out that even a one percent fraud rate -- with upwards of $200 billion being expended by the federal government through various financial aid programs -- will cost the federal government upwards of two billion dollars.

Coronavirus Recovery: The problem faced in opening up the economy and ending self-isolation -- from a public health perspective -- is that the coronavirus has proved to be very aggressive, difficult to contain, and it has not been eradicated. There is a fear that it might remain within the population for several years, and keep causing outbreaks, rather than burning itself out. For the public health authorities the only way to keep the population safe, given that uncertainty, would be to maintain a social isolation policy and a lockdown until a 60 to 70 percent herd immunity is attained through a natural immunity developed by survivors of a coronavirus attack in conjunction the widespread vaccination program once a proven vaccine becomes readily available. In theory, that is ideal, but government are dealing with a practical reality -- the need to get people back to work, while containing the spread of the coronavirus.

Saturday, May 2, 2020

Recovery, Ontario: The Ontario provincial government has produced a list of specific businesses that will be allowed to re-open on Monday, May 4th, in Phase I of the a planned three-phase reopening plan to end the provincial lockdown. The openings are conditional on the businesses concerned complying with provincial heath regulations introduced to combat the coronavirus: viz. the maintaining of physical distancing; the providing of contact-free services; and the avoiding of gatherings of more than five people under current regulations. Moreover, the provincial government is striving to obtain hand-sanitizers and personal protective equipment – presumably, face masks and gloves – with a current emphasis on long-term care homes, presumably for residents, as staffs are now becoming well equipped. (Hopefully, businesses will distribute face masks and gloves to their employees.)

During the Phase I recovery stage, the focus is on enabling businesses to prepare their workplace for a subsequent complete re-opening while continuing to protect the workers, customers, and the public. Garden centres and nurseries can re-open for curbside pickup and deliveries, and lawn and landscaping businesses, as well as construction projects that are needed to support future openings of various goods and services establishments, educational facilities, commercial, industrial, and residential developments. Automatic and self-serve car washes can open, and auto sales departments of dealerships (by appointment only), and golf courses and marinas can begin their preparations for opening but are not open yet to the public. Otherwise, the lockdown will be continued for the immediate future, and is being enforced by municipal bye-law officers ticketing offenders who will have to pay heavy fines.

What is startling about this initial stage in the re-opening of the economy of Ontario is that it appears to be overthought, is excessively detailed, and exceedingly risk adverse – a program designed by bureaucrats in a health department. Premier Doug Ford has distinguished himself for his common sense and decisiveness in providing leadership and direction during the coronavirus epidemic. He has taken control of the government response, has quickly introduced initiatives to curb the spread of the virus, and was the first to contact Canadian industries to 'gear up' to supply sorely needed personal protection equipment. He did not hesitate to punish hoarders who were profiteering in health supplies, and he has been forthright in informing Ontarians of coronavirus developments at every stage of the epidemic. Now, with health authorities harping on a feared second wave of infections -- which has yet to materialize anywhere -- Premier Ford appears to have become overly cautious and hesitant about re-opening the economy of Ontario. However, that perspective can change if a decision is made sometime later this week to allow the specified businesses to fully open, then the initial step can, and will be, viewed as perfectly logical and sensible. Hopefully, all manufacturers and businesses will soon be authorized to open.

In Ontario, testing has reached a rate of over 16,000 tests a day, with 2.5 percent testing positive, which represents a drop in the rate of positive tests. The situation in long-care homes remains grim. There were three new outbreaks in the past 24-hours. Overall, the province has 16,608 confirmed coronavirus cases, 1,121 deaths, and 10,825 cases resolved. The curve is flattening, despite an occasional flare up. On one particularly bad day, the province added 421 new cases. At present, Ontario has 1,017 coronavirus patients in hospitals, inclusive of 225 in intensive care and 175 patients on ventilators.

Recovery, Alberta: Alberta is the first province in Canada to establish a smartphone tracking system to trace the contacts of persons who test positive for the COVID-19 virus. The Alberta re-launch strategy reveals that the Alberta government has learned a great deal from the experience of the several countries that have succeeded in limiting and containing their coronavirus outbreaks. The Alberta re-launching strategy is based on having in place critical public health measures and policies: viz.

- a high level of testing to identify COVID-19 carriers within the general population;

- an effective system of contact tracing, employing modern technology, to identify and test individuals exposed to the virus;

- the isolation of those who test positive to curb the spread of the virus, with the provision of a support system for the individuals in isolation;

- strong international border controls and airport screenings, which will be especially strict for international travellers once bans on international travel are lifted;

- rules and guidelines in place for the wearing of face masks in crowded places, such as on mass transit;

- strong protection and support for the most vulnerable, including those in long-term care, continuing care, and seniors' lodges; and

- a rapid response system in place to respond to any future outbreaks of COVID-19 during the recovery phase.

The Alberta provincial government is also placing a strong emphasis and reliance on individuals to adjust their personal conduct to reduce the risk of becoming infected by the virus.

Public Health Agency & China: Last week, the parliamentary Health Committee of the House of Commons voted unanimously to investigate to what extent the Canadian government had relied on directives issued by the World Health Organization (WHO) in its response to the coronavirus threat. The Committee investigation was undertaken in response to criticism – in the Media, and by Conservative Opposition Leader, Andrew Sheer, and by Conservative MP Derek Sloan – that the Public Health Agency of Canada had mislead Canadians as to the seriousness of the coronavirus threat to Canada. Derek Sloan, in particular, has charged that the Liberal government, on the advice of Dr. Theresa Tam, Chief of the Public Health Agency of Canada, had slavishly followed the directives of the World Health Organization in its response to the coronavirus threat; and that China had deliberately misled the WHO as to the seriousness of the coronavirus outbreak in Wuhan, China, and in denying the highly contagious and deadly nature of the novel virus.

On Wednesday last -- in response to a demand from the parliamentary Health Committee for pertinent government documents on the Liberal government response to the coronavirus -- a collection of documents was tabled in the House of Commons from various government departments. Among the documents were some early planning notes and briefing notes that were prepared by the Public Health Agency for the Health Minister, Patty Hajdu, and for the Prime Minister, Justin Trudeau. The several planning notes and briefing notes pertain to January, February, and early March before Canada closed its border to travellers from foreign countries on March 18th and travellers from the United States on March 21st.

What the government documents reveal is how completely the Public Health Agency of Canada underestimated the threat posed by the novel coronavirus to Canada; how uninformed and unconcerned the Public Health Agency was about the threatening nature of the novel virus in ignoring the ravages of the disease in China and the actions being taken by China, Hong Kong, South Korea and Taiwan to combat the spread of the virus. Not only was the health advice terribly misleading that the Public Health Agency provided to the Liberal government, but the Liberal government accepted that advice without question as it conformed to its belief in maintaining open borders and a free movement of peoples.

One of the earliest briefing notes of January 19th, prepared for the Minster of Health, Patty Hajdu, stated that "Based on the latest information that we have, there is no clear evidence that the virus is easily transmitted between people", and in other supporting documents public health authorities questioned media reports out of the City of Wuhan, China – the epicentre of the novel virus outbreak – that claimed the virus was spreading through human-to-human contact. Despite China imposing a quarantine on the City of Wuhan on January 23rd, and on the surrounding Province of Hubei several days later, the documents tabled in Parliament revealed that 58,000 travellers arrived in Canada from China between January 22nd and February 18th, and 2,030 of them were from Hubei Province. Moreover, only 68 were temporarily detained of whom 65 were giving a pamphlet recommending that they self-isolate for 14-days and three passengers were examined by a quarantine officer – presumably for showing obvious signs of sickness.

(This is a case of criminal negligence on the part of the federal Liberal government in failing to ban travellers from China, or to impose a strict quarantine system on anyone entering Canada, to prevent potential carriers introducing a deadly virus within the Canadian community.

One wonders how many pre-symptomatic, mildly symptomatic, and asymptomatic passengers on those incoming flights from China subsequently circulated amongst the Canadian population.)

In Italy, once the coronavirus outbreak was traced to travellers from China, a ban was imposed on flights from that country as of January 31st. Yet, Canada, in the talking points prepared for the Health Minister, by the Public Health Agency, took the position that preventing the novel virus from entering Canada was "next to impossible"; and that "what really counts is limiting its impact and controlling its spread once it gets here".

(Thus, there was no effort by the Liberal government to close the border to prevent the introduction of the coronavirus from abroad, and thereby limit Canada's exposure, but rather just a faith that Canada's health care system would be able to limit the impact and control the spread of the coronavirus once the inevitable happened. The talking points note, for the Minister of Health, accepts that many Canadians would become sick from the novel coronavirus and that there would be deaths from the disease.)

The only action taken by the federal Liberal government was on February 7th, when a policy was introduced of recommending to the travellers who were arriving from Hubei Province, that they should voluntarily self-isolate for 14-days. By that date, the Canadian media was reporting that South Korean, Italy and Iran all were experiencing an increasing number of coronavirus cases that were traced to travellers from China. Yet, travellers from these countries were permitted to continue to fly into Canada, and the federal Liberal government took no further action. The only concern of the health authorities was about public opinion in Canada.

As of mid-February, a Health department memo warned the Health Minister, Patty Hajdu, that Canadians might question the effectiveness of 'voluntary self-isolation measures' for travellers arriving from China. Yet, the memo assured the Minister that it was best to continue to rely on voluntary self-isolation measures to preclude placing "pressure on public health resources", and that a quarantine would be "difficulty to enforce". As of mid-February, the number of travellers entering Canada from China surged to 20,000 people in one record week, as airports in China were swarming with individuals fleeing the coronavirus disease.

(In effect, the Canadian government through failing to ban travellers from China had lost control of the situation by mid- February -- what is not clear is how many of the travellers from China were Canadians or permanent residents returning home to Canada, as distinct from foreign travellers. However, so many travellers were arriving in Canada from China that any effort to impose a mandatory quarantine would have overwhelmed Canadian health resources. Hence, the implementation of a quarantine policy for new arrivals was no longer possible by mid-February.)

Travel Bans: As of late February, the only policy possible was a complete ban of travellers from China, or preferably the placing of a ban on all foreign travellers. By that time, there were 78,000 reported coronavirus cases in China, and a coronavirus wave was surging in Italy, Iran, and Spain, and a growing number of new cases were occurring in the rest of Europe and in the United States (particularly in New York City). Earlier, on January 31st, President Trump had announced a ban on foreign citizens travelling to the United States from China, in recognizing the virus spread and contagion threat. However, in Canada as late as March 10th, the Public Health Agency of Canada in a briefing note prepared for the Health Minister, Patty Hajdu, claimed that "the risk of spread of this virus within Canada remains low at this time"; and maintained that the public health system was "well-equipped to contain cases coming from abroad" in limiting the spread of the coronavirus within Canada.

On March 13th, President Trump, banned travellers from Europe; and yet the Trudeau government continued to resist demands from the Conservative Party Opposition in parliament, by provincial premiers, and a growing demand by the public, for a ban on foreign travellers entering Canada. Finally, on March 18th, foreign travellers were banned from entering Canada, except for travellers from the United States, and on March 21st travellers from the United States were banned. This was the first, and only ban on travellers from such coronavirus hotspots as China, Italy, and Iran, and it was too late. The coronavirus was already well-established within Canadian communities from coast to coast.

What the documents tabled in parliament reveal is the overriding commitment of the Public Health Agency of Canada, and federal government of Prime Minister Justin Trudeau -- with its Modern liberal globalist mindset -- to open borders and the free movement of peoples, a reluctance to ban foreign travellers from entering Canada, and a rejection of any idea of effectively screening and testing airport arrivals, and the enforcing an effective quarantine.

Travellers vs In-community Transmission: Until February 28th, all of the coronavirus cases in Canada were directly-related to someone who had entered Canada from China, but at the end of February, there were coronavirus cases among travellers entering Canada from Iran and Italy. As of February 27th, there were 33 coronavirus cases in Canada, mainly in Ontario and British Columbia, with a few cases in Quebec. In Alberta, there were several cases related to Canadians who had returned home from a cruise ship that had had an outbreak of the coronavirus.

On March 5th, British Columbia reported the first Canadian case of an in-community transmission of the coronavirus case -- that was not related to anyone who had travelled abroad; and on March 8th, the first coronavirus-related death was record in Canada – a 80-year old man in British Columbia who had pre-existing health problems. As of March 11th, there were 93 confirmed coronavirus cases in Canada. Thereafter, the number began to soar. By March 16th, there were 324 COVID-19 cases in Canada, and eight confirmed coronavirus-related deaths, with more and more cases being attributed to in-community transmission. During the first two week of March, new coronavirus cases were recorded, not only among travellers from China, Iran, and Italy, but including several travellers from Egypt, a traveller from France, and a Canadian who had visited the State of Oregon in the United States.

The delay by the Trudeau government in failing to close the Canadian borders to travellers from China and other 'hotspot' countries until March 18th, has enable a deadly virus to become well established among the Canadian population. It has resulted in the inflicting of a heavy cost on Canadians – in sickness, deaths, and economic disruptions occasioned by provincial lockdowns. By the second week of March, in-community transmission of the coronavirus was well-established in Canada. The coronavirus continued to spread at an accelerating rate: on March 19th, there were 773 coronavirus cases, and nine deaths; by March 27th there were 4,500 cases and 52 deaths; by the end of March, there were 7,448 cases and 90 deaths; and by April 26th, there were 45,354 coronavirus cases in Canada, and 2,465 deaths.

Of course, the Prime Minister, Justin Trudeau, is now claiming that Canada made "the best decisions" with "the information that we have". He is claiming that:

> "Canada has done a good job of keeping on a path that is going to minimize as much as possible the reality we're in right now. As we look back at the end of this, I'm sure people will say, 'You could have done this a few days before'".

Public Health Agency of Canada: Equally egregious is the failure of the PHAC to fulfill its mandated function. The PHAC is responsible for public health in Canada, for emergency preparedness and response, and for infection and chronic disease control and prevention. Following the SARS (severe acute respiratory syndrome, now SARS-Cov-1) epidemic, which originated in China and in 2003 resulted in 438 SARS cases and 44 deaths in Canada – mainly in Toronto – the federal government under Conservative Prime Minister Stephen Harper established the PHAC. At the same time, a Canadian doctor was stationed in Beijing, China, to provide a direct connection with Chinese health authorities, and an independent observer, to report on any recurrence of the SARS virus, or any new virus threat that might emerge there.

Under the Trudeau government that posting was left vacant, with the Canadian government preferring to rely on the World Health Organization (WHO) for warnings of any health threat emerging anywhere in the world, rather than focusing on China. That reliance has proved disastrous for Canada. In June 2017, Dr. Theresa Tam was appointed as Chief of the PHAC, with a responsibility for providing health advice to the Minister of Public Health, and for maintaining Canada's National Emergency Stockpile System (NESS) of medical personal protective equipment and ventilators, among her other duties. Dr. Tam had served on several WHO committees, and was closely linked personally to the World Health Organization.

Personal Protective Equipment: The documents placed before the parliamentary Health Committee have revealed that at the same time China, and the WHO, were re-assuring western nations that the coronavirus outbreak was under control, the Chinese government was pursuing contacts with the Chinese diaspora worldwide, in appealing for personal protective equipment to be purchased and shipped to China. Moreover, while personal protective equipment was being purchased in the open markets of the West and shipped to China, sixteen tonnes of PPEs and ventilators were sent to China, between Feb. 4th to Feb. 9th, by the Liberal government of Prime Minister Justin Trudeau from the National Emergency Stockpile System (NESS) depots. This personal protective equipment and ventilators in the depots were intended for distribution to the provinces in the event of a virus epidemic, and the maintenance was the responsibility of the Public Health Agency of Canada. Whether the PHAC opposed the Liberal government decision to ship the national stockpile of personal protective equipment and ventilators to China, is not known.

Education: During the coronavirus epidemic, with countries closing their borders to foreign travellers, and will Canadian public servants working from home, international students are finding it difficult to secure needed travel and visa documents for travel to Canada for their studies, and to secure work permits to enable them to work part-time, as well as are finding it difficult to secure flights to Canada. What was startling is a report that the percentage of foreign students entering Canadian universities and post-secondary institutions has increased by 95 percent since 2014, and that the number increased by 13 percent from 2018 to 2019, when 642,000 foreign students were present in Canada. The 'open-door policy' of Prime Minister Trudeau, and his 'welcome to Canada' pronouncements, have brought a massive increase not only in immigration to Canada, but of international foreign students. Today, in Canada, foreign students make up more than a one-fifth of the post-secondary student body. Apparently, the largest contingents of foreign students are from India, China, South Korea, and France.

Since the universities and colleges are the embodiment of a nation's culture in what they teach, and the values they inculcate, one wonders if it is a healthy situation to have so many foreign students in our post-secondary education system, and one wonders how many foreigners are in teaching positions at our universities. Are Canadians being squeezed out from entry to specialized study programs, from academic research grants, and from teaching positions?

Modern liberals who believe in open borders, diversity, and a pan-cultural society, have no concerns about such numbers – indeed, Prime Minister Trudeau welcomes that development -- but Conservatives who are concerned about the preservation of Canada's cultural values and national character, and the promotion of the national interests of Canadians, cannot but look askance at the exceedingly large number of foreign students. Foreign students are welcome in Canada, and indeed, have much to contribute to the broadening of the outlook of Canadian students in higher education, but all good things can be taken to an unacceptable extreme. Moreover, in the case of students from mainline China, who are studying in STEM programs and computer sciences, they are being recruited, upon returning to China, for employment in industrial espionage against western companies and research institutes by the Red Army of the Communist government of that country.

The University establishments see only the financial benefit of having international students who pay higher fees than Canadian students, and who bring in a reported $6 billion in tuition fees annually. However, it is Canadians who founded the universities and colleges for the education of Canadians, and Canadians who have paid, and are paying, for the university infrastructure – the buildings, the residences, and campus facilities -- and it is Canadian taxpayers who are funding government financial grants for the education of students in post-secondary institutions. It is a false economy that relies on monies from international students as an economic driver of the economy.

Long-Care Homes: Although there is no vaccine as yet for the coronavirus that is raging through long-care homes in Ontario and Quebec, it is worrisome that only three percent of seniors in long-care home have received vaccinations against common diseases. With seniors having various health problems, and some with an immune deficiency, the crowded situation in these homes is a ripe for disease outbreaks at the best of times. Canada needs to establish a vaccination program for seniors in our long-care homes for common diseases for which there is an existing vaccine, and a program for vaccinating seniors as soon as a coronavirus vaccine is developed and approved for use.

Federal Deficit: The Parliamentary Budget Officer -- a position created by the former Conservative government of Stephen Harper (Federal Accountability Act, 2006) to provide an independent oversight of government expenditures – has reported that the federal deficit may reach a record $252 billion for this fiscal year, and even higher if the temporary financial aid programs are continued longer than planned, or new financial aid programs are established. The economy is expected to shrink by 20 percent in the second quarter, and by 12 percent over the entire year. The Canada Emergency Wage Subsidy (CEWS) -- the payroll wages subsidy for companies -- is expected to cost $75.9 billion, up from the initial estimate of $73 billion; and the Canada Emergency Response Benefit (CERB) wage subsidy payment to laid off worker, is expected to cost $35.4 billion, which is less than the initial estimate of $40 billion.

What these projections do not include is that even further demands will be made for financial aid from the federal government. The Canadian Federation of Agriculture is seeking $2.6 billion in aid to compensate farmers for their financial losses due to processing plant closures; and Canadian airlines are seeking federal financial aid as they are experiencing extremely heavy loses, due to a 90 percent drop in traffic during the travel lockdown.

When asked how the federal government will manage such a massively heavy national debt, Prime Minister Trudeau reportedly refused to speculate. He responded: "There will be time after this is all done as we figure out how exactly this unfolds, where we will have to make next decisions on how the recovery looks, but right now our focus is on getting through this together as a country". Clearly, the federal government of Prime Minister Justin Trudeau is still adhering to its ad hoc, spur of the moment, response to the coronavirus epidemic as it unfolds. No thought is being given to the future recovery and economic well-being of the country. The lack of any sense of fiscal responsibility, or concern about the soaring national debt, is what one would expect from an individual who notoriously proclaimed: "The budget will balance itself".

Drug Treatment: There is a great deal of interest among the medical authorities in the drug Remdesivir, developed by Gilead Sciences, an American biopharmaceutical company. During a trial on a large number of tests of patients, using the drug and a placebo, Remdesivir showed that it can speed recover from the coronavirus disease by upwards of 30 percent faster, but it had no impact on the death rate. Hence, it can result in shorter hospital stays for coronavirus patients, but the drug is not a cure for the disease. Production is being ramped up worldwide at the company factories, one of which is in Edmonton.

(Six days later, as of May 8th, it was reported that the antiviral drug Remdesivir has been approved for use in Japan, just three days after receiving an application from Gilead Sciences. The drug is authorized only for emergency situations where there is no alternative treatment for a seriously ill coronavirus patient. Similarly, in the United States the Federal Drug Administration (FDA) has approved Remdesivir for emergency use on coronavirus patients. To date, it has been found that two-thirds of severe coronavirus cases have improved markedly with the use of the drug.

Two months later, on June 30th, the Department of Health and Human Sciences (NHS) in the United States announced that it had contracted to purchase 500,000 treatments – six vials per treatment – of Remdesivir from the Gilead company for the use of American hospitals in treating COVID-19 patients. That order represents 100 percent of the production capacity of the company for July, 90 percent for August, and 90 percent for September, which leaves little for other countries to purchase to treat their severely ill COVID-19 patients, unless Gilead licenses its patented drug for other companies to produce. Gilead has priced a Remdesivir treatment at $2,340. Such is the nature of the 'wild west', global drug market.)

Sunday, May 3, 2020

Recovery Process: The Canadian provinces are gradually lifting their respective lockdowns in response to not only a flattening of the curve, but a dramatic decrease in new cases of coronavirus. In Quebec and Ontario, the two worst hit provinces, the major areas of increase are the long-term care homes. However, both premiers Legault of Quebec and Ford of Ontario have emphasized that their provinces are facing

201

'two different worlds' in fighting the coronavirus: the long-term care homes where the battle is continuing to rage with major increases in new cases, and the public domain where the virus spread is under control and the instances of new infection cases is falling off. Quebec has already set forth a two- phase plan to completely reopen the Quebec economy outside of Montreal, between Monday, May 4th and Monday, May 11th . Retail stores and supply chain businesses are to re-open in Montreal on Monday, May 11th. (Subsequently, it was decided to maintain the lockdown in Montreal, which is the epicentre of the coronavirus epidemic in Quebec, until at least June 2nd.) Manitoba has announced that it is allowing the re-opening of businesses, stores, restaurant patios, museums, and campgrounds; and Alberta has added medical practitioners, physiotherapists, and dentists to its authorized list of approved re-openings.

The Canadian Federation of Independent Business has cautioned that the opening of some businesses will need to be delayed while safety precautions are being put in place. All provinces are committed to maintaining a social distancing during the recovery phase, and in some provinces a face mask is being required on public transit. However, what is puzzling is how can the Alberta government justify authorizing the opening of dentist offices. Surely, that is an extremely high-risk environment for dentists and dental hygienists in interacting with the public.

Spain, which has suffered greatly from the coronavirus pandemic, is gradually lifting its lockdown, and has made the wearing of face masks compulsory on public transport. The government is going to distribute six million masks at transport locations and intends to provide local authorities with seven million more face masks. In all European countries lifting their lockdowns, social distancing remains in force, and several countries are required face masks to be worn both in shops, businesses, factories, and on public transport.

European countries are still experiencing hundreds of new cases each day, but the number of deaths per day has declined greatly, as well as the rate of new infections. Most countries realize that prolonging the shutdown will inflict an even more devastating damage -- perhaps a lasting damage -- on their national economies; and that, given the economic situation, a continuation of the lockdowns cannot be justified now that the coronavirus curve of new infections is falling appreciably. Moreover, governments now know, based on the experiences of several Asian countries, that social distancing, the wearing of face masks, and hand washing, are highly effective in preventing the spread of the coronavirus. Thankfully, in Canada we are now hearing much less talk from our Prime Minister, and various government ministers, about a need to continue the provincial lockdowns for months more, or perhaps indefinitely until a vaccine can be developed and a widespread inoculation program instituted to develop a projected 'herd immunity'.

Monday, May 4, 2020

Financial Aid Programs: In addition to the 7.3 million Canadians who have applied for the Canadian Emergency Response Benefit (CERB) wage subsidy payment for laid off workers, some 96,000 companies have applied for the Canada Emergency Wages Subsidy (CEWS) payroll support program, and have recalled 1.7 million workers. Upwards of 518,000 small businesses have applied for the $40,000 government-back loan under the Canada Emergency Business Account (CEBA) program. Andrew Scheer has raised a concern, voiced by several leading Conservatives, that the CERB payments and student financial support payments – the Canada Emergency Student Benefit (CESB) -- will discourage recipients from taking the jobs that need to be filled to foster an economic recovery. Scheer proposed a graduated formula be adopted whereby a worker who is in receipt of the CERB, or student who is receiving a CESB payment, could earn more than $1,000 per month without losing their benefit, with the existing payment being reduced only gradually.

(Conservative fears that providing an unconditional CERB payment to workers who have lost their jobs, and unconditional CESB payments to students who are graduating into a locked-down market economy, may well serve as a disincentive for some recipients to avoid taking a job, is well founded. In Finland, a study has found that among unemployed workers who were given unconditional grants of money, a substantial number did not seek to enter the job market to better their condition. The one positive result of receiving a basic income was that it did lead to feelings of 'happiness' and made them feel more financially secure. In response, the government of Finland is rejecting any concept of a universal basic income in favour of a negative income tax that will eliminate the income tax for some low-income workers and even provide a payment to the lowest paid. The emphasis in on providing financial assistance to working people in need – a good conservative policy -- rather than giving a free guaranteed income to layabouts.)

Trudeau Support for WHO: A Conservative Party MP, Derek Sloan, claimed, sometime later, that on May 4th Prime Minister Justin Trudeau committed Canada to contributing $650 million to WHO in declaring that Canadians "take care of ourselves by taking care of others". Why the federal government is making such a large financial contribution to WHO – actually, it is a five-year funding commitment -- when Canada's parliament and other countries are questioning the competence of the WHO, is puzzling. The WHO is being questioned for its misleading initial assessment of the nature of the coronavirus and its transmission potential, and is being blamed for the heavy costs in lives, sickness, and economic dislocation suffered by western countries who followed the wrongheaded directives of the WHO during the early stages of the coronavirus outbreak in China.

The United States has directly accused the World Health Organization of letting its pronouncements on the coronavirus to be influenced by the Communist Party government of China, while other countries have criticized the WHO for its unquestioning reliance on the virus information that was being provided by China during the initial stages of the coronavirus outbreak in that country, viz. the assertion that the novel virus could not be transmitted from human to human, and that it was not highly contagious.

President Trump has withdrawn the annual contribution commitment of the United States to the WHO, which in 2019 amounted to $674.2 million (US) and accounted for 22 percent of the United Nations budget, to which Canada contributed $83.8 million (US), or 2.7 percent of the annual U.N. budget. Yet, now Prime Minister Trudeau in a 'tit-for-tat' has apparently one upped the situation by announcing that Canada will contribute $650 million (US) over five years to WHO. This raises additional questions:

Why is Prime Minister Trudeau treating the Canadian Treasury as his personal bank account? He is not Bill Gates providing funding from his own private Bill & Melinda Gates Foundation; the Canadian Treasury is not Justin's personal trust fund.)

Tuesday, May 5, 2020

Antibody Research: This past Sunday, Prime Minister Trudeau announced that the federal Liberal government is providing $175 million to a Vancouver Company, AbCellera Biologics Inc., which has developed an antibody that provides protection against the COVID-19 virus. The money is for in-human trials of the antibody in July, and for the construction of a technology and manufacturing infrastructure for antibody therapies to be developed against future pandemic threats. Rather than seek to develop a vaccine to prevent a COVID-19 infection, the AbCellera company has been focused on discovering an antibody. The company searched through the natural immune system of a recovered patient of COVID-19 to find an antibody that fights the infection, which it intends to manufacture once the clinical trials are completed and the treatment approved. Rather than a vaccine which triggers the body to develop a natural immunity through the manufacture of antibodies, the AbCellera process takes an antibody already produced by the body of a recovered patient, manufactures it, and then can inject the antibody directly into a recipient in conveying an immunity to the disease. The claimed advantage is that it works immediately, and it does not require a wait period. In contrast with a vaccine, there is a delay in securing an immunity until the body builds up antibodies.

The novel antibody approach sounds good, but a large number of antibodies needs to be administered to a patient to achieve an immunity to COVID-19, which rules out the manufacture of hundreds of millions of doses for a mass immunization program; whereas a vaccine, once developed, can be produced in hundreds of millions of doses. Hence, the AbCellera antibody is suitable for use only in immunizing a select group of persons at risk. That is a major disadvantage. It makes one wonder why the federal Liberal government would give $175 million to a company to produce an antibody that cannot be used in a mass immunization of Canadians. Dr. John Bell of the Department of

Medicine and Biochemistry, Microbiology and Immunology, at the University of Ottawa, is working on the development of a vaccine that will be potentially of much more value in immunizing Canadians, while relying on a private Canadian foundation for a $250,000 government funding grant. Why is a firm, AbCellera Biologics Inc., which has just partnered with an international Pharmaceutical giant, Eli Lilly, receiving $175 million for research when the antibody has already been isolated, and is about to be tested? Surely, Eli Lilly could finance the trials and the establishing of a manufacturing facility.

What we see here is yet another example of the penchant of the federal Liberal government, under Prime Minster Justin Trudeau, for throwing large sums of money at big corporations without thinking through what precisely Canada will receive in return, and whether the expenditure is justified on a cost-benefit basis.

Airlines & Airports: Air Canada has reported a loss of $1.05 billion for the first quarter of the year – as compared with a profit of $345 million in the same quarter last year –and has 20,000 of its 38,000 employees on inactive status. It is expending some $20 million daily to meet its fixed costs. The Canadian government has yet to provide any financial aid to Canadian airlines; although Prime Minister Trudeau has indicated that some financial aid is in the works. In early April, both Air Canada and Westjet, the two major Canadian airlines, recalled their laid off employee in accessing the new payroll wages subsidy plan (CEWS) under which the federal government pays 75 percent of the salary or wages of a laid off worker up to a maximum of $847 per week. Air Canada recalled 11,500 employees, and WestJet recalled 6,400 employees. There is no work for most of the recalled employees, but the intention is to provide them with financial aid. In contrast, the CERB for all workers who lose their job because of the coronavirus lockdown, pays just $500 per week. Airlines are speculating that it might take up to three years to recover economically from the COVID-19 shutdown of international travel. Some are asking for government aid in the form of tax cuts and reductions in landing fees, and reductions in other charges imposed on airlines.

Canadian Media: Canadian newspapers are suffering from a triple blow in an ongoing loss of readership, a continuing flow of advertising dollars online to Facebook and Google, and the loss of their current advertising revenue while businesses and stores are closed during the coronavirus epidemic. To date, over fifty publications have closed in Canada -- inclusive of many local community newspapers -- at a loss of 2,000 jobs, and over 100 newspapers have cut staff. In Canada, Facebook and Google have managed to capture the bulk of a $6 billion dollars advertising market that was once shared by Canadian newspapers. The Canadian Press is arguing for a share of the advertising revenues on the grounds that the content created by the newspapers is being posted by Facebook and Google without paying for displaying that content online with their advertising. In France and Australia, legislation has been introduced that will force Facebook and Google to work out a revenue sharing system based on paying media outlets for their material that is reproduced online. Canadian publishers want Canada to introduce similar legislation, to help them weather the current crisis and enable them to continue publishing.

Canadian Farmers: The change in Canadian eating habits during the coronavirus epidemic in favour of pizza take-outs and baking at home, has created an upsurge in demand for spring wheat (25% rise to $7.25 per bushel), red lentils (76 % rise to 30 cents per pound), and durum wheat (20% rise to $9 per bushel), which in conjunction with a parallel upsurge in global demand, is greatly benefitting Canadian farmers.

Wednesday, May 6, 2020

Coronavirus Impact: As of early May, the statistics pertaining to the coronavirus pandemic are rather grim. Globally, 212 countries have suffered from the impact of the virus, with a total of 3,682,968 confirmed cases, 257,906 deaths, and 1,207,548 recovered cases. In Canada, there are 62,046 confirmed cases, a total of 4,043 deaths, and 26,993 COVID-19 virus patients who have recovered. By far, the worst impact of the coronavirus has been in Ontario and Quebec. As of May 5th, Ontario has 18,310 confirmed cases, 1,361 deaths, and 12,779 recovered cases; and Quebec has 33,417 cases, 2,398 deaths, and 7,923 recovered cases. In Ontario, the number of new cases continues to increase dramatically in the long-care homes. As of May 2nd, long-care home accounted for 59 percent of COVID-19 deaths in Ontario, and by May 6th that figure had increased to 74 percent.

The continued increase in deaths among the elderly residents of long-care homes has occurred in circumstances now beyond control by the existing staff of personal care workers. In response, the Ontario government is dispensing teams of hospital medical personnel to the long-care homes with a high case rate, has banned visitors from long-care homes, has stopped personal care workers from working in more than one long-care home, has secured the assistance of medical personnel from the military – the Royal Canadian Medical Service -- and has recently acquired personal protection equipment for distribution to the nursing staffs and personal care workers in the long-care homes. However, the Ontario government is seeking to gain control of a situation that has had a long gestation.

Even before the onset of the coronavirus epidemic, long-care homes in Ontario and Quebec were chronically understaffed, and when the virus surfaced among the elderly residents, the nursing staffs and personal care workers were totally overwhelmed. When the virus struck, there was a severe shortage of personal protective equipment -- or none in some long-care homes -- to protect the personal care workers. Hence, staff succumbed to the disease, and a number died, which further exacerbated the staff shortages. Initially, no efforts were made to ban visitors, or to stop part-time personal care workers from working at different long-care homes, which increased the transfer threat of a virus infection.

Once residents became sick with the COVID-19 virus, the common dining areas were closed, which required food to be delivered to the rooms, and the sick residents required additional attention and health care, which placed a further strain on already overworked staff. Completely isolating the sick was also an almost insurmountable problem in long-care homes. It was a perfect storm that brought about an unmitigated health care disaster in long-care homes, which was even worse in Quebec. In that province, a significant number of personal care workers refused to continue to work in long-care homes out of a fear of contacting the coronavirus in the absence of any personal protective equipment.

More generally, in Canada the number of new daily cases has been on a sharp downward curve from its height on April 22nd, with but a few intermittent daily spikes. Moreover, the number of positive texts is going down as the number of tests is going dramatically up. As of today, 940,000 Canadians have been tested across the country with a six percent positive rate, down from an earlier seven percent positive rate. Clearly, the coronavirus epidemic is beginning to burn itself out with the enforcement of the lockdown and social spacing, which is preventing its penetration into new areas.

In the Maritimes, several provinces have reported no new cases of the coronavirus over the past four days, and many of the coronavirus patients have recovered. In Western Canada, Alberta has been the hardest hit with the coronavirus, followed closely by British Columbia, with a significantly less impact in Saskatchewan and Manitoba. As of May 5th, Alberta has had 5,893 confirmed cases, 106 deaths, and 3,219 recovered cases, and a total of 167,015 Albertans have been tested.

Inflammatory Syndrome: On May 5th, the Saint Justin Hospital in Montreal reported that somewhere between fifteen and twenty children had been admitted to hospital who were suffering from a mysterious inflammatory disease. It was the first report in Canada of an inflammatory disease among children in Canada. However, in the United Kingdom, France and Spain, there were children who were hospitalized with a similar hyper-inflammatory illness, which seemed to overlap symptoms of the toxic shock syndrome and a Kawasaki-type disease that causes and inflammation and swelling in the blood vessels and the coronary arteries. In Montreal, the children were tested for COVID-19, but in every case the results were negative, and it was concluded that it was a Kawasaki-type disorder. On the same day, Dr. Theresa Tam, Chief of Public Health Canada, declared that there was no known link between the 'inflammatory disease' in children and COVID-19 virus, and inferred that the sick children were suffering from Kawasaki disease. However, that belief was called into question overnight when the New York City Health authority reported on its findings.

The NYC Health authority reported that 15 children, between the ages of two and fifteen, who have been hospitalized that are suffering from the "multi-system inflammatory syndrome". The general symptoms include a persistent fever, rash, abdominal pain, vomiting or diarrhea. Five of the New York City children have required the use of a mechanical ventilator, but no deaths have been reported. Four of the children tested positive for the COVID-19 virus in a nasal swab/PCR test, with ten negatives and one indeterminate. However, when their blood was tested, six of the negatives had antibodies to the coronavirus in their system. In effect, ten of the fifteen sick children are infected with the coronavirus, or have been.

In the Montreal hospital, the speculation now is that the post pandemic virus is possibly causing a delayed, post-infection immunization response that is exaggerated in some children and targeting some of the body's own blood vessels. However, another speculation is that the children were infected with the COVID-19 virus, recovered, and developed the inflammatory syndrome from some other pathogen entirely. In Montreal, the sick children were readily treated and have fully recovered, with only one child having required admittance to intensive care. However, the symptoms in New York appear to have been more severe than in Montreal where the children were reported to have developed pink eye, pain in the hands and feet, fatigue and a 'fussiness' in not wanting to be held. Where coronavirus is concerned, children and youth under the age of 19 account for only five percent of the confirmed coronavirus cases, and they tend to get only mild symptoms.

(Ten days later, on May 15th, an article by a journalist, Elizabeth Payne, in the *Ottawa Citizen* revealed what may well have been Canada's first case of the Inflammatory Syndrome disease that has now become recognize as having infected a number of children in other countries. The following is a précis of the Payne article which provides an excellent description of the symptoms and progress of the disease.)

As related by the mother of the Ottawa patient, the entire family became very ill early in March, at which time her sixteen-year-old son, developed large swollen lymph nodes, began to turn yellow, and broke out in a rash. He was taken to the Children's Hospital of Eastern Ontario (CHEO) where he was initially diagnosed as having mononucleosis. Back at home, his symptoms worsened, he began vomiting blood, and on March 15th was taken to CHEO by ambulance and placed in isolation for four days.

The doctors were unable to determine what was the cause of his symptoms, which continued to worsen. His eyes were an increasingly bright red, two different large red rashes developed which eventually covered most of his body, and he had a high, persistent fever, as well as enlarged organs, including his spleen, pancreas, and liver, together with the persistent of his swollen lymph nodes. He also tested positive for a number of viruses, including chicken pox -- which he had been inflected with as a child and vaccinated against -- as well as for celiac disease -- which he had never had -- and pancreatitis. He was also tested for COVID-19 but tested negative.

According to his mother, the body rash initially consisted of red dots that looked like measles, but then the red dots clustered together in a large rash which was super-hot, "like he was on fire". Her son required cold compresses to ease the heat and the pain. His ears were swollen with the rash, and his lips were cracked. While in hospital, the patient underwent numerus ultrasounds to check on his organs and was biopsied. Once his fever went down, he was discharged from the hospital.

The patient is now waiting to have a blood test. His mother suspects that he was suffering from the inflammatory syndrome, which appears to be related to the COVID-19, and which had brought the hospitalization of almost two hundred children in North American and western Europe to date. Prior to the family becoming ill in early March, they had visited a relative who was suffering from a several case of pneumonia, as well as visited with friends who had recently returned from Japan. At present, two months after the hospitalization, the patient is reported to be well on his way to recovery, although his eyes remain slightly yellow.

The teenager did not test positive for COVID-19. However, that does not rule out a connection as a number of children who have been ill with the inflammatory syndrome have not tested positive for COVID-19, but did have the antibodies present in their blood stream which indicates an earlier infection.

The symptoms of the inflammatory syndrome are now being recognized, as well as the dangers that it poses to the patients who need to be hospitalized. Christine Elliott, Ontario Health Minister, has announced that the province will begin monitoring cases in children of what is now being called "multisystem inflammatory vasculitis". The Ontario case definition of COVID-19 is being updated to include the inflammatory illness as an atypical presentation in children. In the Ontario case definition, some of the symptoms associated with the inflammatory illness are "a persistent fever, abdominal pain, gastrointestinal symptoms, including nausea, vomiting and diarrhea, as well as rash".

Farm Support: Yesterday, Prime Minister Trudeau announced that the Canadian government will provide a $252 million financial aid package for the agriculture and food industries which have been hard hit during the coronavirus lockdown. The amount offered was only one-tenth of $2.6 billion that farm organization were requesting. The financial aid package includes $77 million to enhance the safety of workers in food processing plants by supporting the securing of personal protective equipment and the implementation of physical distancing measures in the plants. (One might ask where are the millions of units of personal protective equipment that the federal government has been ordering helter-skelter from both international and domestic suppliers? Cannot that equipment be distributed to equip packing plant workers? One wonders, if the money is intended to simply improve the bottom line of the financial statements of the packing plants.)

A total of $125 million will be added to the existing Agri-Recovery program, a federal-provincial-territorial program to help farmers during natural disasters. This part of the aid package is intended to help the beef and pork producers -- ranchers and farmers -- who have incurred extra costs in keeping livestock while receiving no revenue during the closures of packing plants. However, the Prime Minister added "if we need to add more, we will".

The final $50 million is to support a novel program to purchase surplus foods to promote Canada's food security. The intention is to help farmers through the government purchasing large quantities of perishable food produce that is going to waste, and to help food producers by purchasing the products of food industry companies, such as the frozen French fries companies which have experienced plummeting sales since the closure of restaurants and fast food outlets. The purchased surplus food is to be distributed where needed, such as to food banks. (How the perishable foods will be purchased, transported, temporarily stored, and quickly distributed to avoid spoilage remains unexplained.)

In addition to the $252 million agriculture and food industry financial aid package, it was announce that the Canadian Diary Commission Act will be expanded to enable the Commission to buy and store surplus dairy products – such as cheese, butter and milk – to put an end to dairy farmers dumping milk; and that the Commission will be supported with a $200 million financial grant from the federal government.

Thursday, May 7, 2020

Face Masks: Yesterday, Prime Minister Trudeau, members of the Canadian Armed Forces -- including the pallbearers at the repatriation ceremony for the six Royal Canadian Navy members who were killed in a helicopter crash during a NATO exercise in the Mediterranean -- were photographed wearing black face masks. Hopefully, this means that the vast amounts personal protective equipment -- face masks, plastic face shields, surgical garments and gloves, ordered by the federal government, are now being received, and are available for distribution to medical personnel, first responders, and personal care workers across Canada.

Testing: Over 970,000 coronavirus tests have been administered across Canada. Overall, the rate of new virus infections is going down dramatically, except for long-care homes – principally in Ontario and Quebec – and a new outbreak among the Dene community at La Loche in northern Saskatchewan where twenty-two individuals have tested positive. Dr. Tam, the Chief of the Public Health Agency of Canada, wants testing to reach a daily rate of 60,000 tests, and be expanded in scope from critical outbreak areas to include people with mild symptoms as well as, eventually, the general public in testing for asymptomatic carriers. Across Canada, the average current rate is 30,000 tests daily. In Ontario, the government has set a target of 16,000 tests per day, which is being exceeded on most days, but when testing failed to reach the target for two days in a row, the Conservative Premier, Doug Ford, called out local health authorities. No slacking off is to be tolerated. According to Premier Ford: "Everyone must be held accountable".

Across Canada, one focus of the testing has been on food processing plants after coronavirus outbreaks occurred at two meat packing plants in Alberta: the Cargill Plant in High River; and the JBS plant in Brooks. At the Cargill plant 946 workers tested positive out of 2,000 meat processors, and at the JBS plant, 566 workers tested positive out of 2,400 meat processers. Testing at other meat processing plants have also found coronavirus infections among the workforce: at Conestoga Meats (Waterloo, ON), and Harmony Beef (Balzac, Alberta), as well as among the workers at poultry processing plants: United Poultry (Vancouver), Lilydale (Calgary, Alberta), and Maple Leaf Foods (Brampton, ON), and at the Olymel hog processing plant (Yamachiche, Quebec). In all cases, the plants were closed for several weeks, were completely disinfected, and efforts made to increase social distancing and personal protection for the workers. Employees who have tested negative for the coronavirus have been recalled. However, a good number of employees are reportedly refusing to report back to work out of a fear of contacting the coronavirus and of passing on the infection to their families. Hence, some plants have gone to a single shift day, from a two-shift production line. Health Canada has reported that there is a less than negligible danger of acquiring the coronavirus through eating processed meats and poultry.

Recovery: With the dramatic decrease in new cases across Canada, the outbreaks in long-care homes are now accounting for 80 percent of the confirmed cases. However, the situation is improving in long-care homes. In Quebec, there are 700 military personnel on site in thirteen of the worst afflicted long-care homes; and in Ontario, outbreaks at forty-one long-care homes have been resolved. With just the exception of Ontario, Quebec, and the La Loche community in northern Saskatchewan, the spread of the coronavirus has been almost halted. The Maritime provinces reported just eight new cases yesterday – seven in Nova Scotia, and one in New Brunswick. There were no new cases in PEI, and of the 27 cases confirmed to date, only one has not yet recovered. Newfoundland-Labrador had reported no new cases for five days in a row. Out west, Manitoba reported only two new cases yesterday, and Saskatchewan had only three new cases in addition to the twenty-two new infections in the La Loche outbreak.

Two weeks ago, Germany was one of the first countries to begin to re-open its economy, and there has been no sign of any second wave of infections. To date, Germany has had 168,655 coronavirus cases, 7,322 deaths, and 139,00 recovered out of a population of 83.74 million. The daily new infection rate has reached a low of 679, or an 0.4 percent increase in new cases nation-wide. The real test will come this month. During the month of May, Germany is allowing restaurants, hotels, stores and pubs to re-open, all open-air sports are to be permitted, but no gyms will re-open, and the Bundesliga soccer league will re-open by the end of the month to play in empty stadiums. One family member will be permitted to visit a resident of a nursing or long-care home. Social distancing will remain until June 4th, and a ban on large public gatherings will stay in place until August. Germany's airports will remain closed to international travel for the foreseeable future. Earlier, it was reported that face masks will have to be worn on public transport. Whether the public in Germany is wearing, or will be required to wear, face masks has not been ascertained.

Aid for Seniors: Treasury Board President, Jean-Yves Duclos, reportedly one of Justin Trudeau's closest top ministers, mentioned that the federal Liberal government intends to provide financial assistance for seniors on fixed incomes who are facing an increase in the cost of living due to the impact of the coronavirus. The government concern is that the increased cost of food and transportation, as well as delivery costs for those who are less mobile is causing a financial struggle for seniors.

Granted, there are seniors on fixed pensions that are struggling to get by under the impact of rising prices. However, one wonders when will the stream of open-ended Liberal government financial aid grants end? Are not the Old Age Security Pension and the Canada Pension indexed to cover the cost of inflation? Do not retired public services employees, teachers, and many retired unionized workers have an additional income source from workplace pensions to bolster the two pensions provided by the federal government? One would hope that the financial assistance for seniors will be targeted to meet the real needs of those who do not have a workplace pension to supplement their federal government pensions, and that the financial assistance program will be based on the income level of seniors to provide assistance to those who are actually struggling financially. Outside of government workers – federal, provincial, and municipal – over 77 percent of retired Canadian workers do not receive a workplace pension to supplement the Old Age Security pension and the Canada Pension payments.

Politics: Well, well! Apparently, a Leger poll this past week has revealed that 77 percent of Canadians are satisfied with the response of the Trudeau government to the coronavirus pandemic. Moreover, the poll indicates that Liberal Party is receiving about 44 percent support, compared to just 25 percent for the Conservatives. One can believe such a result with Prime Minister Trudeau appearing on his TV 'Morning show' each day to dispense billions of dollars to those in need, with parliament effectively emasculated and unable to question and hold the government to account, and with the Liberal Press falling silent on the failings of the Liberal administration. The Liberal government has not been denounced for its irresponsible conduct in sending the National Stockpile of personal protective equipment to China, which resulted in severe shortages that caused unnecessary deaths and hindered efforts to contain the spread of the coronavirus. The Liberal government has received a free pass for its inaction in leaving it up to the provinces to combat the coronavirus without any firm leadership and direction from Ottawa; and the attempted grab by the Liberal government for absolute power and its subsequent emasculating of parliament have been barely mentioned in the Press. Moreover, the Press has ignored how the Liberal government has slavishly followed the pronouncements and directives of the World Health Organization when common sense and the protection of the health of Canadians dictated otherwise.

Now, a columnist has reported that we have machiavellian politicians advocating that the Liberal Party, in its own partisan interest, ought to resign, call a snap election, and appeal to Canadians for a new mandate for a strong majority government to deal with the economic recovery from the impact of the coronavirus epidemic. The intent would be to take advantage of the current good will of Canadians towards the Liberal minority government, before scandals emerge about any massive misspending of government aid monies, and before it becomes necessary to impose heavy taxes on Canadians to pay for the multi-billion dollar financial aid programs. It is a totally cynical proposal, but not beyond belief that it would attract the power brokers of the Liberal Party who are continually focused on attaining and retaining political power with the party leader saying and doing whatever is required to win an election. Indeed, a snap election ploy would probably work for the Liberal Party. The Canadian electorate has not been well informed of the failings of the Liberal government by the Press, and is not particularly astute in seeing through crass, highly partisan, political manipulations.

Friday, May 8, 2020

Oil and Gas Sector: Earlier this week, Prime Minister Trudeau confirmed that the federal Liberal government is prepared to provide financial aid to the oil and gas industry beyond the $1.7 billion allocated earlier for the cleaning up of orphan oil wells, and the $750 million provided for reducing methane gas emissions. In Alberta, the oil industry has suffered a severe double blow. Saudi Arabia flooded global market with oil – driving down the world price by 50 percent – in a price dispute with Russia, which was followed immediately by the shutdown of airlines, industries, and vehicular traffic in response to the coronavirus pandemic. The sale of gasoline had dropped 50 percent, and the demand for aviation fuel is down almost 70 percent. The price of Canadian crude oil had fallen as much as thirty percent which places the price below the cost of production. It has forced Alberta oil producers to seek to cut back their production where possible, to cut costs, and to put oil in storage. Currently, the price of Western Canadian Select crude has rebounded slightly to $22 per barrel, which is still below the breakeven point for small producers. During the first quarter, the major Canadian oil companies – Suncor, Canadian National Resources, Crescent Point, Cenovus, and Husky – have incurred massive losses. There have been massive layoffs in the industry, with the oil companies starved for liquidity with revenue streams drying up. They are in dire need of an immediate financial relief.

In response, Elizabeth May, the leader of the Green Party has declared that the "oil industry is dead", that the government should not provide financial aid to the oilsands companies, but should concentrate on a transition to renewable low carbon emission fuel sources, and should undertake "an ordered shutdown of the oil industry" while providing jobs for oil industry workers in transitioning into a new economy with low-carbon emission industries. The unreality of such a proposal is appalling. That is similarly the case with respect to the comments of Yves-François Blanchet, the Leader of the provincial Parti Quebecois. Blanchet declared that "putting any more money in that business is a very bad idea"; that the oil industry is "never coming back"; and that the federal government should not provide funding to businesses "that will not be self-sufficient in any time in the future". A rather ironic position for the leader of a Quebec political party to take.

Now, that Bombardier has posted a $169 million first quarter loss in its business jet division, will Blanchet oppose the federal government rendering financial aid? Bombardier, which has already sold off its failing passenger jet division and is in the process of selling its train division, has approached the federal government for financial aid. The company has also approached European governments – in Germany and Britain, as well as the European Union – for financial aid for its manufacturing plants in Europe. Bombardier closed its plants during the coronavirus pandemic, and the company is planning to resume operations in Quebec on May 28th.

What Elizabeth May and Yves-François Blanchet ignore, in their heartless attacks on the Canadian oil and gas industry, is that the fossil fuel industry accounts for upwards of ten percent of Canada's gross domestic product (GDP); that the industry, in most years, has contributed $132 billion in value to Canada's total annual exports – the country's single most valuable export – and that the industry supports, directly and indirectly, 530,000 high paying jobs across Canada. Moreover, in recent years the oil and gas industry have contributed $8 billion annually in tax revenue to government.

There will be a huge future demand for oil industry products when the Canadian and world economies revive, and worldwide the demand for crude oil and natural gas – liquified gas – will continually increase as underdeveloped countries become more and more urbanized and industrialized. Whether the needed energy will be provided by a clean burning natural gas – through liquified natural gas exports from Canada -- or the burning of coal with its heavy carbon emissions footprint, will depend on the survival of the Canadian oil and gas industry and the building of pipelines.

The oil industry is far from dead, and thankfully so. What those who want to shut down the oil and gas industry are ignoring is how much that sector contributes to the living standard of Canadians, to the manufacture of many products used by Canadians, and to the financing of social welfare and health services, and how essential the possession of a domestic oil and gas industry is to the achievement of a national self-sufficiency in energy to isolate Canada from devastating financial crises fomented by the OPEC countries manipulating the supply of oil. By all means, let us have the federal government invest in renewable, low-carbon emission, energy sources, but do not starve the oil and gas industry of financial aid in its time of need.

The presence of the oil and gas industry in Alberta, has brought not only prosperity to Albertans, but all Canadians have profited. Since 1961, Alberta has contributed $600 billion more to the federal government than it has received in federal government services; Albertans have paid $28 billion more into the Canada Pension Plan over the past decade than they have received in benefits; and Albertans have contributed $12 billion more to Employment Insurance than they received back between 2007 and 2013. It has been calculated that without Alberta's net contribution to federal finances, the federal deficit in 2017 would have been double what it was. Now, with Alberta's primary industry in need of an estimated $20 to $20.6 billion injection of capital during the coronavirus lockdown and world oil price collapse, it is time for the federal government to put things right and to provide the needed financial aid. What the oil and gas industry is seeking is not the gift of a financial grant, but rather large government loans to allow them to maintain their liquidity until the market rebounds.

Clearly, there are members of the federal government cabinet -- environmental zealots, inclusive apparently of the Prime Minister – who are opposed to the government extending financial aid to the oil companies, and who share the view of Elizabeth May on a supposed need to phase out the fossil fuel industry. However, before opposing financial aid to Canadian oil companies, they ought to consider the economic reality of what the oil and natural gas sector contributes to federal government coffers. Yet, another factor to consider is that Canadian banks have $60 billion in loans invested in Canadian oil companies that will go into default if the oil companies are forced to close through the lack of operating capital. The Canadian banks do not want to end up holding abandoned oilsands properties of no value if the oil and gas sector is obliterated.

A claim by Elizabeth May that Canadian oil is "a product lacking investors" is true only in the sense that international investors and Canadian banks and investment houses are warry of investing billions in large infrastructure projects in the oil fields, and large pipelines projects, when they see environmental protesters occupying private property and blocking transportation routes with no commitment on the part of the federal Liberal government to enforce the law in arresting and prosecuting those who engage in illegal acts. It is not the financial investment factors that have driven international investors away from the Canadian oil and gas sector, but the realization that Canada -- under the present Liberal government of Prime Minister Justin Trudeau -- is no longer a country of 'peace, order and good government'. Currently in Canada, oil industry properties are not safe from occupation or destruction by radical environmental protesters and the vandals who join their cause, or any cause, just to create mayhem.

Recently, there has been several major new developments which are encouraging in terms of the future development of the oilsands, and the economic benefits that will flow to all Canadians. The Irving Oil Company announced last week – Wednesday, April 29th – that it has submitted an application to the Canadian Transportation Agency (CTA) to use tankers to transport western Canadian crude oil from the port of Burnaby, British Columbia, via the Panama Canal, to the Irving refinery in Saint John, New Brunswick. The intent is to enter into long term agreements with Canadian oil companies to achieve a secure source of crude oil that will not be subject to interruption by pandemics and political upheaval in other countries, or price wars launched by OPEC. With the Canadian rail transport system subject to interruption by blockades – to which the federal Liberal government has failed to react in enforcing the law -- and the long-planned Canada East Pipeline in abeyance owing to the lack of federal government political support, the all-sea route to bring western crude oil to Canada's largest refinery is the only viable alternative, at present, to achieve a national energy security.

The project is feasible now that the capacity of the Kinder-Morgan Trans Mountain pipeline is being expanded from Alberta through British Columbia to its terminus in Burnaby, and the last legal challenge to the construction of the Keystone XL pipeline has enable construction to commence on connecting the Alberta oilfields with the American network of pipelines through to the American Gulf Coast. The Keystone XL pipeline will have a capacity of 830,000 barrels per day, and the Irving company has in contemplation the securing of Canadian crude oil from the U.S. Gulf Coast for transport to the Saint John refinery, as well as from Burnaby, British Columbia and from the off-shore oil fields of Newfoundland-Labrador. In future if tariffs are placed on imported oil to reduce Canada's reliance on foreign producers, the Irving Company will have a tariff free Canadian supply.

In London, shareholders of one of Europe's largest banks, Barclays, voted down a proposal from an environmental activist group that the Bank stop investing in Canadian oilsands companies. Barclays shareholders agreed to cease lending to the coal industry and arctic drilling companies, but supported continued investments in the Canadian oilsands on the condition that carbon emissions, per barrel, are lower than the global median by the end of the decade.

Rejection of Globalism: The coronavirus pandemic has had a major impact on the psyche of Canadians. It in making Canadians much more aware of the dangers posed by, and the extent of their vulnerability in relying on foreign sources for critically needed goods, services, and supplies. Globalism may be fine in economic theory, but in times of crisis – war, pandemics, economic depressions, and shortages of materials – governments worldwide will invariably make sure that the needs of their own peoples are addressed, and will not hesitate to restrict exports from their countries of any and all goods and products – such as drugs, medical supplies, and personal protective equipment -- that are badly needed by their own populations. Hence, there is a need for the Canadian government to introduce a national economic policy of self-sufficiency in basic goods, products and services on which Canadians rely for their health, well-being and their common good – a characteristic Tory conservative policy.

Chapter Seven

Friday, May 8, 2020 (continued)

Pandemic Prognosis: Now that the number of new coronavirus cases is flattening in all provinces of Canada, except for Ontario and Quebec, epidemiologists are predicting that the virus will remain within the general population for another 18 to 24 months. There are three different theories concerning what to expect concerning the future impact of the virus: 1) that there will be a series of small waves of infections during the summer and fall and into 2021; 2) that there will be a second major wave of infections in the fall of 2020 which will be worse than the first wave, with the virus burning itself out in smaller outbreaks during 2021; or 3) that there will be simply a series of smaller outbreaks occurring well into 2022.

What the two wave theories fail to take into consideration is that western nations are now aware of the contagious nature of the coronavirus. Canada now has a testing capacity in place with domestically manufactured testing kits, smartphone tracking systems are being developed in Canada, and the country will soon have ample supplies of personal protection equipment manufactured by domestic manufacturers. Hopefully, never again will Canada rely on the global market for the resources needed to fight a virus epidemic. Another critical factor is that Canadians are now aware of the terrible toll of the disease, and will quickly adopt to social spacing, the wearing of cotton face masks, and an increased washing of hands. Stores and industries will quickly enforce the wearing of face masks and gloves by their employees, and perhaps in some businesses or practices involving close contact – by dentists, doctors, or dental hygienists -- even the wearing surgical gowns and goggles, in addition to a combination of a face shield and face mask when in close contact with a patient.

When new outbreaks occur, governments at all levels are well positioned to concentrate on testing to identify and quarantine infected individuals, will use smartphone technology to track, test, and isolate any contacts found to be infected, and hopefully will spray and disinfect public areas where there are clusters of infections. Ultimately, a vaccine will be developed, which may be sooner rather than later. At present, there are two potential vaccines being clinically tested, and research institutes in Canada, and other developed nations, are now well-funded by government and private foundations in pursuing different avenues of research to develop an effective vaccine.

No doubt, there will be future outbreaks of the coronavirus, but they can and will be quickly isolated as all levels of government now know the nature of the virus threat and what needs to be done. South Korea, Taiwan, and Hong Kong have shown the way, and the Canadian government and Canadians will no longer be ignorant of the dangerous contagion threat posed by the coronavirus. In January and February, through early March, western governments were misinformed by the Chinese government and the World Health Organization in downplaying the danger posed by the coronavirus and its highly contagious nature. Governments lacked the personal protective equipment needed by medical personnel, first responders, personal care workers, and the population at large, to prevent the spread of community infections. Countries were relying on a global supply system focused on a China – and India for drugs – that failed to function as China and India banned exports to ensure that the needs of their own citizens would be met. Canada cannot let this situation happen again!

Hopefully, even the Modern liberals of our current federal Liberal government have opened their eyes, in being chastised and exposed for their blind faith in globalism -- in global supply chains for supplying the nation's basic needs, and in their reliance on the United Nations for directives. Canadians have paid a terrible price in sickness, deaths, social and economic dislocations, and a heavy national indebtedness, for the failures of the federal Liberal government. It is a government that failed to take command of the situation to protect Canadians early on, that failed to exercise an independent judgement of what needed to be done based on what observers on the ground were reporting from China, and that failed to act immediately in a forthright manner to protect the health and well-being of Canadians against a foreign virus threat.

Social Distancing: Local businesses in Ottawa are showing ingenuity in finding ways to help themselves and others to keep their businesses open which maintaining social distancing in dealing with customers during the ban on in-store shopping. A butcher's store has temporarily replaced its entrance door with a sheet of plexiglass, incorporating a double door box, like a small air lock chamber. The customer can phone in an order and drop by for the pickup. The store employee opens one door of the box, places the meat order inside, and closes the door, and then the customer opens the outside door of the box to retrieve the meat. As an added service, the butcher shop employs a virtual connection so that customers can view the meat products and select what they want from their smartphone.

Testing Booth: An Ottawa manufacturing company, the Honey Group. has developed a portable booth for COVID-19 testing. Rather than coming close to the person being tested, the healthcare worker stands in the booth and places his or her arms through two-holes in the plexiglass into two long rubberized gloves to perform the nasal swab. The two gloves are disinfected after each test. The booth not only protects the health care worker from exposure to a coronavirus infection, it eliminates the need for a large supply of personal protective equipment – face masks, gowns, and gloves. The practice at testing centres -- that may test upwards of 500 individuals per day -- is for the healthcare workers to discard their personal protective equipment after each test, to prevent any cross infection of the persons being tested. Hence, the testing booth represents a major saving in the purchase of personal protective equipment. The concept originated in South Korea, where booth-style units are part of a mass testing program.

Respiratory Masks: The federal government effort to procure the N-95 respiratory mask for use during the coronavirus epidemic has suffered a major setback. Eleven million N-95 respiratory masks -- ordered from a Montreal distributor and manufactured in China -- have arrived in Canada for testing before being distributed. However, eight million of the face masks have 'failed to meet specifications'. (The standard N-95 respiratory mask generally is capable of screening out 95 percent of virus particles and of completely screening out the larger coronavirus.) Only one million masks in the shipment have been deemed acceptable, with tests ongoing on the remainder of the shipment.

The federal government department of Public Services and Procurement Canada has declined to name the Montreal distributor. However, back in March 21st it was announced that the federal government had ordered 11.3 million N-95 respiratory masks from a Montreal distributor, Medicom. The problem in procuring personal protective equipment in China is that many companies have sprung up to fill massive orders from western companies and governments, and there is no uniform system of quality control over the Chinese companies. Moreover, some of the face masks were reportedly found to be 'contaminated' – perhaps a Chinese 'entrepreneur' recycling used face masks? Yet another problem has been the long delays in obtaining personal protective equipment -- six weeks or more during the height of the coronavirus epidemic in Canada -- owing to China having banned the export of personal protective equipment while its battle with the coronavirus was raging. This episode illustrates, once again, the need for a national self-sufficiency in medical supplies, with domestic manufacturers in place capable of gearing up quickly to meet Canadian needs in response to national health crises. The federal government has refused to pay for the faulty face masks and has disassociated itself from the Montreal company. Why the federal government is refusing to name the company, remains a mystery.

Personal Care Workers: The federal government and the provincial governments have established a $4 billion fund to top up the wages of minimum-wage personal care workers who have been risking their lives in long-care homes ravaged by major coronavirus outbreaks. The federal government is contributing $3 billion and the provinces $1 billion, with the provinces to allocate the funds in deciding who will get paid and how much. Previously, Ontario, Quebec, and Saskatchewan topped up the wages of personal support workers in long-care homes with some limited financial aid from the federal government.

One wonders if the establishing of multi-billion-dollar financial aid packages is getting out of hand. How many personal care workers are there in Canada to divide up that amount of money? With the glaring exception of long-care homes in Ontario, Quebec, and several long-care homes in British Columbia, personal care workers across Canada have not been facing the coronavirus each day at work. The staffs of long-care homes of other provinces may well be understaffed and overworked, but they are not working amongst a coronavirus outbreak raging through their workplace.

What of the personal care workers, principally in Quebec, who refused to report to work out of a fear of becoming infected, and who left their fellow workers critically short of help during a life and death crisis. Are they to receive additional monies on top of their CERB payments? At present, there are even calls for grocery store workers and delivery vehicle drivers, and other low pay workers, to be financially compensated by the federal government for continuing to work during the coronavirus. If the Liberal government keeps up its largesse, soon there will be a financial grant for anyone who ventured outside their home to perform a public service during the coronavirus epidemic.

Tracking Systems: When it comes to tracking apps that can be download to a smart phone to track the movements of an individual, there are two basic types: an open access app that everyone is required to have on their smartphone, and a private voluntary app for recording contacts. With the open access app on all smartphones, as soon as an individual tests positive for a coronavirus infection, the public health authorities can access the smart phone app of the infected individual to identify all contacts who were exposed to a possible infection, can located them by their own smartphone app, can test them and quarantine the individuals who test positive. With the private voluntary app, it is up to the infected individual to inform the contacts of their exposure to a potential infection and to encourage them to be tested

The federal, provincial, and territorial privacy commissioners have issued a joint statement that participation in a smartphone app for tracking contacts should be voluntary; that the personal data collected should be kept secure; and that the personal data should be destroyed once the crisis is over. One can readily agree about the need for security for personal data and its destruction when no longer needed for tracking potentially infected persons, but the insistence on a voluntary participation in the tracking program is ludicrous. However, the system will not work effectively in controlling the spread of the coronavirus, if individuals are not required to download the smartphone tracking app, and if public health authorities do not have a direct access to the app.

The tracking of potential infections is critical to preventing local outbreaks, and cannot be left to a haphazard system when some individuals may chose not to download the tracking app, and others who become sick may neglect to contact the individuals who were exposed to the coronavirus to encourage them to get tested. Why some people are so obsessed with keeping their public activities private is beyond understanding, unless they are up to no good in which case the authorities ought to be aware of where the individual has travelled.

United Nations Appeal: In March, the United Nations asked for the developed nations to donated $2.8 billion to a global humanitarian response plan to support poor countries in combatting the coronavirus threat, and as of May 5th, a total of $1.3 billion had been donated. Now, the United Nations has appealed for a total of $9.4 billion to combat the spread of the coronavirus and mitigate its impact on 63 states, mainly in Africa and Latin America. To date, Brazil, with a population of 212.3 million, is the most effected with 148,670 cases, 10,100 deaths, and 52,297 recovered. African and Latin American nations and poor nations elsewhere have already suffered economically during the coronavirus pandemic, which has devastated their export earnings, remittances, and tourism revenues.

What the U.N. appeal has raised is a serious question as to how much can the developed countries be expected to give. Their economies have been devastated by lockdowns, their governments are paying out billions of dollars in financial aid to their own peoples, and governments are racking up multi-hundred billion-dollar deficits for the current fiscal year. Moreover, developed countries now face the need for government to pump billions of dollars into recovery programs and infrastructure projects to re-start the economy and stimulate employment, and their peoples are faced with years of heavy taxation to service, if not to begin to pay down, their national debt. The economies of the developed countries are bleeding enough without imposing an additional financial burden on their peoples through the donation of billions of dollars to African and Latin American countries, and poor countries elsewhere.

These countries can learn from the experiences of the developed nations in dealing with the coronavirus threat. It is now known that there is a low tech approach that is effective in limiting the spread of the coronavirus: viz. the wearing of cotton face masks and gloves in public, avoiding touching the face, the practice of social spacing whenever practicable, the avoiding of large gatherings, the encouraging of families to stay home who can do so, the frequent washing of hands when able to do so, the quarantining of the sick, and the disinfecting of public areas where outbreaks occur. What the developed countries can provide in aid of African, Latin American, and poor countries elsewhere, is a commitment to donate and distribute a vaccine to these countries as soon as a vaccine is developed and in production – a willingness to share a vaccine immediately, rather than confining the initial use of vaccine strictly within the developed countries that can pay for it.

Saturday, May 9, 2020

Statistics Canada: The April survey of Statistics Canada has revealed that Canada lost 2 million jobs in that month, on top of the one million jobs lost in March. Moreover, an additional 2.5 million Canadians have reported that they are working substantially reduced hours. Nationally, the jobless rate reached 13 percent, which jumps to 17.8 percent with the inclusion of the unemployed who have given up searching for work. The unemployment rate in the three largest metropolitan centres ranges from 10.6 percent in Vancouver, to 11.1 percent in Toronto, to 18 percent in Montreal. Among the hardest hit sectors since February are the wholesale/retail with 615,000 jobs lost (employment down 22 percent) and restaurants and hotels with 583,000 jobs lost (employment down 44 percent). (What this diarist finds confusing is that with a total of three million workers having lost their jobs to the coronavirus impact by the end of April, why are there 7.5 million Canadians who have applied for, and are receiving, the Canadian Emergency Response Benefit (CERB)? What is missing in that equation?)

Long-Care Homes: In response to the high infection and the soaring death rates in long-care homes from the coronavirus, there is a growing demand in Ontario for the provincial government to investigate the situation. Moreover, it has become obvious that it is the privately-owned, long-term care homes that have had by far the worst rates of infection; that they are responsible for the soaring death rates from the coronavirus; that they are unacceptably understaffed; that they were bereft of personal protective equipment for their staffs; and that they failed to institute proper health precautions to protect their residents from the threat of infection. This has led to a questioning of whether it is the profit motive inherent in privately run long-care homes that is the underlying cause of the severe shortcomings in the privately-owned and operated long-care homes. That line of thought has resulted in some demands, from the public, that the Province of Ontario take over the responsibility for operating long-care homes.

Recovery Policies: In a further easing of the provincial lockdown, the Ontario government announced that professional sports training facilities will be allowed to re-open on Monday, with leagues required to have 'coronavirus-specific health-and-safety rules' in place. Ontario has also extended its temporary State of Emergency to May 19th. It was initially introduced on March 17th.

Today, the Province of Quebec accounts for 35,150 coronavirus cases (over half of the Canadian total), and for 2,725 deaths related to the virus (over half of the total of 4,471 coronavirus deaths in Canada). However, there is a stark difference between the high concentration of coronavirus cases and deaths in the greater Montreal area – the epicentre of the coronavirus epidemic in Canada – and the rest of the province. In the province outside of Montreal, there is a low to moderate rate of infections and deaths, except for a small number of long-care homes. Hence, the paradox that Quebec with the highest number of cases, deaths, and new cases in Canada, is the first province to begin to open up its economy, which it is currently doing during the first two weeks in May. However, the explanation is that in the greater Montreal area, schools, daycares, businesses, and stores are being forced to stay closed until June 6th. Moreover, even that latter date is conditional on the coronavirus epidemic being brought under control in the greater Montreal area.

The Quebec provincial government has added its voice to the Conservative complaint that the Canada Emergency Student Benefit (CESB) payment is making it difficult for the agricultural sector to attract students to work in the fields for the summer months. Under the CESB, students and recent graduates who are Canadian citizen or permanent residents of Canada -- but not international students -- can apply for the $1,250 payment per month between May and August. As finally acted into legislation, the CESB took account of the earlier Conservative view -- as expressed during the parliamentary debate -- that a simple payment would serve as a disincentive for students to seek summer work. Hence, the Act, as finally passed, encourages students to continue to search for work and allows a student to earn up to $1,000 more per month through part-time work while continuing to receive the CESB. Apparently in Quebec, the receipt of the $1,250 monthly payment has resulted in students declining to work in agriculture for the summer.

Sunday, May 10, 2020

CEWS Extension: Yesterday, Prime Minister Trudeau announced that the federal government will extend the payroll wage subsidy – the Canada Emergency Wage Subsidy (CEWS) -- past the June 6th termination of the original program for 'months more', as yet unspecified. The twelve-week financial aid program was introduced on April 27th to run from March 15th to June 6th. To date, the Canada Revenue Agency has received 132,481 applications from companies, of which all but 9,000 have been approved. To date, the CEWS has been used by companies to pay 75 percent of the wages of 1.7 million workers, who would otherwise have been laid off. Payments can range up to $847 per week from CEWS, with the employer responsible for the paying the remaining 25 percent of each employee's wages.

With the provinces now beginning to lift their lockdowns to get the economy re-started, and employers anxious to put their employees back to work, why is it deemed necessary to continue the CEWS program for 'months more'? The current estimate is that the federal deficit will soar to $252 billion for the current fiscal year. If there is an economic argument for extending the CEWS program, it is probably that it is being viewed as a means of easing the capital demands on companies that are transitioning to a fully-operation status, and that are starved for capital after having sustained a drastic loss of revenue since the mid-March lockdown of the economy.

(A week later, on Thursday, May 14th, it was reported that economists see the CEWS as having "a vital part" in the re-opening of the economy in that it will enable companies to afford to hire all of the workers that they need, and people who are making, and spending money, will be a driver of the economic recovery. Economists are recommending that the CEWS be continued until at least September, and that the CERB wage subsidy to workers who have lost their job due to the coronavirus lockdown should be gradually phased out.)

Elective Surgeries: After a two-month hiatus in scheduling elective surgeries – during the provincial lockdowns – hospitals are now beginning to tackle a backlog of surgeries and procedures that were postponed, and which some hospitals are saying might take a further two years to clear. That situation has been investigated by Tom Blackwell, a health care reporter with the *National Post*. In mid-March, hospitals began to cancel non-emergency operations to preclude recovering patients from being exposed to the coronavirus, and to free up beds, as hospitals expected their ICU's would become overwhelmed with severe cases of the coronavirus disease. It was a fear based on observations of the situation in northern Italy where the coronavirus was raging through the population. However, the expected wave of coronavirus cases did not materialize. The provincial lockdowns and the stay-at-home policy effectively prevented the spread of the virus throughout the Canadian population.

During the cancellation of elective surgeries, 72,400 fewer surgeries were performed in Ontario than during a comparable period last year, and in British Columbia 30,000 surgeries were cancelled, with perhaps as many as 189,000 cancelled across Canada. Only emergency surgeries were performed where there was a critical need. However, when the wave of coronavirus patients failed to materialize, Ontario hospitals alone have only a 69 percent occupancy with 11,200 free beds. Among the surgeries and procedures cancelled were elective cancer surgeries, elective heart surgeries, MRIs, CT scans, and diagnostic tests for cancer, and regular screening tests – mammograms, pap smears, and colon-cancer tests. The major exceptions were chemotherapy and radiation treatments which were continued.

In Ottawa, hospitals are working together to prioritize postponed elective surgeries based on the conditions of the patients, the availability of alternative treatments, and an evaluation of the risk in imposing a further delay, as well as an assessment of the resources available for each procedure.

Another unexpected phenomenon during the coronavirus epidemic was that visits to Emergency departments by individuals suffering from other diseases declined greatly. The sick are apparently avoiding going to the hospital out of a fear of contacting the coronavirus. Emergency department visits have dropped by 30 percent in Ontario, and by 40 percent in British Columbia. Those who are being admitted to hospital are far sicker than would be normally the case, which is another indicator that the sick, and those in seriously ill health, are putting off going to hospital for as long as possible. Now, hospital emergency departments are declaring that they are ready to welcome those with health problems that need to be addressed.

Monday, May 11, 2020

Long Care Homes: In British Columbia, there have been outbreaks in 34 provincial long-care facilities, and over 400 residents and staff have tested positive for the coronavirus. However, the situation is under control as more than half of these long-care facilities no longer have any cases. Public health authorities in British Columbia learned about the nature of the coronavirus threat by observing what was transpiring in Ontario and Quebec long-care homes and in Italy. As soon as an outbreak occurred in a long-care home in British Columbia, all residents and staff were tested regardless of the presence of any symptoms, staff were extensively equipped with personal protective equipment, visitors were banned, and individuals who tested positive were placed in isolation. Tests were conducted to check for contaminated equipment and areas in and around each facility, and the buildings were deep cleared and disinfected. Moreover, the public health authorities were aggressive in tracing and testing the contacts of known cases, and the medical personnel on site were continually monitoring residents and staff for symptoms.

What the British Columbia experience highlights is that at the onset of the coronavirus threat to Canada, what Canadians needed was not theorizing and modelling by experts of the potential impact of a virus epidemic by public health authorities and epidemiologists. All such modelling was based on unknowns and pure speculation with respect to the nature and potential impact of the coronavirus.

What was, and is, needed is more of a commonsense approach to dealing with the actual virus threat. The federal government ought to be basing its approach to combatting the virus threat on observations of the earlier experiences of other countries that were experiencing the highly contagious nature of the coronavirus and struggling to combat its spread. Based on the experiences of other countries, the federal Liberal government should, and could, have quickly deduced what restrictions were required on foreign travel to prevent the virus from being introduced into Canada, and what practical steps were effective in containing its spread once introduced within a community.

In Canada, the possibility of taking such a practical approach was hamstrung by the initial resistance of the federal Liberal government to the closing of Canada's borders to foreign travellers, the unquestioning reliance by Public Health Canada and the Liberal government on the misinformation contained in the communiques and directives of the World Health Organization (WHO), and the inexcusable -- verging on criminal negligence -- decision by the Trudeau government to ship Canada's National Stockpile of personal protective equipment to China just as the coronavirus was making its initial penetrations into Canada. Another highly questionable decision was taken by the provinces in imposing a total lockdown, which although effective in combatting the spread of the coronavirus, exacted an extremely high cost from Canadians. There were other highly effective practical measures that could have been mandated by the federal government had it chosen to invoke the Emergency Measures Act.

Any close observation of what had been, and was being, done in Hong Kong, Taiwan and South Korea, would have revealed the practical effective measures that could have been taken to combat the spread of the coronavirus without imposing a lockdown of the Canadian economy and all social functions: viz., the immediate closing of Canada's borders to foreign travellers from infected countries, the testing of all returning Canadians and the mandatory quarantining of the sick and asymptomatic returnees, the mandatory wearing of cotton face masks, the enforcing of physical distancing measures in all establishments and businesses and, once an infected person was identified, the tracing and testing of all contacts followed by a mandatory quarantining of any contacts who tested positive and the self-isolation of the other contacts for 14-days.

Moreover, these practical measures, should have been bolstered by encouraging the practice among the public of disinfecting of surfaces commonly touched in stores, businesses and workplaces, and a municipal program of spraying, with a disinfectant, any urban public areas with a cluster of infections. Had these practical measures been widely adopted, with personal protective equipment readily available for medical personnel, first responders, and personal care workers, there would have been no need for a lockdown in Canada to prevent the spread of the coronavirus. For Canadians, it has been a highly costly learning process made more difficult by the abject failings of the Public Health Agency of Canada and the federal Liberal government in their response to the coronavirus threat.

Recovery Phase: A survey has been conducted to ascertain the response of Canadians to various methods that might be adopted to prevent an upsurge in coronavirus cases with the re-opening of stores and businesses. Anywhere from 75 to 80 percent of the respondents are okay with a variety of physical distancing requirements. The survey group was supportive of having quotas on the number of people let into a store or restaurant based on the square footage of floor space – with restaurants, for example, being required to have table at least 1.5 metres apart with a limit of four persons to a table. There was also an equally high level of agreement on limiting the size of public gatherings to eight persons, with public parks fully open but with no sports, games, or use of children's play equipment, and with the wearing of face masks being required in public both out-of-doors and for entering any public building.

Body temperature screening was equally acceptable, but just 57 percent agreed with a random testing for COVID-19 by public health officials.

Second Wave: Public health authorities are worried about a second wave of coronavirus infections, but are failing to distinguish between minor outbreaks on the re-opening of the economy in various countries, and a true wave of infections. At present, some health authorities are warning that we are seeing the beginning of a second wave in South Korea, with a report of 34 new inflections. However, the outbreak was at several Seoul nightclubs that had been visited by a highly contagious young man infected with the coronavirus, and at least 24 of the new infections were traced directly to him. What this episode reveals is not the beginning of a feared second wave. Rather it reveals the danger of an early re-opening of nightclubs where people are drinking, and talking, and associating close together in abandoning the wearing of face masks. (Subsequently, South Korea announced that it was rescinding its authorization for nightclubs and bars to re-open.) Similarly, a high-risk rating and warning of the beginning of a second wave in the Chinese city of Jilin, is an overreaction. It is based on a single coronavirus case – a woman who infected eleven members of her immediate family.

What is evident is that the coronavirus has not been, and cannot be, totally eradicated in any country, and that additional small outbreaks are unavoidable. In Germany, as the lockdown is being gradually lifted, new cases surged to high of 933 on one day from a previous daily low of 357. However, Germany has rejected any talk of a second wave of infections. The German Chancellor, Angela Merkel, advised Germans simply to stick to the rules of social distancing and the wearing of a face mask. Germany has simply re-imposed a lockdown in the several areas of the country experiencing a cluster of new cases. What has been well established is that local outbreaks can be readily contained with contact tracing, testing, and quarantining of the infected persons with medical support. To classify each small outbreak, which health authorities are capable of handling, as the beginning of a second coronavirus wave is irresponsible.

Sports: The Canadian Football League (CFL) is facing the prospect of either having a shortened season in the fall, or cancelling the entire 2020 season, and is in a financially precarious position as it depends on gate receipts to stay in business. A $50 million TV contract divided among nine teams does not begin to cover operating costs. The League has appealed to the federal government for financial aid. What the League is asking for is a $30 million grant to cover immediate expenses for coaches and team employees on contract, a $70 million grant if it plays a shortened season, and $150 million grant it has to cancel its entire season because of the coronavirus impact. This poses a quandary for any government.

Sports teams ought not to receive government monies, but in this case the League is a business that has suffered because of an external factor, the coronavirus lockdown, the same as any other Canadian business. It was government that deliberately shut down the economy, and caused the dire financial situation faced by the Canadian Football League. Another troubling aspect of this issue is that some of the teams are community owned, and the stadiums – which were funded to some extent by the public through providing financial support in various ways -- will have no major tenant if the Canadian Football League folds. The stadiums will require upkeep by government at a continuing major cost.

Apparently, some members of the Liberal government are concerned that the CFL has not specified how a federal financial grant would be used. The League reportedly lost $20 million last season, and there is a concern that a financial grant will be used by the League to pay its accumulated debts, rather than for providing aid to the football players who are unable to play, and have been deprived of their income, because of the coronavirus lockdown. There is also a resistance within the federal government to providing a financial aid plan that benefits American players who live in the United States and come to Canada only to play during the football season. However, American players do pay Canadian income tax on their earnings while in Canada, and they are not eligible to apply for the Canada Emergency Response Benefit (CERB) which is restricted to Canadian citizens and landed immigrants. Stay tuned!

The National Basketball Association (NBA), which depends on gate receipts for 40 percent of its revenue, is thinking of concluding its 2019-2020 season by gathering the teams, coaches, and support personnel at two sites where the teams can play in empty areas before TV cameras, with the players housed and isolated nearby and continually tested for the virus. The two sites being considered are Orlando (the Disney World Sportsplex) and Las Vegas.

The UFC (Ultimate Fighting Championship company) became the first organization to stage a sports event before an empty area for TV viewing on Saturday night, May 9th, in Jacksonville, Florida. Fighters and their cornermen were tested for COVID-19 when they arrived in Florida with the taking of nasal swabs for laboratory testing and blood tests for coronavirus antibodies, each fighter and his cornermen were isolated in a hotel, and worn face masks at all times inside and outside the arena. The media personnel who attended were also tested for the coronavirus and encouraged to wear face masks. The two fighters only shed their masks upon entering the octagon to fight. The event was staged without any setbacks, and at least one additional 'fight night' has already been scheduled for Jacksonville. Within two weeks, test results will reveal whether any of the fighters contacted the coronavirus during the initial fight card in Jacksonville.

Excess Deaths: In assessing the death rate from an coronavirus pandemic, one problem is the number of confirmed coronavirus deaths is known, but in calculating the "excess deaths" during an epidemic what is not known is the number of deaths indirectly caused by the impact of the virus epidemic on society. Among the excess deaths which are not directly attributable to the virus, might well be those who died because of surgery delays, those who delayed in going to hospital for treatment out of a fear of contacting the virus, and those who suffered from a medical condition that was neglected during the period of self-isolation. In British Columbia, one of the few provinces that reports the cause of all deaths, the number of "excess deaths' during March and April was 170 of which 111 were coronavirus cases. In effect, there was an excess of 59 deaths -- over the same period of the previous year -- that are probably indirectly attributable to the coronavirus epidemic. In New York City, currently one of the worst hit cities in the world, there were over six times as many deaths as would normally be expected during March and April, but the number of indirect deaths is not known. For epidemiologists, the total number of 'excess deaths' is the true indicator of the impact of the COVID-19.

Quebec Schools: Elementary Schools have re-opened in the Province of Quebec, except for the greater Montreal area which still has a high rate of new coronavirus cases. School attendance is voluntary. Parents were required to indicate ahead of time whether their child or children would be attending. A survey of English school boards in western Quebec and the Eastern Townships revealed that only 15 percent and 35 percent, respectively, of pupils have returned to school. There is a maximum limit of 15 pupils per classroom, and the desks have been placed two metres apart. Teachers are monitoring the drop off and pick up of pupils at the school to ensure that they do not mingle together, and a teacher is assigned to disinfect the hands of pupils with a hand sanitizer upon their entering or leaving the school building. Parents are not allowed to enter a school.

Sanitation stations have been placed near washrooms, and janitorial staff are continuing disinfecting the common areas. There are arrows on the floor of the hallways to direct pupils to remain in a straight line on one side or the other depending on the direction they are going. Common facilities like the library, gymnasium, laboratory, and science rooms are remaining closed. In the play yards, teachers have laid out cones to direct the children to walk in a line in one direction for outdoor exercise while keeping a two metre spacing between the pupil ahead and the pupil behind, and the pupils are not being allowed to engage in team games or use play equipment.

Both teachers and bus drives have been issued with personal protective equipment – primarily face masks and gloves -- and school buses will carry only one child per seat. One wonders why the Quebec government is not issuing a face mask to each pupil upon the initial arrival at school. That is the ultimate protection against the spread of a virus where social spacing is not consistently possible. Cotton face masks could be manufactured quickly in the Montreal garment industry for school pupils. In Quebec, the elementary school openings are being regarded by teachers, school boards and the provincial government as a trial run for September when the school will be open to the full school enrollment. Secondary schools in Quebec will not open until September, and elementary schools in the greater Montreal area will not open until June 2nd, if then, depending on the coronavirus threat level as defined by the daily number of new coronavirus cases.

What is surprising in the reports concerning the elementary school openings in Quebec was a mention of regret that the school breakfast and lunch programs, which "many students depend on for adequate nutrition", have not been restored. It is unbelievable that in Canada elementary school pupils are arriving at school hungry or ill-nourished. Rather than blaming society, why are the parents not being called to account?

Parliament: Rex Murphy, a *National Post* columnist, is a lone voice in questioning why, during the greatest crisis that Canada has faced since the Second World War, there is no concern among the Press, or Canadians at large, for the restoration of parliament. What he finds equally surprising is that the NDP, the Block Quebecois, and the single-issue Green Party, have willingly acquiesced in the muting of the voice of the people. Only the Conservative Party is standing up for the rights and prerogatives of parliament and demanding its recall – in a reduced proportional representation during the coronavirus crisis. One might add is parliament to continue to be regarded as superfluous during the recovery phase, as it has been regarded during the coronavirus epidemic by the Liberal government?

Murphy maintains that rather than shutting down most of the functions of parliament during the coronavirus crisis, the emphasis should have been on: how can we maintain parliamentary sovereignty, parliamentary debate, and accountability, which are the very foundations of our democracy? He questions: Why are Canadians acquiescing in government via a daily zoom session during which the Prime Minister announces government policies followed by a twenty-minute press session with parliament reduced, for the most part, to a virtual conference chat-show? Canada, under Prime Minister Justin Trudeau, is the only country that has suspended, or muted, its parliament during the coronavirus pandemic.

To which one might add: Why are Canadians so ignorant of how a true democracy functions, and the crucial role of parliament -- the elected representatives of the people -- in questioning the government, in holding the government accountable to the people, and in overseeing the expenditure of public monies? Why was there no public outrage at the recent attempted coup d'état of the Liberal government in seeking to establish an absolutist form of government for an initial period of two years? One suspects that it is the product of the poor education received by Canadians in our schools where the history and traditions of parliamentary government are not being taught because it is viewed as being too British, and passé. What we have in Canada is a people ripe for the imposition of an elective dictatorship under a charismatic leader, supported by a toady Liberal press.

Tuesday, May 12, 2020

CERB & EI Fraud: In Canada, workers who have lost their job can apply for EI (Employment Insurance) to receive a $500 a week payment during their period of unemployment, and the claims are processed, and payments approved, by the Service Canada branch of the Employment and Social Development Canada department. Service Canada also processes many CERB (Canada Emergency Response Benefit) applications as under the existing legislation, applicants can apply for the CERB payment to either Service Canada, or directly to the Canada Revenue Agency (CRA) which makes the payments. To date, during the coronavirus epidemic, Service Canada employees have 'red-flagged' a total of upwards of 200,000 applications as possibility fraudulent because of a dubious claim of past-employment or other suspicious factors. One would expect that payments would be withheld in these instances pending a further review, but such is not the case.

It has just been revealed that in late April an Employment and Social Development department memo was circulated to employees that, in effect, called for an approval of a payment to every and all EI applicants no matter how dubious the claim: viz.

"Effective immediately, while processing a claim, if an agent uncovers information that suggests potential abuse of the EI system by a Client, an employer or a third party, they do not impose a stop pay and do not refer the file to integrity [Integrity Operations] unless it is considered an urgent investigation".

Now, the kicker is that the Department has not only suspended claimant information sessions, in-person interviews, and on-site visits, to screen applicants for EI – which was rendered necessary by the coronavirus epidemic -- but the memo informed staff that the department had suspended "all Integrity Operations activities for compliance and enforcement of the EI program". In effect, there is no longer an investigative unit to which staff can refer 'urgent cases' of suspected fraud. Normally, 'urgent cases' are those that involve applications on behalf of a dead person, the use of a dormant social insurance number or a social insurance number that was never been used before with respect to any employment, and fraudulent records of employment. However, these suspected fraudulent applications are no longer to be investigated, payment is simply to be made to every EI applicant. Moreover, a number of government employees -- who understandably wish to remain anonymous -- have indicated that the same unquestioning payment of claimants policy is also being applied by Service Canada in processing applications for the CERB (Canada Emergency Response Benefit), which pays $500 a week to workers – employees and self-employed -- who are out of work because of the coronavirus lockdown, and had an income of at least $5,000 in 2019 or in the twelve months prior to their application.

Carla Qualtrough, the Liberal government Minister of Employment and Social Development Canada, is defending the unquestioning approval by the Liberal government of all EI and CERB applications submitted to Service Canada. She claims that the government anticipated "a heightened risk of fraud with pandemic-aid program'". The emphasis was placed on getting the money, as quickly as possible, to Canadians in need. That the government would be "working later to claw back any unwarranted payments". (Apparently, the Minister does not recognize that applicants who submit false claims to secure a financial payment from the government are engaging in criminal fraud! They are not just innocents in receipt of 'unwarranted payments'. What we have here is yet another example of the Modern liberal psyche which is punishment adverse and does not believe in forcing individuals to follow the rules, or in vigorously enforcing the rule of law.)

Departmental employees have reported that there are known cases where a CERB payment is being made to workers who have not lost their jobs but are working and being paid by their employers 'under the table'; that applicants are fabricating employment records to qualify for payments, and are making false claims about earning over $5,000 in a previous twelve- month span, and that international students, who according to their visas are allowed to work only 20 hours a week, are applying for EI and claiming to have worked 40 hours a week while attending classes. (International students are not eligible for the CERB but are not excluded from EI coverage and payments.)

A departmental spokesperson for the Minister has emphasized that the payments system has "backend safeguards" which will ensure that any payments made to ineligible recipients will be eventually repaid. That the department intends "to regularly conduct file reviews and investigations to identify and address cases of error, fraud, and abuse", and will do so through "using computer tracking, data analytics and linked data systems to detect mis-payments and fraudulent activity".

It sounds good, but what is truly off putting about this whole situation is that the Liberal government is instructing public servants to authorize payments in spite of clear evidence of a potential fraud, and that the projected future investigation will require a heavy investment of resources and is unlikely to recover much money. Many of those who are cheating the system appear to be part-time workers, workers in low-paying occupations, and international students who will be long gone when, and if, the government tries to recover the money.

Yet another problem with the CERB and EI programs is that the government has found that a significant number of Canadians -- who have lost their jobs during the coronavirus epidemic -- have applied to both programs, and are receiving a double payment. Given the close relationship between the two programs, one wonders why the government did not institute a systematically cross-checking of the names and addresses of applicants to either program, with that of the individuals approved to receive payments under the other program. It is basic common sense and the right thing to do, but one of the things that the current Liberal government appears to lack is common sense in setting up the guidelines for the administration of financial programs. Nonetheless, one must recognize that Canadians, who lost their job and who were desperate to secure some source of income, might well have applied in good faith for both the CERB and EI benefits in not being sure which program they were entitled to apply to, and trusting that the government would sort it out.

Services Canada is now in the process of contacting Canadians who are receiving a double payment to inform them of the need to repay the CERB payments. (The EI payments are ongoing, whereas the CERB payments are of a four-month duration.) The Canadian Revenue Agency has established an online portal through which the repayment can be made, or the cheques can be mailed directly to the CRA.

Large Company Loans: Finance Minister Bill Morneau, announced yesterday that the federal government intends to establish a Large Employer Emergency Financing Facility (LEEFF) to provide liquidity to large companies that cannot secure loans from a bank during the lockdown to keep their operations going. The objective is to enable large companies to avoid bankruptcy, and thereby to protect Canadian jobs. Only companies in real need will be eligible for a government loan at a low interest rate.

The LEEFF program will be open to large for-profit businesses as well as not-for-profits, such as airports, that have annual revenues of over $300 million, but excludes financial institutions. To qualify companies must be seeking loans of $60 million or more, have a significant workforce and operations in Canada, and be currently solvent. The program will require the cooperation of private sector lenders who will be encouraged to provide access to capital for Canadian businesses in the oil and gas sector, and major companies in other sectors of the economy across Canada. That failing, the federal government being the lender of last resort. The program will be administered by the Canada Development Investment Corporation (CDIC), with the support of Innovation Science and Economic Development Canada (ISED) and the Department of Finance. To obtain a LEEFF loan, the applicant must first have approached banks and the financial market and have been unable to borrow the needed monies.

Companies that are approved for a loan, must agree not to use the monies to pay executives and/or dividends, or to fund buy-backs of their own stock, and must agree to respect collective bargaining agreements and to protect workers' pensions. Companies that have been convicted of tax evasion will not be eligible to participate in the program. How the loan program will shake out is unclear. The government has been made aware that the oil and gas sector needs upwards of $20 billion to maintain liquidity during the current drastic drop in crude oil prices, in market demand, and in revenues, caused by OPEC flooding the market with oil and the coronavirus lockdown, and the major airlines have been seeking substantial financial support to maintain their liquidity as well. Smaller airlines will be unable to participate in the LEEFF support program as they do not have an annual revenue of over $300 million, even in the best of years.

Where the oil and gas sector is concerned, the Finance Minister had promised financial aid as early as March 25th, and there was talk of the Finance Department preparing a $15 billion financial aid package for the oil and gas sectors, but nothing materialized. Rumours have persisted that the federal Liberal cabinet is divided on whether to provide aid to the oilsands industries. The news of the LEEFF program is encouraging, but there is a concern over the lack of details as to how the program will work. Nonetheless, the LEEFF has been well received by the oil and gas sector. The Canadian Manufacturers and Exporters association cautioned that their member companies cannot afford to take on more debt during the present crisis, and that the association was looking for non-repayable measures that would help their temporary cash flow problems. What is disturbing, as John Iveson, a National Post columnist, has pointed out is the politicization of the new LEEFF program by the Liberal cabinet, which contains zealous environmentalists who would "prefer to see the industry wither".

Apparently, when the proposed financial aid program – as prepared by the Department of Finance – reached the Cabinet a rider was added which requires that any company seeking LEEFF support must include in its application an assessment of how its future operations will support environment sustainability and the achievement of national carbon emissions goals. Whether or not an environmental assessment of the operations of an oil or natural gas company will be a required criterion for receiving approval for financial support through the LEEFF program remains unanswered. Hopefully, the Liberal government will not inject its environmentalist political ideology into an economic rescue plan for Canadian industries in desperate need of greater liquidity to stay in business. Prime Minister Trudeau has been under pressure from environmental activist groups to refrain from aiding the oil and gas sector, and to put federal monies into emission reduction technologies and green energy sources. In announcing the new credit facility, the Prime Minister was careful to note that the federal government was providing "bridge loans, not bailouts".

The LEEFF program is critical to the survival of the oil and gas industry in Canada. Given the lack of any announcement of an amount of federal government monies to be committed to the credit facility, it appears that the intent of the program is to provide some form of lines of credit for loans from either the federal Treasury or from Canadian banks with the federal government providing an interest payment guarantee; yet, how the new credit facility will operate is unclear. What is clear is that during the present crisis, the banks will not loan billions of dollars to a fossil fuel industry that the federal government has been deliberately strangling through its inordinately demanding and virtually endless environmental reviews, its lack of support for the construction of pipelines, and its prohibition of tanker traffic off the northern coast of British Columbia. Canadian banks have already invested $60 billion in the oil and gas industry, and do not want to greatly increase their level of risk and the prospect of acquiring unwanted oilsands properties from bankrupt companies.

LEEFF Update: Nine days later, it was announced that LEEEF program would be open for applications on Wednesday, May 20th; that the government would be taking an ownership stake or a cash equivalent in the companies taking out a loan; and that all companies would be treated equally in a strictly commercial transaction. Publicly traded companies, and their private subsidiaries will have to issue warrants to the government which will enable the government to purchase shares worth 15 percent of the loan or to receive its equivalent in cash. (Warrants convey a special right to purchase stock at a fixed price for a specified period, and they can be converted into equity or cash if the loan is not repaid.) The reason given for opting for warrants was to ensure that Canadian taxpayers will share in the gains made by any company taking out a loan. (One assumes as well that the securing of warrants is intended to keep the government at arms length to avoid the government being both a shareholder and the regulator of a company.) Privately held companies will pay the same amount as the warrant values in fees.

There will be no limit to how much a company can borrow beyond the $60 million minimum. The loan is intended to keep major company operational during the coronavirus lockdown and early recovery phase, to help maintain their employees on their payroll, and to avoid bankruptcies of economically viable company during the market collapse resulting from the coronavirus lockdown. (One wonders whether taxpayers would have preferred the federal government to take direct equity in any large company receiving a massive government loan with the government being recognized as a secured creditor if the company should fail. But that is not to be.)

The loans will be offered for only the next twelve months, and will be structured so that the first 20 percent will be "Senior debt" secured through existing lenders, and the remaining 80 percent will be unsecured loan, with an interest rate of 5 percent the first year, and 8 percent the second year, with the interest rate to rise 2 percent a year over each year thereafter until the loan is repaid. The unsecured loan portion must be repaid within five years.

(These are exorbitant, and uncalled for, interest rate charges, and an unreasonably short repayment period for potentially billion dollar loans by large companies with an existing heavy debt load, who are currently struggling to survive in a stagnant economy that is just beginning to be re-opened. While this Liberal government has not hesitated to give billions to every sector of the economy and everyone in need without any strings attached, one wonders if this loan program for large companies is designed to cripple the oil industry with debt payments, and render it unable to invest in new production facilities and pipeline construction. Clearly, the environmentalist lobby and the environmentalists in the federal Cabinet, inclusive of the Prime Minister, are adhering to their policy of 'strangle the oil industry' as reflected in the terms of this financial aid program for large industries. What happened to the 'low interest' loans mentioned by the Finance Minister, Bill Morneau, in the original announcement of the large company emergency loan program?)

BCAP Loans: To provide large amounts of needed capital to mid-sized Canadian companies, the government has expanded the Business Credit Availability Program (BCAP) to enable companies to obtain loans of up to $60 million, and even up to $80 in some cases. The BCAP, in cooperation with Export Development Canada (EDC) and the Business Development Bank of Canada (BDC), will work with private sector lenders "to provide access to capital" for mid-sized Canadian companies in all economic sectors and regions across Canada. The Conservative Party strongly supports the BCAP initiative, but questioned why financial aid was not made available to mid-sized companies a month ago when financial aid was promised by the government, and why, after such a long delay, there are few specifics as to how the credit facility will operate.

Oil Industry Investment: To add to the economic perfect storm striking the oil and gas industry worldwide, the Norges Bank Investment Management (Norway) fund – the world's larges sovereign wealth fund which held a $1.15 billion in stock in two Canadian oil companies – announced that it had sold its stock and would no longer invest in oil producing company worldwide. It would no longer invest because of the "market situation, including liquidity in individual shares" of the companies, as well as their "unacceptable greenhouse gas emissions".

Had the federal Liberal government, and other governments, provided an adequate financial support to the oil and gas sector in late-March, when the critical need for liquidity became apparent amidst plunging oil prices, its doubtful that international investors would be looking for an exit. As to greenhouse gas emissions, one Canadian oil company, Cenovus, has cut its carbon emissions by 30 percent over the past 15 years, and is introducing new initiatives that will reduce its carbon emissions by a further 30 percent over the next ten years. More generally, Canadian oil companies have already reduced their carbon emissions by 28 percent in response to the global warming concerns raised by environmentalists. The oil and gas industries in Canada are acting responsibility, but their environmentalist critics want to take advantage of the current economic crisis to strangle and shutdown a major segment of the Canadian economy while it is economically vulnerable.

Recovery Policies: In viewing the age profile and health condition of those who have been afflicted the most by the coronavirus, and the significant decline in new cases, Diane Francis, a columnist with the

Financial Post, is arguing that the most sensible approach to dealing with the aftermath of the COVID-19 epidemic would be to fully re-open the economy everywhere in Canada – except for Quebec, which still has a high rate of infections – with precautions being taken to protect the most vulnerable members of society. The argument is that anyone over 65 years old should remain in isolation, as well as people with underlying heath conditions that render them a high-risk element of the population. Support efforts would continue for these two groups remaining in isolation, while the rest of the population returns to work. The argument is that the general population, particularly those under 50 years old, has nothing to fear from the virus other than a small number getting cold-like symptoms. In any case, the provincial health care units are more than adequate to deal with any small outbreaks that might occur with businesses, stores, and factories reopening.

To which one might add, any risk in fully re-opening the economy can be greatly reduced through the wearing of face masks, continuing to practice social distancing where practicable, and providing the full range of personal protective equipment to workers in close proximity, while continuing the frequent washing of hands, and a regular attention to disinfecting common areas. What is feared is that if the lockdown is continued any longer, it will have consequences for Canadians far worse than any remaining COVID-19 disease threat.

According to figures cited by Francis, 90 percent of the COVID-19 deaths in Canada were people over 60 years of age, with the heaviest toll among people over 75 years of age who were living in close proximity in nursing homes and long-care homes. In New York City, the worst-hit city in North America, 75 percent of the deaths from COVID-19 were of persons over 65 years of age, with a heavy concentration of deaths among those over 75 years of age. Moreover, within the general population most of the deaths from COVID-19 occurred among people who were already suffering from heart diseases, cancer, diabetes, or other chronic health conditions.

Wednesday, May 13, 2020

Payments to Seniors: Deborah Schulte, Seniors Minister, has announced that all Canadians who are receiving the Old Age Security

(OAS) pension will be receiving a one time, tax free, grant of $300, and all Canadians who are receiving the Guaranteed Income Supplement (GIS), in addition to the OAS pension, will receive an additional tax free grant of $200, in addition to the $300 special payment. The payments are intended to provide a temporary financial assistance to Canada's 6.7 million seniors during the coronavirus lockdown; and it will cost at total of $2.5 billion. Seniors will not need to apply for the special payment. It will be deposited to their bank account or mailed to them. The Minister has justified the extra payment as being needed to relief the financial stress of seniors who are paying extra fees for the dispensing of drugs and higher food costs, and who are incurring extra cost for delivery services and taxi fees during the lockdown. The federal government is investing another $20 million in an existing program for seniors, the New Horizons for Seniors Program, which funds community-based activities that benefit the health and well-being of seniors.

The Treasury Board President, Jean-Yves Duclos, declared that the announced special payments to seniors would be made within a few weeks because "they will not require parliamentary authority". This is a puzzling statement. How can $2.5 billion be expended on a one-time payment to seniors without parliamentary approval? Moreover, why is the special payment to seniors being made now as the lockdown restrictions are beginning to be lifted?

One wonders whether the Liberal government is listening to the crass politicos who are recommending that the minority Liberal government resign, and appeal to the Canadian people in a snap election for a strong majority government to deal with the recovery phase. The intention would be to take advantage of the popularity of the Liberal government that is announcing the dispensing of millions of dollars each day – totaling the expenditure of billions of dollars -- during the 'morning show' TV appearances of Prime Minister Trudeau. It is an expenditure blitz with the only guiding principle being to make sure that every Canadian receives some form of Liberal government largesse, in addition to the truly sorely needed financial support provided for laid off workers and businesses facing financial ruin. Is the groundwork being laid by the Liberal Party for a snap federal election?

(The next day, the social media was full of protests from seniors stating that they do not need the $300 special payment; that seniors in receipt of pensions have not experienced any reduction in income; and that financial aid monies should have been targeted for low-income seniors who are receiving the Guaranteed Income Supplement (GIS). What is ironic about the indiscriminate special payment for all Canadian seniors – upwards of 6.7 million seniors in total -- is that during the coronavirus lockdown, with millions of Canadian workers losing their job (their sole source of income), the most secure element of the population are the healthy seniors who are receiving the Old Age Security pension and the Canada Pension Plan pension (based on employment contributions) and, in addition, in many cases, a workplace pension.

In Canada, all Canadians citizens and legal residents of Canada who are over 65 years old, who have lived in Canada for at least ten years after the age of 18, and who have an annual income of less than $128,137 (2020 limit), are eligible to received the Old Age Security (OAS) pension which is geared to income. The Old Age Security pension is indexed and taxable, and it currently pays a maximum of $613.53 per month or $7,352.36 per annum, per person.

The Guaranteed Income Supplement was introduced as a temporary program during an economic recession in the late 1960s and made permanent in 1971. The purpose of the Guaranteed Income Supplement is to raise low income seniors out of poverty. Single seniors with an annual income of $18,600 or less, and senior couples with a combined income of $45,720 or less, who are receiving the Old Age Security pension, are eligible to apply. Under the Guaranteed Income Supplement program, a single senior can qualify for a maximum payment of $916.38 per month ($10,996.56 per annum), and a senior couple can qualify for a maximum payment of $551.63 each (or combined GIS income of $13,239.12 per annum.

In effect, single seniors who receive the full Old Age Security pension, and the maximum Guaranteed Income Supplement, are receiving an income of $18,348.92 per annum from the federal government, and senior couples who are in receipt of the full Old Ages Security pension, and the maximum Guaranteed Income Supplement, have a combined income $20,591.48 per annum from the federal government, exclusive of provincial government financial aid programs. In Canada, the base poverty line is defined as having an income of less than $18,000 per annum to secure accommodation and basic goods and services.)

Thursday, May 14, 2020

Recovery Phase: Now that lockdown restrictions are being relaxed in the Province of Ontario, many Canadians are anxious to open their cottages during the coming Victoria Day weekend, May 16th -18th. However, a rife has developed between cottagers who want to spend this coming weekend at their cottage and the permanent residents of the villages in cottage country who do not want crowds of people descending on their village and potentially bringing a coronavirus infection into their community. Some villages are telling cottagers to stay away for the present; whereas other villages are advising cottagers to bring all of their needed supplies with them to avoid having to go into the village, and to isolate themselves at their cottage during the weekend. That latter approach appears to be a reasonable solution to the problem. Hopefully, cottagers will comply with what is being asked of them.

One segment of the oil and gas sector that boomed during the coronavirus lockdown was the petrochemical industry of Alberta the produces the polyethylene used in plastic products. During the lockdown, the demand for plastic packaging for food items, for plastic face shields, and for surgical gloves has soared. Moreover, during the recovery phase, it is anticipated that the demand for plastic wraps for food, plastic packaging, face shields, and gloves will increase greatly among retailers. At present, it is estimated that 30 percent of the general population are wearing cotton facemasks when entering grocery stores, although that number appears to be increasing.

Free Trade Farce: Without tariff protection, the Alberta petrochemical industry will soon face a fierce competition from China. At present China is establishing a $1 billion plant in the Philippines, and within China is spending billions of dollars in establishing a major new petrochemical complex. The government of China has an economic plan to greatly expand the Chinese petrochemical industry and to modernize the production facilities. With the Chinese government targeting the production of plastics, the free trade with China policy of the federal Liberal government will leave Canadian industries highly vulnerable to losing market share, to large layoffs, and ultimately a takeover by a Chinese-government affiliated corporation. Free trade is a farce when the Chinese government targets an industry for a takeover and puts the financial, technological, and marketing resources of the Chinese government into the competition for market share!

Drug Supply: The coronavirus has created a fear among the public that has resulted in a rush to acquire any drug that is reputed to provide an antidote to the virus. When President Trump declared that hydroxychloroquine -- an anti-malaria drug used in treating autoimmune diseases -- appeared to be an effective antidote to the coronavirus, sales of the drug skyrocketed. In March, 9.5 million doses of the drug were sold in Canada, almost double the normal level. The result was a shortage of the drug for the treatment of patients with autoimmune disorders, a problem that was made decidedly worse when India -- the largest producer of the drug -- placed a ban on exports of hydroxychloroquine and 23 other standard drugs. To date, there is no convincing evidence that the anti-malaria drug provides an effective treatment for COVID-19. However, what the episode does reveal is the danger implicit in relying on the global market for drugs that are critical to the health of Canadians.

GAVI: The international vaccination organization, GAVI -- an affiliate of the United Nations and UNICEF that administers vaccination programs in Third-World countries -- has repeatedly expressed its concern that there be 'an equitable use' of any vaccine developed. The concern is that the initial use of a coronavirus vaccine ought not to be confined to the developed countries that can afford to purchase it, but that the vaccine should be distributed and administered -- by GAVI – in inoculating the poor of Third-World countries in tandem with inoculation programs in the developed nations. Currently, there are two different viewpoints as to how a vaccine should be initially distributed, once developed, tested, and approved for use: the nationalist versus the universalist.

The nationalist viewpoint is based on the argument that whatever country develops a successful vaccine, should initially administer the vaccine to its own people. In effect, the argument is that the initial use of a successful vaccine should be to inoculate and save the lives of the people of the country that funded and undertook the research that led to the successful development of a vaccine, until production can be ramped up sufficiently to supply other countries, and to provide for inoculation programs for the Third-World poor. The nationalists do not question that the developed countries will fund the purchase of the vaccine and the costs of administering vaccination programs, for the poor in Third-World countries. What the nationalists are maintaining is simply that the initial priority, when the vaccine is in limited supply, ought to be to secure the inoculation of the population of the country that financed and developed the successful vaccine.

The universalist viewpoint is that science is not national, but universal, and that a vaccine once developed and in production, should be 'equitably distributed' to all countries with a priority being given -- during the early limited production phase of the vaccine -- to inoculating peoples in the areas of the world that are experiencing a soaring rate of new coronavirus cases. In this scenario, the developed nations who have funded and undertaken the coronavirus research, and who will be funding the vaccination programs in the Third-World countries, would be the last to receive the vaccine.

Under the universalist approach, the developed countries will be deprived of an initial access to the vaccine because they have successfully contained the spread of the virus and have greatly reduced the incidents of new infections, at a terrible economic cost through national lockdowns. They will have to wait in line for a future vaccination program for their peoples, which will be dependent on production of the vaccine being ramped up sufficiently to provide the massive number of doses required to treat the threatened populations in Third World countries. In effect, the Third-World countries that have contributed nothing to the development of a successful vaccine, or have failed to systematically combat the spread of the coronavirus within their countries, will have their people given the vaccine on a priority basis.

One can see the rationale of the universalist viewpoint – from a world health perspective -- in advocating the focusing of vaccination programs immediately on major outbreaks that occur anywhere in the world. Moreover, eventually a world-wide vaccination program will be necessary to control the spread of the COVID-19 and minimize its impact. Health authorities do not expect that the coronavirus can be eliminated totally through a world-wide vaccination program. However, it will be controllable with a vaccine – once developed -- as are other viruses that remain active among the world population, such a measles.

Despite the arguments of the universalists, once a COVID-19 vaccine has been developed, it is only right and just that the developed nations focus initially on protecting the lives of their own peoples through the implementation of national vaccination programs; and that whichever country develops the successful vaccine gives an initial priority to vaccinating its own citizens.

(Nine days later, on May 23rd , GAVI reported that its efforts to vaccinate 80 million children in some 68 Third-World countries against diphtheria, measles, and polio, is in jeopardy because of international travel restrictions, vaccine delivery delays, and parents fearing to leave their homes during the coronavirus pandemic to go to vaccination stations.)

Chapter Eight

Thursday, May 14, 2020 (continued)

Recovery Process: The Province of Ontario is taking a quite cautious approach to Phase II of its recovery plan. Schools are to stay closed until at least May 31st. For the Victoria holiday weekend – May 16-18 -- golf courses can re-opened – but only washrooms and take out food facilities within the clubhouses – marinas, boat clubs and public boat launches can re-open as well, together with private parks and campgrounds for trailer and RV owners who are regular summer residents. On the following Tuesday, May 19th, all construction work is authorized to resume, retail stores with a street entrance can re-open – in limiting the number of customers admitted to maintain social spacing – and maintenance, repair and property services can re-open, as well as veterinary clinics by appointment only, pet grooming, pet sitting, and pet training, libraries requesting books and pickups, housekeeping services and babysitting.

One problem for retail businesses is that Ontario's emergency legislation remains in effect which limits public gatherings to five persons.

In proceeding to Phase II of the recovery plan, Premier Ford reiterated that there is a real possibility that coronavirus cases will spike as people emerge from their self-isolation at home and begin to interact in public. He exclaimed: "The truth is, we can't fully predict where things will go, so we need to be ready to react if we see a sudden increase in cases". At present, the Province of Ontario is engaged in talks with the federal government to secure financial support for urban transit authorities whose ridership revenues have plummeted during the coronavirus lockdown.

What is surprising is that the province has not made it compulsory for workers in the re-opening businesses to wear face masks and gloves, and for businesses to institute a program of disinfecting common surfaces. It appears that a reliance is being placed solely on social spacing to prevent the spread of the coronavirus by asymptomatic carriers. One suspects that bars and nightclubs, and restaurants with indoor seating, will be the last businesses permitted to re-open. The Premier mentioned that he is "waiting for the word from the chief medical officers before restaurants can open".

Restaurant owners have voiced a concern about government relying solely on social spacing capacity as the critical factor in allowing a business to re-open. Many in the restaurant business are stating that they cannot run a restaurant successfully on a fifty percent occupancy, which would be the effect on many dining establishments if a two-metre spacing between tables were enforced. Moreover, a Restaurant Canada survey has revealed that half of Ontario's independent restaurants will not be able to re-open if the restaurants are forced to remain closed for another three months. There is a need for government to look at other means to protect diners in restaurants. The solution -- as advocated herein -- is the compulsory wearing of face masks and gloves by kitchen and serving staff, the wearing of face masks by diners except when seated in eating and drinking, and a regular program of disinfecting common surfaces. In late March, the Ontario government amended the Liquor License Act to allow restaurants to sell liquor through their takeout service to increase their revenues.

International Border Closures: The Trump administration has announced that the border closure ban on non-essential travel between the United States and Mexico, which was introduced for 30 days on March 21ˢᵗ and extended for a further 30 days on April 20ᵗʰ, will be extended indefinitely. Critics are charging that the Trump administration is using the public health law to stop illegal migrants from crossing from Mexico into the United States. (And why is that objectionable?) Since March 21ˢᵗ, some 20,000 migrants have been apprehended in trying to enter the United States illegally; they were quickly processed and returned immediately to Mexico, or to their country of origin in Latin America. Only two persons were granted asylum as legitimate refugees seeking asylum from persecution. To date, Mexico will not reveal the death rate from the coronavirus among its population, and the Trump administration is adamant that they will not allow illegal migrants, who may be coronavirus carriers, to enter the United States.

Canada is currently in negotiations with the United States concerning the extension of the ban on non-essential travel across their common border. Both Premier Ford of Ontario, which is adjacent to New York State, and Premier Hogan of British Columbia, which is adjacent to Washington State, have gone on record as saying that they are strongly opposed to any relaxation in the ban on non-essential travel across the Canada-United States border. New York is currently the major epicentre for coronavirus cases in the United States and Washington State is a major centre of infections. Overall, the United States has 1,431,993 confirmed cases, 85,601 deaths, and 246,972 recovered cases, with new coronavirus cases continuing to soar upwards to the most recent total of 11,282 new cases in a single day.

Canada Emergency Commercial Rent Assistance: The joint federal-provincial rent relief program – which provides a temporary financial relief to landlords who reduce the rent of small business tenants -- has not proved as popular as anticipated. Under the Canada Emergency Commercial Rent Assistance (CECRA) program -- which was announced on April 25, 2020 -- the federal government has projected paying upwards of $1 billion to match an equal $1 billion in funding, in total, from the provinces. The program is open to landlords with small business tenants who pay less than $50,000 a month in rent, have been forced to close their business because of the coronavirus lockdown, and have been paying less than 70 percent of the rent owed to their landlord because of their business being closed with no revenue stream.

The intention of the CECRA program is to provide landlords with forgivable loans to cover up to 50 percent of the monthly rent of any of their small business tenants who are experiencing a financial hardship and unable to pay their full rent. The program is open to landlord who agree to reduce the rent of their small business tenants by 75 percent -- to just the 25 percent of the regular rent level -- and who agree to refrain from evicting their small business tenants for non-payment of their full rent. In effect, the financial aid to landlords will required small business tenants to pay only 25 percent of the amount of rent normally paid, with the joint federal-provincial forgivable loan covering 50 percent of the rent owed.

It appears to be a win-win situation for landlords as they will definitely receive 50 percent of their rent for the three month duration of the program – April, May, June – with the possibility of receiving a total of 75 percent of the regular rent if the small business tenant can pay 25 percent of the monthly rent. The alternative in the case of small business tenants who cannot operate their business during the coronavirus lockdown, and who have no revenue coming is, is bankruptcy with the landlord receiving no rent and having to search for new small business tenants during a lockdown. As of May 14th, only 30 percent of the expected number of commercial landlords with small business tenants, have applied for the non-repayable loan under the CECRA program. The program is being administered by the Central Mortgage and Housing Corporation, a Crown corporation of the Government of Canada.

Among the reasons cited for the moderate level of interest in the CECRA program are: the program has just become operational in mid-May, by which time many landlords have already made arrangements with their commercial tenants to reduce or defer rent payments; landlords prefer to receive 100 percent of the rent due through deferred payments rather than a guaranteed 50 percent plus 25 percent under the CECRA program; and many small businesses, in being poorly capitalized, cannot afford to pay even a reduced 25 percent rent during the coronavirus epidemic lockdown with no revenue coming in.

It is expected that a significant number of small businesses will default on their rent and not have the capital to re-open. Others will go bankrupt during an extended recovery period. The small businesses that are particularly vulnerable to bankruptcy are those that cannot readily accommodate social spacing: viz. restaurants, bars, and all types of entertainment organizations that bring together large crowds of people.

(Six days later, on Wednesday, May 20th, Prime Minister Trudeau announced that starting on May 25th, all landlords with commercial tenants will be able to apply for the emergency commercial rent assistance, and that payments would be processed quickly. Moreover, the Prime Minister mentioned that the federal government was working on a new financial support system for larger retailers.)

Real Estate: In the Toronto, real estate market home sales have plummeted by 66 percent during the month of April, and fell by 56.8 percent across Canada during the coronavirus lockdown. In the greater Toronto area prices have remained surprisingly stable and have even inched slightly upwards, and elsewhere across Canada the Home Price Index has increased by 6.4 percent over home prices in April last year. The explanation appears to be that not only has demand collapsed, but also the supply of units to buy, and the shortage of housing stock has sustained prices. What will happen, once the lockdown is lifted, has brought forth two decidedly different analyses. On the one hand, some major relators have expressed a belief that the pent up demand will drive prices upwards when the market resumes normal activity; but, on the other hand, there are predictions that the weakness of the recovery of the labour market could bring a five to ten percent decline in price for residential housing. What these diametrically opposed prognoses reveal is that no one knows how the economy will respond as the lockdown is lifted.

(Several days later, a Canadian bank study revealed that between 75 and 90 percent of Canadian renters paid their May rent on time, which was about the same percentage range as in April. One oddity is that although most of the job loses have been concentrated in low-wage occupations, the collections of rent has been higher among low-income renters. The explanation appears to be that laid-off workers are using their CERB income -- $2,000 per month, for four months – to pay their rent; although one wonders how these laid-off workers are managing to meet their living expenses for the month after their rent is paid. What this situation reveals is that landlords are benefitting indirectly from the CERB financial aid for laid-off workers.)

Across Canada, apartment rents fell 3.2 percent during the previous month of April, ranging from a drop of 1.1 percent on average in the greater Toronto area to a drop of 5.6 percent in Vancouver. The condo rental rate fell 4.6 percent. During the lockdown, the existing rental market has been stable with renters staying in place.

Schools & Day-Cares: In Quebec, the provincial government has now postponed the opening of daycare centres and elementary schools in the greater Montreal area until September. They were scheduled to open on June 2nd, two weeks after the rest of the daycare centres and elementary schools elsewhere in the Province. However, the coronavirus threat in the greater Montreal area remains unacceptably high.

In Canada, only the elementary schools in Quebec -- outside of the Montreal areas -- are open, and British Columbia plans to open elementary schools on June 1st. All other provinces and the territories have closed their schools until September. A major problem that has emerged in the projected re-opening of businesses, shops, and industries is: how are parent going to return to work when schools and day care facilities remain closed? Where can parents place their children while at work?

COVID-19 Status: Across Canada, coronavirus outbreaks appear to be well under control and a general flattening of the number of new coronavirus cases.

Quebec: In the Province of Quebec, a total of 21,236 coronavirus cases have been reported, with 1,765 deaths, and 15,845 recovered cases. As a province wide testing continues, the number of new cases reached a low of 329 yesterday. The Provincial government has just empowered itself to impose a temporary provincial management on any long-care home that is continuing to struggle to recover from a coronavirus outbreak.

Across the province, there are thirteen long-care homes and seven retirement residences that are struggling with a coronavirus outbreak, despite receiving aid from intervention teams comprised of medical personnel and support workers from local hospitals.

To date, three-quarters of the provincial deaths from the coronavirus have occurred among elderly residents in long-care homes, with a significant number of personal care workers on staff having also become infected at these homes. What has become evident is the great differences in staffing levels, and personal health care, in the different long-care homes across the province.

Ontario: The Ontario government has declared that it intends to launch an investigation into the management and health situation in long-care homes that have experienced major outbreaks. To date, private operators of long-care homes are not eligible for any government funding to refurbish and update inadequate facilities. However, the personal care workers staffing the long-care homes are eligible for the federal-provincial pay supplement during the coronavirus epidemic. In Ottawa, the nation's capital, two-thirds of the coronavirus deaths have occurred in just four of the twenty-eight long-care homes in the City.

Friday, May 15, 2020

COVID - 19 Status: At this point, with the Canadian provinces entering into the first phase of a re-opening of the economy, an overview of the coronavirus situation in the respective Canadian provinces will serve as a benchmark for what comes next in the recovery phase.

Ontario: As of Friday, Ontario has recorded 437 new cases of COVID-19 and 27 more deaths over the past 24 hours. Overall, the provincial total has reached 21,922 coronavirus cases, and a death toll of 1,825, with 16,641 recovered cases. Clearly, the number of COVID-19 cases and deaths continues to increase, but the overall trend is downwards, and the public health situation is considered manageable. Five days later, on May 20th, Premier Ford announced the appointment of an independent commission to investigate the long-care home situation in the province. To that date, more than 1,400 elderly residents and five staff members of Ontario long-care homes had died from a coronavirus infection out of a total of 1,919 coronavirus related deaths in the province.)

Quebec: Today, Quebec recorded 50 coronavirus-related deaths, the lowest daily total since mid-April, but 696 new cases were reported. The number of new cases in Quebec is by far the worst rate of new infections anywhere in Canada, although it represents a decrease of thirteen over the total yesterday in the province. Quebec has a total of 41,420 confirmed COVID-19 cases, has recorded 3,401 deaths, and has 11, 039 recovered cases. At present, there are 1,822 coronavirus patients in hospital, inclusive of 192 coronavirus patients in intensive care. The new cases are mostly in the greater Montreal area, and in long-care homes which the Quebec government is considering 'nationalizing'.

To impede the spread of the coronavirus, the provincial government has distributed one million face masks, mostly to transit users in Montreal. There are 1,700 members of the Canadian military providing medical and personal care support in twenty-five long-care homes in Quebec, and at five long-care homes in Ontario. The federal government is considering providing hazard pay to the military personnel who are deployed in long-care homes to fight a coronavirus outbreak.

Alberta: The Province has had 58 new COVID-19 cases over the past 24 hours, and four deaths have occurred in a long-care home. Overall, since the beginning of the impact of the coronavirus in mid-March, Alberta has had 6,515 coronavirus cases and 125 deaths. There are currently 1,073 active cases, and 62 patients in hospital of whom nine are in intensive care. Alberta is well advanced into its recovery phase, except for the cities of Calgary and Brooks where a local lockdown remains in force owing to a major COVID-19 outbreak, each at a major packing plant employing thousands of workers and among the community adjacent to the plant.

British Columbia: The Province has fifteen new cases and five additional deaths in the last daily report. The province currently has 369 active cases, 2,407 individuals who have tested positive for COVID-19, and a total of 140 deaths. At present there are 15 outbreaks being dealt with in long-care homes. Most of the coronavirus cases in British Columbia have been in the Vancouver area, with the major outbreaks confined to long-care homes.

Maritimes: In the Maritimes, New Brunswick has had only 120 confirmed cases of COVID-19, no deaths, and 119 recovered; Nova Scotia has had 1,034 confirmed cases, 55 deaths, and 918 recovered; and Prince Edward Island has had 27 confirmed cases, no deaths, and 27 recovered. Newfoundland-Labrador has had 260 confirmed cases, 3 deaths, and 248 recovered. In the West, the province of Manitoba has had 289 cases, seven deaths, and 254 recovered, and Saskatchewan has had 590 confirmed cases, six deaths, and 408 recovered, with a report of five new cases within the past 24 hours.

Territories: In the far north, the Nunavut Territory had had no confirmed cases of COVID-19; the Northwest Territories has had five confirmed cases, no deaths, and five recovered; and the Yukon Territory has had eleven confirmed cases, no deaths, and eleven recovered.

Indigenous Peoples: The federal government has little reliable data concerning the number of coronavirus cases among Indigenous peoples on the reserves across Canada. As of May 13th, it was reported that there were 465 coronavirus cases among Indigenous peoples in forty-two communities across Canada, and seven virus-related deaths. Two days earlier, there were 183 cases on the reserves in five provinces, 18 hospitalizations and two deaths. There is presently a major outbreak among Indigenous peoples in northern Saskatchewan at the village of La Loche, where the residents are mostly of the Clearwater River Dene Nation and Métis.

Clearly, the coronavirus is beginning to penetrate Indigenous communities on some reserves, but the reporting is only partial. Several Indigenous communities are refusing to report on their number of coronavirus cases. The Minister for Indigenous Services, Marc Miller, has declared that "out of respect" the Liberal government will not investigate the reserves that fail to report coronavirus cases. That politically correct attitude is deplorable. With Canada's Indigenous peoples on the reserves facing the potential prospect of the coronavirus sweeping through their communities, the federal government should have feet on the ground in providing testing and health care services regardless of whether the leaders of a community wants aid or not. It is imperative that the government institute measures that will halt the spread of the coronavirus on the reserves that have a local community infection.

(Oddly enough, there is a concern among the government officials to know how many Indigenous people living off the reserve have contacted the coronavirus. To date, Indigenous peoples, who are living off the reserve, have received the same attention in testing and health care as anyone else in the community where they reside. Only Ontario and Quebec use a testing form that enables an individual being tested to voluntarily self-identify as First Nations, Inuit, or Métis. Perhaps someone will explain why this is considered pertinent information during a national virus epidemic.)

Canada: In Canada, the worst outbreaks of the coronavirus were, and are, in Quebec and Ontario, followed at a distance by Alberta and British Columbia, with the other provinces having a comparatively small number of coronavirus cases, and a very low death rate. As of May 15th, Canada has had 74,662 confirmed COVID-19 cases, 5,562 deaths, and 36,895 recovered. Moreover, the rate of new infections has turned dramatically downward.

WHO Prognosis: After downplaying the seriousness of the original coronavirus outbreak in China, the World Health Organization (WHO) has now gone completely the other way in response to the easing of the lockdowns in western Europe. Dr. Hans Kluge, Director of the European Region for the World Health Organization is now calling on Europe to brace for "a second deadly wave" of the coronavirus as the western European nations ease their lockdowns. In a publish statement, he stressed that although the number of coronavirus cases was falling in the western European countries, the pandemic was not over. Moreover, he warned that the second wave could well coincide with an outbreak of other infectious diseases. Why the WHO is engaging in what might well be called 'fear mongering' is beyond comprehension. Has not the competence and credibility of the WHO -- for making prognoses of potential virus threats -- been long since discredited? Europeans now know how their public health authorities need to respond to prevent the spread of the coronavirus when any secondary outbreaks occur. The emphasis now needs to be on lifting the national lockdowns as soon as it is deemed prudent, to avoid the more immediate threat of a complete economic collapse.

As of today, the epicentre of the coronavirus pandemic in Europe has shifted to the east with severe outbreaks in Russia, Ukraine, and Belarus. Hopefully, the leaders of the European Union have learned a lesson from their past errors and will recognize the necessity of keeping the eastern borders closed to strictly quarantine the countries now at the epicentre of coronavirus pandemic. It is critical to the health and well-being of western Europeans to tightly enforce a ban on travellers from eastern Europe to keep them from entering the West.

Coronavirus Research: Scientists at Cardiff University in Wales have found that low amounts of ethanol can disrupt the outer fatty membrane that envelops the coronavirus. In particular, the study found that exposure of the virus to a 21.6 percent ethanol solution produces "a near 100 percent reduction of infectivity". Now, the critical question is: what is the ethanol level in the hand-sanitizers being marketed? (A commercial hand sanitizer in the household of the diarist has a listed 70 percent ethyl alcohol content.)

National Debt: There are serious concerns being expressed by financial analysts that the federal deficit could reach $350 billion, or 20 percent of the GDP, during the current fiscal year. It is a situation made worse by the irresponsible spending of the federal Liberal government under Prime Minister Justin Trudeau who appears to relish distributing billions of dollars to all Canadians, regardless of need. The federal debt has ballooned from $685 billion in 2018 – after two years of a heavy deficit spending by the Trudeau government -- to the new estimate of $962 billion. Some analysist are predicting that if the temporary emergency financial aid programs -- which were introduced during the lockdown to ease the economic distress of laid off workers and distressed industries -- are extended during the recovery process, it could add another $400 billion to the national debt.

Currently, it costs Canadian taxpayers $23 billion per annum to service the national debt, which monies could be betters used to support social programs and infrastructure construction. What is equally worrisome is that the massive national debt is manageable only because interest rates are at an historically low level. The federal government is currently able to borrow money at a very low rate of interest – less than one percent interest -- but that will not last.

What is equally worrisome, is that Canada may lose its AAA borrowing rating if the economy does not recover rapidly over the summer. At present, analysts maintain that the national debt is manageable at the very low rates of interest being paid, but that could change rapidly if interest rates rise appreciably, or if Canada loses its AAA credit rating. If the heavy spending is not curtailed by the Justin Trudeau government, with the temporary financial aid programs allowed to terminate on their fixed date, former Prime Minister Stephen Harper has warned that Canada could well face a debt crisis that will require the imposition of "brutal austerity measures".

What these figures neglect is the level of indebtedness being incurred by Canadian provincial governments, and the deficits that were run up by municipal governments during the coronavirus lockdown. The City of Ottawa – with a population of 900,000 – is forecasting a deficit of $66 million by the end of June, and if lockdown restrictions remain in force until the end of the calendar year, the municipal deficit might well reach $186 million.

CERB Fraud: The fraud story, with respect to the processing of applications for Canada Emergency Response Benefit (CERB) payments, is getting worse and worse. The memo -- from the Employment and Social Development Canada depart to its Services Canada branch – that ordered staff to process and pay all applicants for the CERB payment while disregarding and ceasing to red flag flagrant cases of potential fraud for investigation, has even broader implications than anticipated. One commentator has pointed out that the federal government in giving its approval for the payment of fraudulent claims, has deprived itself of any legal grounds for seeking a future repayment. In effect, the fraudulent claim payments have been 'authorized'. Another negative aspect of this whole sorry situation is that it is undermining the respect of Canadians for the honesty, integrity, moral character, and fiscal responsibility of the federal government as an institution. What is quite revealing in this situation is the character of the Modern liberals of the Trudeau government who are discipline adverse, and who have a free spending mentality unrestrained by common sense, by any sense of fiscal responsibility, or by any feelings of moral indignation on the discovery of evidence of a potentially massive fraud in a government program.

The 'look the other way' Liberal government policy in the processing of CERB applications, is reportedly having a devastating effect on the morale of Service Canada employees. An important part of their job is to root out ineligible and fraudulent applications for government financial grants, and they are being directed to dispense with that critical function. On his part, Prime Minister Trudeau has defended the position of his government --that all CERB applications be approved for payment -- on the grounds of necessity. He dismissed the number of fraud cases as being not that extensive: just "a few people" among upwards of eight million applicants.

The Prime Minister declared that his government was willing to accept that "one or two percent might be fraudulent claims" out of a need to get payments out quickly to 'the 99 percent of Canadians who were truly in need'. The government did not want to risk "paralyzing the system" and preventing Canadians from getting the financial aid that they need. To which he added that "there will be consequences for engaging in fraud"; and that the government intends to pursue any inappropriate payment – presumably to seek a repayment.

The claim of 'necessity' rings hollow. How Service Canada employees in upholding the legislation passed by parliament that governs eligibility for CERB payments, and red flagging obvious cases of fraud for investigation, would paralyze the payments system was not explained by the Prime Minister. The House of Commons Finance Committee was informed that there were 200,000 questionable cases pertaining to applicants who were receiving the CERB payments of $2,000 per month, "mistakenly or not". In effect that constitutes $400 million a month in possibly fraudulent payments identified to date, or a potential total of $1.6 billon fraudulent CERB payments over the course of the four months duration of the wage subsidy program for workers laid off due to the coronavirus epidemic.

Moreover, the level of fraudulent payments may well be far greater as both Service Canada and the CRA are processing CERB payments and Service Canada is also processing some of the EI applications under the same 'look the other way' directive of the federal Liberal government. (EI applicants can apply either to Services Canada, or directly to the Canada Revenue Agency (CRA) to have their application processed. However, it the CRA that pays the EI benefit.)

Subsequently, it was revealed that CERB payments are going to applicants who voluntarily quit their jobs, or were fired for misconduct, which directly contradicts the legislation governing eligibility for a CERB payment, as enacted by parliament.

Fishing Industry Support: Prime Minister Trudeau has just announced a new $469 million financial aid program for the benefit of fish harvesters (fishermen). It includes a $267.6 million benefit to cover up to 75 percent of the losses incurred by fish harvesters – presumably inclusive of companies, associations, and captains -- that expect a twenty-five percent of more drop in income this year. It also includes a $201.4 million non-repayable grant to pay up to $10,000 to self-employed fish harvesters who own their own business – their own fishing boat. (Fishermen who have been laid off by their employer during the coronavirus lockdown, are eligible to apply for the Canada Emergency Response Benefit (CERB) wage subsidy payments.)

The new financial aid program is in addition to the $62.5 million Canadian Seaford Stabilization Fund (CSSF) that was announced on April 25th to provide financial aid to the fish and seafood processing sector to modernize their plants, increase their storage capacity, and adapt to new market demands while introducing new health and safety measures to protect their workers.

A question was raised as to whether fish and seafood would be included in the Agriculture and Food Industry financial aid program -- announced on May 6th, -- which included a $50 million grant to the existing Agri-Recovery program of the federal government to purchase and store surplus food to provide Canadians with food security. When announced, that program was aimed at farmers in the dairying, cattle, hog, and poultry sector of the food industry to preventing the wasting of food

-- such as the dumping of milk – that cannot be sold. Including fish and seafood in the new Agri-Recovery mandate to purchase and store surplus foods makes sense in view of the current situation in the fish and seafood sector. The immediate problem is the lack of sufficient cold storage capacity.

With the coronavirus lockdowns, the seafood market collapsed with the closure of restaurants, the loss of the America market, of the cruise ship industry demand, and other food service markets. This coming Friday, over 3,000 lobster fishermen will be placing their lobster traps with the opening of the spring lobster season in the Gulf of St. Lawrence and in the Atlantic near Cape Breton, Nova Scotia. Lobster fishermen regard the new program as an insurance policy which they hope will not be needed, if their traditional markets revive. Questions remain. Some fish harvesters are worried that with a truncated fishing season, they will not be able to generate enough income to qualify for Employment Insurance (EI) payments during the off-season, and fish packing plans are worried about a potential labour shortage, if temporary foreign migrant workers are unable to come to Canada with the international travel restrictions in place.

The Liberal government has responded to the EI concerns by proposing to allow self-employed fish harvesters to access EI benefits based on their insurable earnings from previous seasons. To address the potential labour shortage, the Conservative Party opposition has called for the launching of a new government job creation program to match students and other youth with jobs in the agriculture and agri-food sectors, inclusive of the fish harvesting and seafood industries. (An effective incentive might be to make it plain that anyone who is offered a summer job, and refuses to take a job that they are competent to perform, will have their government financial benefit payment cancelled from whichever program they have accessed; and that those who accept a seasonal job will have their benefits extended.)

In response to President Trump imposing restrictions on seafood entering the United States, Prime Minister Justin Trudeau called on Canadians to purchase Canadian produced foods to help the dairy industry, farmers, fish harvesters, and the seafood industry. This is an interesting turn on the part of the Prime Minister. For the most part, Modern liberals are champions of universal free trade and open borders, and the free movement of goods and people, and services and capital. However, in a time of crisis even Modern liberals can see the necessity of developing a domestic market in basic food stuffs, although the domestic market that young Trudeau envisages has a voluntary basis. It rests on the willingness of Canadians to give a priority to purchasing Canadian produced foods rather than a government commitment to developing a domestic food supply security as part of a national economic policy.

U.N. Security Council: It was reported today, the Liberal government has been pushing forward in a relentless effort to secure for Canada a seat on the United Nations Security Council. Canada is currently competing with Norway and Ireland (Eire) for votes among the members nations in the General Assembly to gain one of the two non-permanent seats to be filled on the Security Council. In February 2020, Prime Minister Trudeau went on a jaunt to Africa to visit and lobby African governments for support for Canada's Security Council bid, and other international jaunts were planned for the same purpose before his travels were cut short by the coronavirus crisis. Yet, during the height of the Coronavirus epidemic in Canada, he has been busy in contacting twenty-eight heads of state in lobbying for support for Canada's bid for the Security Council seat. Among heads of government contacted were those of several island nation members of the United Nations -- Fiji, Saint Lucia, and Tuvalu -- as well as the prime ministers of Kenya, Rwanda, Senegal, Columbia, Chana, Sudan, Jamaica, and Ethiopia. One wonders how many tens of millions of dollars in foreign aid have been promised. The heads of government of Sweden and the State of Qatar were contacted as well; although one doubts that Sweden can be weaned away from supporting Norway, a fellow Scandinavian country, in the U.N. vote, and Qatar has no need of foreign aid.

At first glance, one might wonder why the Trudeau government would devote so much time and energy, and funding, to an effort to secure a U.N. Security Council seat while the coronavirus pandemic is raging worldwide. Why not just let the June vote of the General Assembly – a secret vote – simply go whichever way it will go? Either Norway or Eire would be a highly acceptable and responsible representative of traditional western values, and a voice of common sense and reason, on the Security Council. What would be lost, other than an ephemeral sense of prestige, if Canada were to lose the appointment to either country? However, that is not the mindset of the Modern liberals of the Trudeau cabinet, and of Justin Trudeau himself. They have an ideological agenda to propagate on the world stage, as François-Philippe Champagne, the Foreign Affairs Minister has made plain.

While Prime Minister Trudeau -- according to an earlier statement -- has not had the time to think about the future development of Canada following the COVID-19 epidemic, and claims that his government is totally focussed on meeting the day-to-day challenges posed by the impact of the coronavirus on Canadians, apparently that is not the case with respect to the United Nations where his government is firmly focused on future developments.

The Foreign Minister has declared that the Prime Minister and his Cabinet "absolutely want a seat on the U.N. [Security] Council"; and that Prime Minister Trudeau had made it a top priority of his government. According to Foreign Minister Champagne, the Trudeau government is looking to the future, and wants "to keep an eye on the future that we want, and how we want to shape it." Since the Security Council is where "the most consequential decisions are taken", it is imperative that Canada has a seat "because it's a chance to shape the world's response on any number of issues".

Now, one might ask, what is the ideology that the Trudeau Liberal government wants to bring to bear in shaping "the world's response on any number of issues"? The ideology is that of Modern liberalism. Indeed, Justin Trudeau himself is the personification of Modern liberalism. He embraces globalism (economic, social and political), open borders and immigration (migrate to whichever country you please), moral relativism (choose your own values), pan-nationalism (loyalties and cultural values that transcend the nation-state), and multiculturalism (which denies that immigrants ought to adopt Canadian values and define themselves as being Canadians). More broadly, Modern liberals embrace naturalism (a philosophy that denies all religious belief and the religious foundation of the traditional moral values of western society), and post-nationalism (which denies any continued validity of the nation-state as the embodiment of the common interests, freedoms, and cultural values of a people).

Domestically, Modern liberals believed in identity politics (a new form of tribalism that is destructive of any concept of a common national good that transcends individual and group interests), and political correctness (a confining of free speech to innocuous subjects that cannot possibility offend anyone's personal, racial, gender identity, religious, or cultural sensibilities.) Moreover, all differences in beliefs and values among peoples of the world are held to be beyond comment or reproach. They are regarded as equally acceptable or are viewed with indifference. The focus of Modern liberals is on a new world order.

Internationally, Modern liberals look to the United Nations as the precursor of a homogenous universal state which they believe will promote social equality, human rights, peace, happiness, and material prosperity, with a common sharing of humanity in the benefits of modern technology. In theory, the Modern liberal ideal of an egalitarian world, with everyone sharing in a common material prosperity, can be quite appealing. However, it fails to take account of the real practical problems in governing such a mass of people, of human nature, historical developments, cultural values, and national loyalties. People have a strong innate desire, and a commitment to retaining their own peculiar identity -- their religious and cultural distinctiveness and values, their nation-state and, for the majority, their social status. The peoples of the world do not want to blend into a homogenous egalitarian mass under a universal, Big brother government imposing Modern liberal values and politically correctness on humanity.

In addition to personifying the values and mindset of Modern liberalism, Justin Trudeau is a self-proclaimed and committed feminist, a promoter of a LBGTQ special rights agenda, and a fervent environmentalist who is dedicated to a reduction of carbon emissions to the levels called for in the U.N. Paris Agreement of 2016, regardless of the economic and social costs to Canadians. The securing of a seat on the Security Council of the United Nations is a personal goal for Justin Trudeau. He sees himself as the leading spokesperson for feminism, for the LBGTQ special rights agenda, and for environmentalism on the world stage; and he needs a platform at the United Nations to fulfill his personal ambition. What is ironic in the extreme is that Justin Trudeau himself may be the biggest obstacle to Canada obtaining a seat on the Security Council. The heads of the African and Latin American states cannot but be aware of his commitment to a feminist, LBGTQ, and environmentalist agenda.

(Five days later, Prime Minister Trudeau spoke openly about Canada's bid for a seat on the Security Council. He maintained that with the world emerging from the coronavirus pandemic, there is a role for Canada to play "in creating a better, and fairer world", as Canada had done following the Second World War in the founding of the United Nations and multilateral organizations such as the North Atlantic Treaty Organization (NATO). According to the Prime Minister, for Canada to play that role, it needs to be a member of the Security Council – "the United Nations' most powerful body". Clearly Justin Trudeau and the Modern liberals of the Liberal Party government, have a universalist, pan-national vision focussing on the establishing of a new world order. If history teaches any lesson, it is to beware of zealots who want to establish a new world order, whether on the Left or the Right of the political spectrum.)

Saturday, May 16, 2020

Air Canada: Today, there was a shocking indicator of the true depth of the damage that the coronavirus lockdown policy has had on one particular sector of the economy, and why many industries and businesses cannot just shift into a recovery mode without financial support from the federal government. Earlier, Air Canada had accessed the Canada Emergency Wage Subsidy (CEWS) program and had begun recalling its laid off employees. Under the CEWS payroll wage subsidy, the federal government pays 75 percent of the wages of the recalled workers for four months, with the company paying only 25 percent of the wages. The intention of the program is to provide an economic boost for a company until it can become fully operational again in a recovering economy, and to encourage the company to recall is furloughed workers.

Such was the plan, but with President Trump extending the ban on non-essential travel into the United States for an indefinite period, and the

European Union deciding to extend its ban on nonessential international travel to Europe for a longer period, Air Canada had to re-examine its business plan in the face of that new reality.

During the coronavirus pandemic lockdowns, Air Canada lost 95 percent of its business. Now, it faces an unforeseeable future in not knowing when flights can resume on traditional international routes, and the prospect that it might take months more beyond that for passenger traffic to rebound after international airports are reopened. Hence, Air Canada cannot afford to pay 25 percent of the wages of its recalled staff with no prospect of getting its fleet in the air for the foreseeable future. Under the CEWS financial aid program, bridge financing is also available to any company in need – up $60 to $80 million in repayable loans, but that is a negligible sum to a major company like Air Canada.

The airline is currently losing $20 million a day with most of its 258 planes grounded, and its normal volume of traffic -- 51 million passengers a year – having been lost for the most part with the international lockdowns. It appears that international travel may remain banned until the late fall, if not for the rest of this calendar year. Hence, the abrupt reversal, and the current decision of Air Canada to downsize with a projected layoff of anywhere from 50 to 60 percent of a 68,000 workforce. The current plan is for 19,000 staff to be laid off on June 7th, with perhaps as many as 22,800 layoffs in total. It is not a coincidence that the Air Canada layoffs are scheduled for the end of the week during which the CEWS payroll wage subsidy program is scheduled to terminate on June 2nd.

When questioned by the Press about the drastic Air Canada layoffs, Prime Minister Trudeau refused to comment on whether the Canadian government would provide a bailout for the airline. To date, the Prime Minister has repeatedly emphasized that his government is offering financial aid grants and loans to companies in need of a temporary financial support during the lockdown, and that his government has no intention of offering bailouts to companies on the verge of bankruptcy, or with little prospect of an immediate economic recovery once the lockdown is lifted. In contrast, in the United States as early as April 29th, the United States government set aside $29 billion for loans to American airlines at a low interest rate, and Congress designated $50 billion for direct financial aid to American airlines. The German government has provided a nine billion Euros financial aid package for Lufthansa.

Among business spokesperson in Canada, there is a palpable fear that other major companies may find themselves in a similar situation where a severe downsizing, and the laying off of a major component of their workforce, may well be the only alternative to going out of business, if markets do not open quickly or are not accessible immediately.

(A week later, a major blow was struck against any quick recovery of international air passenger traffic. On May 22nd, the British government announced that after June 8th all international travellers arriving in Britain will have to self-isolate for 14 days and provide information on where they will be staying. Anyone breaching the isolation period will be fined £1,000, and spot checks will be carried out. Whether the isolation requirement will remain in place is doubtful as it is being denounced by airlines, business groups, and public figures in Britain and Europe.)

The International Air Transport Association (IATA) has expressed concerns that if air passenger traffic fails to quickly return to pre-pandemic levels during the recovery phase, that a significant number of airlines may well go bankrupt owing to their heavy indebtedness. Globally, governments have provided $123 billion in total for the support of airlines – in loans and equity arrangements – and the banks have loaned a further $52 billion, which will need to be repaid. Canada alone has declined to provide any substantial financial aid to its national airlines. (Presumably, the environmentalists in the Trudeau government are happy as the grounding of airlines will appreciably reduce carbon emissions.)

Parliamentary Government: Thomas Klassen, a professor in the School of Public Policy and Administration at York University (Toronto) has written an interesting piece on how decision making in government has migrated to government bureaucrats during the coronavirus epidemic. Dr. Theresa Tam and her 2,400 staff at Public Health Agency of Canada, are exercising a decisive influence on government policy decisions based on the specialized knowledge they possess with respect to communicable diseases and their supposed knowledge of how the spread of the coronavirus can be contained. In the words of Professor Klassen:

> "Canadian politicians have relied exclusively on the advice of bureaucrats in designing responses at the federal, provincial, or municipal level. Politicians of every stripe have adhered to the instructions of public health bureaucrats. All speeches by politicians and government statements highlight that "the government is acting on the best advice of public health officials"".

Traditionally, public service mandarins and public agencies are supposed to supply evidenced-based options and recommendation to government, and the elected representatives of the people – the government ministers -- make the decisions. Yet, as the welfare state has brought government interventions into to more and more areas of the economy, power has flowed to bureaucrats. Ministers no longer have the knowledge to understand public policy in all its ramifications. Yet, as Professor Klassen remarks the allowing of public health experts, educators, engineers and planners and other unaccountable officials to determine government policy is fundamentally undemocratic – a travesty of the principles of parliamentary government. In the words of Professor Klassen: government leaders need to "have the fortitude to set aside, at times, the specialized and rational calculations and recommendations of their officials".

A Tory conservative could not have said it any better. During the coronavirus epidemic, the abject submission of the Trudeau Liberal government to the supposedly knowledge-based pronouncements and directives of the World Health Organization and the Public Health Agency of Canada, without question, or any common sense appraisal and observation of the actual situation on the ground, is inexcusable. One can readily understand why a Prime Minister who has never managed anything in his life, might feel overwhelmed in a national crisis and be prone to listen and act upon so-called 'expert advice' without question, but that does not constitute an excuse.

The lack of competent political leadership at the top has been compounded in Canada by a relatively new practice of a periodic wholesale reshuffle of cabinet ministers, with a minister rarely serving more than two years in any portfolio. As a result, ministers have little opportunity to master their portfolio and become familiar with the policies of the department. They are absorbed in familiarizing themselves with, and carrying out, their day-to-day departmental responsibilities and duties. The negative effect of periodic cabinet shuffles has been further compounded by the feminist and multicultural agenda of the Trudeau government. That policy has resulted in a large number of novice ministers being appointed, on the basis of their gender, race and/or ethnicity, from among new parliamentarians who had little or no experience in management either in government or in the private sector. It was, and is, a recipe for bureaucrats taking over the running and direction of a department from a novice minister, and for the minister to be under the thumb of the Prime Minister's Office (PMO) with no power to question, influence, or dissent from any government action.

In times of crisis, there is no need to set aside parliament -- which has the function of questioning government decisions and overseeing government expenditures on behalf of the people -- solely because a government does not want to be hampered or criticized for its dispensing of public monies in support of the unemployed, distressed sectors of the economy, and social groups that the government wants to aid. The Parliament of Canada has shown, on two occasions during the coronavirus epidemic, that it could debate, improve, and expeditiously approve major spending programs in a one-day session; yet its role has been circumscribed by the manipulations of a Liberal government that does not want its policies and expenditures to be publicly questioned in parliament, and examined by parliamentary committees. In effect, Canadian democracy has suffered a double blow: unelected bureaucrats are directing government policy during a national crisis; and the representatives of the people have been effectively deprived of their powers, rights, and prerogatives of parliament in overseeing government programs and expenditures.

CEWS: Yesterday, Prime Minister Trudeau announced the Canada Emergency Wage Subsidy (CEWS) payroll support program is going to be extended from its original termination date of June 2nd to August 29th, a three month extension that effectively doubles the duration of that emergency program. It pays companies 75 percent of the wages of workers recalled to work, up to a maximum payment of $847 per week. Moreover, the eligibility requirements are going to be loosened to extend the benefits of the program to five new categories of employers: partnerships that are 50 percent owned by non-eligible members; Indigenous government-owned corporations that operate as businesses; registered amateur athletic organizations; registered journalism organizations; and private colleges and schools. Apparently the loosen of the criteria has been made in response to these businesses and organizations complaining that they were being excluded from the program due to various 'technicalities'.

Moreover, the Finance Minister, Bill Morneau, has revealed that the Liberal government has in contemplation the reduction of another CEWS eligibility requirement: that a company must have experienced a 30 percent or greater gross revenue loss due to the coronavirus lockdown. In effect, not only is the life of the temporary CEWS payroll subsidy program to be doubled, but the basic eligibility criteria for participating in the payroll subsidy program -- as approved by parliament -- are being watered down by the Liberal government. It appears that the Prime Minister Trudeau does not want to exclude any business or organization from the financial benefits of the program. The CEWS is being totally distorted from its original purpose which was to provide government financial aid to companies that had suffered a major financial loss owning to the coronavirus lockdowns, to encourage them to recall their workers and place them back on the payroll.

(Presumably, the Liberal government was hoping that the extension of the CEWS program would influence Air Canada to rescind its planned massive layoff of employees on June 7th. However, a week later, on May 22nd, Air Canada announced it would not be applying for the CEWS payroll support under the program extension. Upwards of 20,000 employees are being given the option of unpaid leave, resigning, or working reduced hours. Air Canadas workers who are laid off are eligible to access the Canada Emergency Response Benefit (CERB) of $2,000 per month. Air Canada intends to recall its employees only when border closures are relaxed and quarantine restrictions are no longer deemed necessary in the countries that it serves.)

Lockdown Panacea: An open letter from an Ottawa think-tank, the Macdonald-Laurier Institute -- dated May 14th and signed by twenty-four leading health professionals and business leaders -- is questioning the reliance of the federal Liberal governments solely on a national lockdown as the panacea needed to combat any further outbreaks of the coronavirus. While the provinces have been struggling to reopen their economies, Prime Minister Trudeau has been issuing warnings that the lockdown might have to be continued into July. Moreover, the letter accuses the Prime Minister 'of shifting the goal posts' in changing the metrics established for the re-opening of the economy.

Initially, the key metric for re-opening the economy was the ability of hospitals to respond to any new outbreak, but hospitals are now well below capacity and welcoming patients to their emergency departments. Yet, the federal government has changed the metric for re-opening the economy from a capacity to manage an outbreak, to a 'flattening the curve' and a policy of encouraging everyone to 'stay at home' to prevent the coronavirus from infecting anyone at all. Moreover, not only is the Prime Minister speaking of pushing the timeline for a return to full economic activity into the summer, he is claiming that the Canadian economy will not return to normal for a year or more.

The open letter accuses the federal Liberal government of "contributing to an atmosphere of fear" in maintaining that any premature lifting of the national lockdown may well result in a 'second wave' of infections; and that it will undo all that Canadians have sacrificed to achieve in enduring the lockdown. Moreover, the Liberal government insistence on social distancing as a panacea for preventing the transmission of the coronavirus during any re-opening of the economy, and as the only away to prevent the spreading of virus infections and fomenting another coronavirus wave, is too simplistic. Such a policy will greatly inhibit any economic recovery. There are other means of preventing infections and the spread of the virus.

The open letter is arguing that what is needed is a cost-benefit analysis of the cost of the economic damage being done in totally closing down the economy for a long term to avoid any serious risk of infection, and the risk of infection that would be incurred by keeping the economy going and employing more personal methods of reducing the threat of acquiring an infection. To date, the total lockdown of the Canadian economy has inflicted a severely heavy cost on Canadians with business, stores and industry shutdown, a massive unemployment with stock markets plummeting, and the Canadian, provincial, and municipal governments drowning in an unprecedently heavy debt load.

(Among the 'other means' for controlling the spread of the coronavirus, without the resort to a national lockdown, are: the maintenance of a ban on travellers from any country where there is a severe coronavirus outbreak, the wearing a face mask or face shield at work, the use of hand sanitizers, the disinfecting of common touch surfaces, the wearing of surgical gloves, and the placing of plexiglass panels between workers at stationary workstations, together with the avoiding of large crowds, the quarantining of the sick, a widespread testing program to identify asymptomatic carriers, and a tracking system to trace down, test and quarantine any infected contacts. These 'other means' can be used to control the spread of the coronavirus while re-opening the economy and getting people back to work.)

The open letter maintains that it is imperative for Canadians to get back to work without delay, and for businesses, shops and industries to re-open; that a national lockdown is no longer necessary, if indeed it ever was; that hospitals are now equipped to handle any local outbreaks; and that more limited lockdowns can be introduced in threatened areas to keep the local health-care system from being overwhelmed. Moreover, the letter notes that there is a "growing chorus" of medical professionals who are now questioning the necessity of maintain a strict national lockdown over several months as the panacea for combatting the spread of the coronavirus.

Whether the open letter will have any impact in influencing Prime Minister Justin Trudeau to abandon his belief in the need to prolong the Canadian provincial lockdowns, remains to be seen. The sad thing is that a national lockdown, and the terrible social and economic damage it has inflicted on Canadians and the Canadian economy, was avoidable to a large extent. The imposing of an immediate ban on foreign travellers entering Canada from countries where the coronavirus was raging, a limited lock down of any area in Canada with an outbreak, and a concerted effort to test, trace, to test, and quarantine any infected contacts, would have prevented the virus penetrating other areas of the country. Canadians could have continued to work and socialize in being isolated from an imported disease.

Research Funding: Prime Minister Justin Trudeau announced a new $450 million funding program to aid research institutions to stay open and keep their employees. According to the Prime Minister 'many labs were closed or at risk of imminently closing' and were in dire need of federal government financial support. The money will be provided through a federal grant programs, and is expected to act in the same manner as the CEWS payroll wage subsidy in paying up to 75 percent of the costs for "essential research-related activities" during the coronavirus crisis. This new laboratory research program appears to be rather ad hoc, and not well thought out, or clearly focussed. How does one define 'essential research', who will make that judgement, and has any account been taken of existing financial grants from government and private trusts that support laboratory research? Did anyone investigate the claim that 'many labs were closed or at risk of imminently closing'?

Income Tax: Prime Minister Trudeau has just announced that government benefits will not be cut off for anyone who does not file their income tax return by June 1st. The income tax filing deadline had already been extended from the traditional April 30th date to June 1st, and now the Prime Minister is saying do not worry about filing your income tax on time. He promised Canadians that all Canada Child Care Benefit (CCB) payments, and HST and GST tax refunds will continue to be paid until September, regardless of whether the individual has filed an income tax return by the June 2nd deadline. How is government going to continue to function with such a casual attitude on the part of the Prime Minister towards the responsibilities of the citizen and legal requirements of the Income Tax Act?

Sunday, May 17, 2020

A quiet day on the Victoria Day weekend.

Monday, May 18, 2020

Vaccine Development: A Massachusetts biotechnical company, Moderna, has announced an initial successful Phase I trial of a new coronavirus vaccine, called mRNA-1273. Forty-five healthy adults were given a low dose 25 micrograms) and eight adults were given a moderate dose (100 micrograms). The eight given a moderate dose produce large amounts of antibodies equal or greater to the blood level of virus-fighting antibodies in recovered COVID-19 patients. The drug has proven safe. The only side effect was found in three of the moderate dose cases displayed a fever, muscle pain, and headaches which disappeared after 24 hours. The second phase of clinical trials will start in July with 600 healthy volunteers, who will receive either a 50-microgram dose, a 250-microgram dose, or a placebo. That phase will test how the vaccine performs against COVID-19 outside of the laboratory and will enable the company to decide on the proper dose of vaccine. The Phase III clinical trial will be a test on thousands of patients. If all goes well, the "creditable objective" is to have doses of the vaccine available for emergency use by the fall of 2020, with a commercially available vaccine in 12 to 18 months.

The Moderna vaccine has been developed in collaboration with the National Institute of Allergy and Infectious Diseases (NIAID) in the United States. However, there is some skepticism among the scientific community regarding the effectiveness of mRNA-1273 as it does not activate the T-cells, and it is not clear that the level of antibody response is capable of providing a complete immunity to COVID-19. Based on its early promise, financial analysts are speculating that the vaccine could generate $10 billion per annum for the Moderna Inc. (Hopefully, the assessment of the financial return -- to the company and its investors – is based on being sold at moderate prices, rather than through price gouging.)

Tuesday, May 19, 2020

Child Care Support: It was reported today that the Social Development Minister, Ahmed Hessen, has been making calls for several weeks to childcare experts to determine how federal spending on child care can be targeted to aid in the restart of the economy. There is a concern as well of the health risk to children that needs to be addressed in helping child-care centres to re-open.

WHO Accountability: On Monday, during a virtual conference of the World Health Assembly, a coalition of 120 countries -- led by Australia and the European Union – supported a motion calling for an independent comprehensive examination of how the WHO coordinated the global response to the COVID-19 threat with respect to the accuracy of the information that was being received from China during the early outbreak of the coronavirus in Wuhan. Before the meeting, the proposed resolution was circulated and signed by 62 countries, including Canada, rather belatedly. Among the contentious issues demanding investigation are: how did the coronavirus originate in humans, did China deliberately cover up the dangerous nature and high level of contagiousness of the coronavirus during the early stages of the Wuhan outbreak, and did the World Healthy Agency willingly, or unwittingly, repeat the misleading diagnoses being provided by China?

On the one hand, the U.S. administration has repeatedly charged that the coronavirus was developed in the laboratory of the Wuhan Institute of Virology in a study of potential viruses, and that it subsequently leaked into the adjacent wet market in Wuhan which has been established as the source of the original coronavirus outbreak. To the contrary, there are scientists who are saying – speculating – that the virus spread from bats to human in the wet market of Wuhan, possibility through a transference through another animal, such as the pangolin.

Secondly, President Trump and the American administration has repeatedly accused the WHO leadership of concealing the extent of the coronavirus epidemic within China during its early stages, and of initially downplaying the highly contagious nature of the virus which left the developed countries unprepared for what was to come. Surprisingly, France, South Korea, South Africa, and Germany have expressed support for the WHO, and the European Union has refrained from criticizing the WHO leadership.

An oversight advisory committee established by the United Nations to look into whether the WHO warning system for alerting the world to outbreaks, is "inadequate", concluded that the member states might need "to reassess" the role of the WHO in providing travel advice to member countries. Yet, the report concluded that such an investigation should not be undertaken "in the heat of the moment". (This is a typical bureaucrat response – blame no one, infer that the system may be inadequate, and suggest that there may be a need for a reassessment but at some time in the future.)

The Director-General of the World Health Organization, Tedros Adhanom Ghebreyesus – an Ethiopian public health researcher and former Minister of Foreign Affairs for that country – declared that he welcomed such an investigation. He stated that he will personally lead an independent evaluation of the response of the WHO "at the earliest appropriate moment". (Does that look promising? Tedros is offering to lead an investigation of his own conduct and competence.) On its part, China has called for a comprehensive review of the global response "based on science and professionalism and conducted in an objective and impartial manner", to be led by the WHO. (It sounds good, but how 'objective and impartial' would an investigation be of the WHO by the WHO?)

To its credit, China has announced that it will contribute $2 billion dollars to the WHO to help control further outbreaks in Third-World countries, and to aid in their economic recovery. China has begun shipping medical supplies to over fifty African countries threated by the coronavirus, and currently has forty-six medical teams on the ground in African countries to combat the virus. However, the United States government has allocated $9 billion to coronavirus containment efforts worldwide. Moreover, the United States has been contributing over $400 million (US) a year to the WHO – the largest contributor – which accounts for one third of its budget. President Trump has threatened to withdraw the United States financial support of the WHO, but he has not done so to date.

(With China promising $2 billion over two years to the WHO -- which has a $2.3 billion per annum budget -- it is highly unlikely that any investigation by the WHO into its early response to the COVID-19 outbreak in Wuhan, China, and its relationship with China, will ever be thoroughly investigated and reported on. Australia, which played the leading role in promoting the resolution calling for an investigation of the WHO response to the coronavirus threat, is now paying the price. Two days after the World Health Assembly meeting, it was announced that China has imposed an embargo on Australia beef imports and is threatening to place a substantial tariff on barley imports from Australia.)

More generally, Director-General Tedros has commented that 'lessons have been learned' during the coronavirus pandemic, but he has yet to explain what specific lessons have been learned. He did exclaim that the coronavirus pandemic has exposed "the fault lines, inequalities, injustices and contradictions of our modern world. And geopolitical divisions have been thrown into sharp belief". One suspects that what we have here is a thinly veiled resentment – when speaking of 'injustices' -- felt by a Third-World politician at the material wealth and prosperity of the developed countries of the world and the well-being and high standard of living of their peoples. This language of 'injustice' ignores the facts that the peoples of the developed world created their wealth through their own efforts, and that the billions of dollars in economic aid and health services is being provided to Third-World peoples through United Nations agencies is largely funded by the developed nations. (All too often, whatever the magnitude of the aid given to the Third-World nations by the developed nations, it is never regarded as being enough, and there is little gratitude publicly expressed by the recipient governments.)

One of the motions passed by the World Health Assembly during the virtual conference, contained wording about giving poor countries the right to waive patent rights. (What we have here in embryo is an international organization, dominated by Third-World countries, moving towards giving poor countries a right to pirate the property of private companies.)

Vaccine Development: At the virtual conference of the World Health Assembly, the Who expressed a concern that a global agreement be forged to achieve a fair and affordable manufacture and distribution of any coronavirus vaccine that might be developed. The European Union proposed that a voluntary patent pool be established to encourage pharmaceutical companies to surrender their patents to enable all countries to be able to manufacture and distribute an affordable vaccine. This is noble thought on the part of the Modern liberals of the European Union leadership. However, as was the case with the 19th century socialists, Modern liberals are quick to espouse an equitable sharing of the products of the developed countries, as long as it is the property of someone else that is to be taken and distributed. (One doubts that these EU representatives would sell their own property to help finance the purchase of vaccines for the peoples of the poor nations.)

Patent property rights need to be respected. However, that does not preclude governments from bringing pressure to bear -- on any private pharmaceutical company that develops a successful vaccine -- to have the vaccine sold at a moderate price to avoid profiteering, and to make the vaccine available at a low price and for a rapid distribution to any poor Third-World country that experiences a major coronavirus outbreak in future.

Personal Protective Equipment Inquiry: A House of Commons Committee investigating why there was a critical shortage of personal protective equipment during the coronavirus epidemic has questioned a Vice-President of Public Health Agency Canada (PHAC), which is responsible for maintaining the National Emergency Strategic Stockpile (NESS) of supplies that the federal and provincial governments might require during national emergency In her testimony, the representative of the PHAC declared that the National Emergency Strategic Stockpile was not meant to back up the provincial health care system; that the PHAC did not focus on personal protective equipment "because we count on our provinces, within their respective authority, to maintain their stockpile; and that the focus of the PHAC is on responding to natural disasters or terrorist attacks, as well as on stockpiling vaccines for rare diseases and antibiotics for dangerous chemicals.

The PHAC representative stated that the NEES is run by eighteen people; that it has a $18 million budge per annum, and that the stockpile is stored in eight warehouses in six centres across Canada. The Committee demanded to know why two million N-95 respiratory masks were thrown out at the end of last year. They were told that the masks were nearly ten years old and beyond their useful date. When a Committee member asked what supplies the NESS currently has in stock, the members were told that there is no up-to-date inventory. Committee members found it incredible that a detailed up-to-date inventory of the NEES stockpile did not exist. (The more likely explanation is that PHAC is denying that it has an up-to-date stockpile inventory to prevent having to reveal to the Committee the actual depleted state of the national stockpile.)

In reviewing newspaper accounts of the testimony of the Vice-President of the Public Health Agency Canada, one cannot help wondering why the parliamentary Committee did not demand to know what types and volumes of supplies were held in the national stockpile depots prior to the 16 tonnes of personal protective equipment and ventilators being removed and shipped to China in February 2020, and whether the Public Health Canada Agency protested that political decision by the federal Liberal government. Secondarily, one wonders why the parliamentary Committee did not consult the Canadian government website that sets forth the mandate and responsibility of the Public Health Agency Canada for maintaining and restocking the National Emergency Strategic Stockpile, to verify or discredit her testimony.

National Emergency Strategic Stockpile: According to the Government of Canada website, the National Emergency Strategic Stockpile (NESS) "contains supplies that the provinces and territories can request in emergencies, such as infectious disease outbreaks, national disasters and other public health events, when their own resources are not enough. These supplies include a variety of items such as: pharmaceuticals, and social service supplies, such as beds and blankets.

The Public Health Agency of Canada (PHAC) maintains the NESS, and PHAC continuously assesses the composition of the stockpile and refurbishes the supplies that are distributed.

NESS facilities consist of a central depot in the National Capital Region; and warehouses strategically located across Canada."

According to the Government of Canada website, the NESS stockpile includes "medical equipment and supplies, such as ventilators, stretchers, x-ray machines, mini-clinics for triage and minor treatment, and personal protective equipment, including masks, gloves and disposable gowns".

(Enough said! The effort of the House of Commons Committee to determine why there was a critical shortage of personal protective equipment during the coronavirus epidemic, is clearly being thwarted by the obfuscations and deliberately misleading statements being introduced through the testimony of the Public Health Agency of Canada representative.)

Lockdown Lessons: A National Post journalist, Richard Warnica, has produced an overview of the response of the Province of Ontario to the coronavirus epidemic and the lessons to be learned. With the Ontario entering the first phase of the re-opening of the economy after a two-month lockdown, and with coronavirus cases on a downward trajectory, there remains a major problem in continuing to contain the coronavirus and prevent future outbreaks. (The Warnica article summarizes the conclusions already reached by the author in previous diary entries, but it presents a useful summary framework based on the independent research of Warnica. (For the author's earlier conclusions, see the diary entry on South Korea, Chapter Three, April 18, 2020.)

Infectious disease experts are concerned that Ontario has yet to set forth clear benchmarks in a plan to identify and isolate infected personals before they can cause a cluster of infections, or a major outbreak, during the re-opening of the economy and the restoration of social activities following on the gradual lifting of the lockdown. Elsewhere, such as in South Korean and Australia in particular, a four-layered plan has been developed which consists of: testing, contact tracing, isolation, and support.

Initially, Ontario locked down the province -- as did the other provinces and many countries worldwide -- to get the outbreak under control, with the intention of lifting the lockdown when the daily number of new coronavirus cases began to follow a consistently downward daily trend. However, that next stage requires a plan to quickly identify and isolate any new case of infection. In the words of a University of Ottawa epidemiologist: "The goal is to prevent one case from becoming an outbreak and to prevent an outbreak from becoming an epidemic".

The first step is proactive testing for the coronavirus. In Ontario, the worldwide shortage of testing kits, has forced the province to be reactive in confining its testing to individuals showing flu-like symptoms and frontline workers and personal care workers and residents of long-care homes who are highly vulnerable to the coronavirus. The intention is to isolate the coronavirus among these groups working in environments where they could rapidly spread their infection if asymptomatic. However, what is needed is a surveillance testing that randomly tests a large segment of the provincial population to proactively track down infected individuals and clusters of infection.

The second step is contact tracking to identify, locate, and test any individuals who may have been exposed to the virus through contact with an infected individual, so that those who test positive can self-isolate and receive health care support if they develop symptoms of the disease. Ontario has established teams to engage in contact tracking, but as yet there have been no reports on the contact tracking work of these teams, and no reports as to whether Ontario is developing, or adopting, a smartphone tracking app to trace contacts with an infected person. The province has declared that it has a goal of identifying and reaching all contacts of a confirmed case within 24-hours so that they can be tested. Currently, the Ontario government maintains that the goal is being reached by its local tracking units, most of the time, but there is no central Ontario database recording the contacts and whatever follow-up support is being provided.

The third step is to isolate the infected and any of his or her contacts that test positive, but problems remain in that the self-isolation is voluntary and many individuals are unable to completely self-isolate. Persons who test positive for the coronavirus may live with a family in a small house with a common bathroom and dining room where self-isolation from family is impossible, and homeless people have nowhere to isolate. What is needed is a program to establish quarantine stations, such as in empty hotels, where infected persons could be isolated in a separate room with separate washroom facilities.

The last step is to provide medical and personal care workers to tend to the infected persons in isolation, with a system of providing them with needed foods and medicines, so that they can remain in isolation and do not have to venture out into to procure them. Having established quarantine stations in empty hotels would facilitate the providing of a support system.

Currently, Ontario is struggling to greatly expand the scope of its testing into the broader population, and has tracking units employed in tracking the contacts of infected persons, but the province has not provided any quarantine facilities for those who cannot self-isolate at home, and no dedicated medical support teams to provide support for infected individuals in quarantine.

(Three days later, on Friday, May 22nd, Prime Minister Trudeau announced that the federal government would fund provincial efforts to test Canadians for COVID-19 and to support provincial tracking programs.)

Ontario has been focusing its testing and tracking on front line medical support personnel and is about to commence a second round of testing on staff and residents of long-care homes with teams of trackers deployed to identify contacts exposed to an infected person. However, Ontario is currently failing to meet its goal of 16,000 tests per day. To date the Statistics Canada has staff employed as interviewers, who are making calls -- in working with the Ontario tracking teams – to contact person at risk who have been exposed to an infected person.

Chapter Nine

Wednesday, May 20, 2020

Border Closures: Canada and the United States have extended the ban on non-essential travel across their common border for another thirty days until June 21st. Only essential trade, commerce and essential employees are currently able to cross the border. Canada sought the extension of the border crossing ban as the United States is currently 'a source of vulnerability' for the spread of the coronavirus. Currently, the United States has 1.5 million active COVID-19 cases – 42 percent of the world's active cases. It has recorded a total of 90,000 coronavirus related deaths, and the death rate has reach 1,000 per day and continues to grow. Moreover, many U.S. states are ending their lockdown and re-opening their economies, which will result in asymptomatic persons freely circulating within that country.

When it will be deemed safe to re-open the U.S.-Canadian border remains a matter of pure conjecture. Dr. Theresa Tam, Chief of the Public Health Agency of Canada, has commented that travel restrictions will have to be eased within Canada first, to gauge the impact before the international border is reopened. It is the policy that the European Union is currently following in reopening borders within Europe -- among its western member states -- while maintaining a ban on international travel into Europe. It makes good sense with the coronavirus now spreading to eastern Europe and Third-World countries.

General Recovery: Italy, which recorded 226.699 coronavirus cases, 32,169 deaths, and 129,401 recovered cases – currently the third highest death total after the U.S. and Britain -- has experienced a significant decline in new cases and is lifting the lockdown that was imposed in March. After a ten-week lockdown, Italy has opened cafes, shops, outdoor patios, bars, restaurants, beauty salons, hairdressers, and churches, as well as beaches. Over 60 percent of the people, and most of the children, are wearing face masks in public, people are practicing social distancing, and restaurants have table two metres apart, and bars are urging their patrons to stay a metre apart. Travel between regions is banned until June 3rd, when the Italian borders will be open to European visitors. Italy is one of the first European countries to re-open its economy after the coronavirus pandemic and, to date, there has been no second wave outbreak of the coronavirus.

Oil Industry: With the lifting of the lockdown in China, and Chinese transportation and manufacturing industries returning almost to their pre-coronavirus pandemic levels of economic activity, the Chinese demand for oil soared to 13 billion barrels a day, which all but matches the pre-pandemic level of Chinese purchases. Russia and Saudi Arabia are maintaining their agreed lower levels of output, which is enabling oil prices to begin to recover in North America. In India, the sale of diesel fuels is 75 percent higher than it was during the first two weeks of May; and an oil tanker has recently left British Columbia for China with a load of Canadian crude oil transported to the coast along the Trans-Mountain Pipeline.

The oil industry is showing signs of a revival with crude oil prices in the United States reaching $30 U.S. per barrel, a level at which oil companies can avoid operating losses. It puts Canadian oil companies in a sustainable holding pattern, until demand returns, and prices rise with the recovery of the North American market.

However, the twin blows of the plummeting of world oil prices, and the collapse of domestic oil demand during the coronavirus lockdown, has severely damaged the Canadian oil industry. Planned expenditures have been cut by 40 percent, or $10 billion in total, for this year; the cash flow of the industry has been reduced by $25.3 billion; and the industry is facing $6.5 billion in debt maturity by the end of 2021.

Face Masks: One of the most contentious issues in the response worldwide to the coronavirus threat, according to the Ontario Medical Association, is the wearing of non-medical face masks. The crux of the issue for health authorities is that there is no positive scientific evidence that face masks "prevent even a limited amount of transmission of COVID-19". Nonetheless, the OMA is recommending the wearing of home-made and non-medical face masks for whatever good they might do in preventing the spread of the coronavirus, together with social spacing, and the practicing of good hygiene, during the recovery phases.

What we have here is a reference to the 'lack of scientific proof' argument used at an earlier date by Dr. Theresa Tam, Chief of the Public Health Agency of Canada. She had maintained during the initial stage of the coronavirus outbreaks in Canada, that Canadians in good health and asymptomatic Canadian did not need to wear face masks when in public. In defence of her position, she cited the lack of any scientific studies proving the efficacy of non-medical face masks in preventing infections. Yet, the physical evidence of the effectiveness of face masks in preventing coronavirus infection is overwhelming in countries where the wearing of the face masks was made compulsory during the early stages of the COVID-19 pandemic. As of early April, even Dr. Tam came to realize the value of face masks when she reversed herself, and proclaimed that non-medical face masks were "an additional measure that you can take to protect others around you".

Today, it was announced by Dr. Tam that Public Health Canada is recommending that people wear face masks – the medical or cotton face mask – in situations where a physical spacing is not possible or practicable. Although Dr. Tam has cautioned that the wearing of a face mask does not negate the need to continue to give a priority to social spacing and to hand washing. Public Health Canada is recommended that these measures be continued throughout the remainder of the spring and through the summer.

South Korean, Taiwan and Hong Kong have proved beyond a doubt that the compulsory wearing of non-medical face masks over an entire population can very effectively limit the spread of the coronavirus, and there is a lot of anecdotal evidence as well. A letter to the editor, in the Ottawa Citizen newspaper, has pointed out that in Berkeley, California (population 122,000) where face masks were made compulsory on April 17th, only 67 cases of coronavirus have been reported since and but one death; whereas in the City of Ottawa (population 900,000) -- where only a very small proportion of the community are wearing face masks -- there are currently 1,692 coronavirus cases and 178 deaths have occurred.

The wearing of face masks has been made compulsory in the City of Los Angeles outside of the home, in France on the metro transit and high schools, and on public transit in European countries. In the United States, the State of Maine has taken the lead in making it compulsory to wear a face mask in grocery and retail stores, pharmacies, parking lots, and line ups for takeout food and for taking a ferry, bus or train. Germany has made the wearing of a face mask compulsory in public. In Ontario, the provincial government is 'urging' all public transit riders to wear a face mask or covering, except for children under two years of age.

Social Promotion in Education: On May 20th, Premier Ford of Ontario announced that the opening of elementary schools in the province would be postponed until September, when the secondary schools will re-open as well. Where the re-opening of the elementary schools is concerned, Premier Ford exclaimed: "I'm just not going to risk it". At the same time, the Premier announced that report cards will be prepared for the present school year and students will be allowed to pass to the next school year, and those in their final year of elementary school or high school, will be allowed to graduate. Some students are being home schooled during the coronavirus lockdown, and others not, but there will be not tests to determine how far they have advanced in keeping with the curriculum. There has been a mention of the first month of school in September being devoted to reviewing what should have been learned during the present school year.

Apparently, no consideration is being given to having students repeat their school year to learn the skills, to gain the requisite knowledge, and to understanding the concepts, that they would have been taught according to the curriculum for their current school year. Owing to the coronavirus lockdown, students will miss upwards of 65 school days to the end of June – almost one-third of the minimum requirement of 194 days of school each year under the provincial Education Act. The assumption that all students ought to be promoted each year regardless of whatever they have learned, or have not learned, and regardless of their level of achievement and intellectual development, is based on a 'social promotion' policy that has become established in the Province of Ontario.

For decades Ontario has followed a politically correct social promotion system where every child is promoted into the next grade each year regardless of their intellectual development, comprehension of the curriculum, grade appropriate knowledge, or application in class. The aim seems to avoid any child being labelled as a failure. It sounds good but the reality is that promoting children who have not mastered the basic learning of the previous grade curriculum condemns them to continually falling behind, to their becoming increasingly frustrated and sullen, and distanced. It almost invariable leads to low self- esteem in their being unable to match their fellow classmates in their school assignments. It turns classrooms into a breeding ground of discontent and anger against the school and teachers among an ever-growing minority of students who are disengaged, frustrated and angry against the system which is evident in the growing number of attacks on teachers.

If educators are looking for the source of the growing turmoil in the classroom, and the disrespect and anger directed towards teachers by frustrated students, they might start looking at the social promotion policy and the students who have been promoted beyond their learning competence and the basic knowledge requisite at each level of school. Another detriment of the social promoting by age policy is that it precludes intellectually gifted students from skipping a year to be exposed to a more challenging learning environment. Intellectually gifted students who are bored, can be just as disruptive in a classroom as the weak students who have been promoted beyond their learning competence.

In a letter to the local newspaper, a writer provided personal information on the catastrophic impact of the social promotion policy of pushing students forward based on their chronological age, rather than basing promotions on the extent to which a student has acquired the knowledge, skills and concepts that will be built upon at the next grade level. The writer cited the case of an elementary school student who was placed in Grade Six, after missing upwards of 30 days each year during the previous school years. Unable to cope, a tutor was hired for the student. It was found that the student was functioning at a Grade Three level. Hence, the tutor went back to the Third Grade curriculum which served as a base for an accelerated learning program that taught the content and inculcated an understanding of the subsequent curriculum subjects each year, until the student could function at the Grade Six level. Promoting a student beyond his or her level of competence and learning ability can only lead to behavioural problems, poor school performance, and psychological problems, and result in the student becoming a dropout.

Some years ago in California, the parents of a student who had graduated from high school sued the School Board for derelict of its educational responsibilities. Their son had attended school each day, year by year, had benefited from a social promotion system, and after his graduation from high school, it was discovered that the son had never learned to read and write. It was an extreme case, but all too revealing of the lack of attention to whether each and every student is actually learning anything in class and developing the requisite skills. Another phenomenon that covers up the failure of the social promotion by age policy, is the lack of testing. The author can remember having spelling tests and arithmetic tests each week in elementary school, as well as having in class reading assignments – passages of stories to be read out loud in class with different students reading different sections. If a student were struggling, and in need of extra help, the teacher quickly became aware of it. Streaming of students according to their level of advancement also benefitted the more advanced students who need more challenging assignments, as well as the poorer students who need to advance at a slower pace with more attention and learning support from the teacher.

In Ontario, the problem posed by students lagging far behind their prescribed level of studies, and the learning required to advance to the next higher grade -- as a result of missing upwards of four months of schooling this year due to the COVID-19 closure of the schools -- will be masked by promoting all of the students together. However, when these students arrive at a higher level of education -- whether high school, college, or university -- the real problems will emerge. It would be better to have elementary and high school students repeat this school year, as yet another harsh consequence of the coronavirus pandemic, than to just promote them, or let them graduate to go on to a community college or university where they will arrive ill-prepared and prone to failure.

Canada Emergency Business Account: Yesterday, Prime Minister Trudeau announced a modification in the eligibility rules governing access to the $25 billion Canada Emergency Business Account (CEBA) program, which provides a $40,000 interest-free loan to small businesses who apply. To encourage repayment, 25 percent of the loan is forgivable, if repayment is made before the end of 2022. (The logic here is rather odd. Why would anyone bother to repay a loan when there are no interest payments required to service the loan? A better approach to secure repayment would have been to grant a two-year interest free grace period, followed by the imposition of an escalating interest rate charge on the loan until it is repaid.)

The Canadian Federation of Independent Business had complained that the eligibility rule requiring that a small business must have a payroll and a business bank account to qualify for the CEBA program, was blocking many small businesses from securing the business loan. In response, the two eligibility requirements have been removed. Among the small businesses that are now eligible for the program, are self-employed, independent contractors and professionals such as physiotherapists, hair dressers who rent a chair, contract trainers in health clubs and gyms, and personal trainers, etc., who were put out of business by the coronavirus lockdown, and many of whom use a personal bank account for their small business. Similarly, small family-run businesses that pay their members through dividends, are now eligible for the CEBA program loan.

Critics are pointing out that the loans are better than nothing, but that outright grants to small businesses are what is needed. That loan repayments will add to the financial burden faced by small businesses -- many of which are heavily indebted –and will impede their recovery from the lockdown.

Among the remaining eligibility requirements are that the small business applicants must have an active bank account, a Canada Revenue Agency business number, a 2018 or 2019 tax return, and an employment income of between $20,000 and $1.5 million per annum, and non-deferrable overhead expenses such as rent, property taxes, utilities and insurance. Unions, charities, and religious or fraternal organizations, as well as small businesses owned by members of Parliament are not eligible for the CEBA program assistance.

Among the other benefits of the CEBA program are the deferral of Sales Tax remittances and customs duty payments on imported goods. As expressed by Prime Minister Trudeau, eligibility rules for accessing the program needed to be modified to aid the small businesses who were 'falling through the cracks'. The intention of the $40,000 loan benefit is to enable the borrower to meet non-deferrable operating expenses during the coronavirus lockdown.

Airports: The Ottawa Citizen newspaper has a story on the changes that are being introduced at the Ottawa International Airport in anticipation of the recovery of air travel. At present the airport has only ten scheduled daily flights, mostly to Toronto, with 200 passengers using the terminal as opposed to a maximum of 7,000 daily passengers in normal times, and 5.1 million per annum. Airport management sees its major task in a recovery process being to convince travellers that airports and planes are safe, and to assuage any fears of contacting the coronavirus. At present, 60 percent of the people surveyed in Canada and the United States are not prepared to fly just now.

Among the steps taken to protect and reassure the public are a Transport Canada mandated wearing of face masks by all staff and passengers, and the enforcing of spacing at check-in counters, restaurants, bank machines and taxi queues, and plexiglass shields at service counters. Pre-boarding temperature checks will be made -- with anyone recording a temperature of 37.6 Celsius or above being advised to obtain a medical certificate clearance. Passengers will have to fill out a health questionnaire, and anyone displaying COVID-19 type symptoms will be denied boarding of the plane.

Airport authorities are predicting that there will be a post-pandemic emphasis on the efficient and expeditious processing of air travellers at airports to avoid line-ups; that there will be fewer flight options for the accommodation of fewer passengers; that there will be longer turnaround times owing to the need to clean and disinfect airplane cabins after each flight, and that the planes will be smaller. During the coronavirus epidemic, the Ottawa International Airport authority has borrowed money to maintain its limited services, has halted new capital spending projects, has decreased employee wages, and has greatly reduced its energy consumption and costs.

(There was no mention of limiting the number of tickets sold for each flight to maintain a social spacing of passengers on the plane. Clearly, the consensus is that airlines cannot survive financially if they fly at one-third or one-half of their capacity to adhere to a social spacing policy.)

CERB Fraud: The Canada Emergency Response Benefit (CERB) is a financial aid program that all parties in the House of Commons have enthusiastically supported as a means of providing financial support to the millions of Canadians in need who lost their jobs with the coronavirus shutdown. However, now concerns are being publicly expressed on all sides as to who is getting the CERB payments, and suspicions are being expressed that there is widespread fraud being tolerated through a lax administration by the Liberal government.

According to a Statistics Canada report published on April 18th, two million Canadians had lost their job during the coronavirus lockdown, and 2.5 million were working less than half of their normal house since the lockdown – a potential of 5.5 million individuals who could qualify for a CERB payment. However, as of April 19th, 6.73 million Canadians were receiving a CERB payment with $19.8 billion having been paid out for under that program. In effect, there is an obvious discrepancy of a million payments per month between those who could legitimately qualify for the CERB payment and those who are receiving it. With the standard CERB payment of $2,000 per month, a potential one million fraudulent claims could be costing the government $2 billion which, over the four months of the program will result in $8 billion in fraudulent payments made with borrowed money. Moreover, the number of CERB payments by mid-May is now close to eight million.

What several critics of the Liberal government are pointing out is that when you declare publicly that everyone who applies for the CERB program with receive the payment without question, you are inviting people to commit a fraud. It invites people to apply for the CERB payments regardless of whether they meet the eligibility criteria or not. As one former Statistics Canada economist commented: "the capacity for abuse or opportunistic behaviour in this program is enormous".

Auditor-General's Office: Karen Hogan, the former Assistant Auditor-General for Canada, has been nominated for the post of Auditor-General, with the appointment pending approval by Parliament. She declared that with financial aid programs, such as the CERB, there is a need to have a mechanism in place to allow the government to identify fraud and recoup the money. However, Hogan declared that a shortage of funds has hampered the ability of the Auditor-General's Office to fulfill its function to conduct a proper audit of government programs. Moreover, with the reports of fraud in the CERB program, the sample size for an audit of that program will have to be expanded beyond what would normally be investigated in auditing any government program. Hence, the Auditor-General's Office will need more funding to expand the scope of the audit of the CERB – the costliest financial aid program in Canadian history.

Hogan called also for the establishment of an independent funding mechanism to avoid the Attorney-General's Office having to ask the government, which it audits, for a budget increase to conduct the necessary audits. Currently, the Attorney-General's Office reports directly to the Minister of Finance. (One can foresee the CERB audit being derailed at some point! Those in power never let their mistakes, miscalculations, and stupidities be investigated and exposed to public scrutiny.)

Thursday, May 21, 2020

Sweden: Today, it was reported that Sweden has overtaken the United States, Italy, the United Kingdom and Belgium, with the highest per capital death rate in the world during the coronavirus pandemic. Currently,

Sweden has an average daily death rate of 6.08 per million inhabitants per day, versus the U.K(5.57), Belgium (4.28), and the U.S. (4.1). In Sweden, the government was more worried about the impact of the coronavirus on the economy and welfare costs, and has relied basically on the health care service and the encouraging of the practice of social distancing and basic hygiene, to combat the coronavirus. Sweden relied on the common sense of Swedes to self-isolate if they felt endangered, and to take precautions against unnecessarily risking exposure to the virus; a secondary strategy was to protect the 'vulnerable'.

Gatherings of more than 50 persons were banned, high schools, colleges and universities were closed, and citizens over 70 years of age, and those with underlying medical conditions that rendered them highly susceptible to the coronavirus were urged to self-isolate. Elementary schools, most restaurants, businesses, workplaces, shopping malls, and gyms remained open. A ban on foreign nationals entering Sweden was imposed on March 19th, with an exemption given to citizens of the European Union, and the associated European Economic Area countries (Iceland, Liechtenstein, and Norway). Swedish citizens have been allowed to return from abroad, and the border has remained open to diplomats, health care workers, and the workers employed in the transport of goods in supply chains.

To date, Sweden (population 10.10 million), has 32,809 coronavirus cases, with 3,025 deaths, and 4, 971 recovered. Despite refusing to resort to a national lockdown, Sweden was not struck by a wave of coronavirus cases far beyond that of any other country, has not suffered any major economic dislocations, and has not accumulated a massive national debt in providing financial aid to its citizens and businesses. Over 70 percent of Swedes support the non-lockdown policy, including politicians, the media, and the public health agency. Young people are reportedly pleased that the economy has not been destroyed or a heavy national debt incurred, and that they have been allowed to get on with their lives. The point being made is that 'everyone was told of the risk'. To date, opposition to Sweden's approach to the COVID-19 pandemic has been confined, for the most part, within the academic and the science communities.

How could Sweden have done better, while still avoiding the imposition of a lockdown, comes down to several basic shortcomings. There was a lack of awareness that asymptomatic persons could be virus carriers, which could not be remedied until known. Moreover, there was no pre-influenza preparedness in strictly applying the approaches taken years earlier to contain the Spanish flu (wearing face masks, social distancing, avoiding crowds, washing hands, and self-isolating if sick) and the more recent Swine flu (travel restrictions, avoiding visiting high risk areas, disinfecting breakout areas, and directing the sick to self-isolate and contact a doctor). Nonetheless, without the imposition of a nation lockdown, the number of coronavirus cases in Sweden has not been excessive by any measure.

Canadian Lockdown: In Canada, several generations of Canadians will be paying for the potential $400 billion deficit for the year 2020 in spending incurred through providing financial aid to Canadian citizens, businesses, and industries during the COVID-19 lockdown. Moreover, despite the national lockdown, to date Canada has 81,765 coronavirus cases, 6,180 deaths, and 41,986 recovered, within a population of 37.7 million people. Canadians have suffered severely health wise, in job losses, and in damage to their businesses and industries due to the failure of the federal Liberal government to impose -- in February -- a ban on foreign nationals entering Canada, and a screening and testing of returning Canadians and permanent residents and a mandatory quarantining of anyone testing positive. Instead the Liberal government let political correctness hold sway in not wanting to single out foreign travellers of a particular ethnicity/race – initially Chinese nationals, and subsequently Italians and Iranians -- as being potential carriers of the coronavirus and who needed to be immediately banned from entering Canada.

One can only conclude that the governments who imposed a national lockdown on their economies in forcing their citizens to stay home, were engaging in a drastic overreaction to the coronavirus threat, and needlessly badly damaged their national economy and the social and economic well-being of their people. To the contrary, an immediate ban on the entry into the country of foreign nationals from infected countries, together with the introduction of elementary safe health practices –

social distancing, an emphasis on the washing of hands, an enhanced disinfecting and cleaning of common areas of contact by the public, and the wearing of face masks, together with the introduction of a tracking system to identify and test all contacts, with the testing and a mandatory quarantining of all who tested positive, would have sufficed to prevent the spread of COVID-19 when detected. All of these approaches were known to be effective in preventing the spread of a virus -- historically from the Spanish flu experience and, more immediately, with respect to the protocols successfully implemented in Taiwan and South Korea to curb the spread of the coronavirus.

Restaurants: The City of Ottawa is seeking to address a critical problem that restaurants are anticipating during a re-opening phase: viz. that it will be uneconomic and unstainable for restaurants to maintain a two-metre social spacing between diners, which will cut their potential income from one-third to one-half. The City is now proposing to allow restaurants to use the adjacent street space for outdoor patios, whenever they will be allowed to re-open. It is not clear whether that proposal envisages the closure of city streets in restaurant areas, or merely a narrowing of the road width, or both options. Another proposal is that the city allow the setting up of temporarily roofed patios for weather protection, and the use of propane heaters to extend the patio dining season well into the fall. One major problem identified by the local restaurant owners' organization is the shortage of personal protective equipment for their serving and kitchen staffs. At present, restaurants owners are competing with large companies to secure personal protective gear for their employees.

Personal Protective Equipment: With Canadian companies now producing high-quality personal protective equipment, and the vital importance of plastic face shields, face masks, and gloves in protecting staff, business professionals, workers, customers and clients, in re-opened businesses, industries, shops, and private practices, why has the federal government not directed the Canadian Standards Association (CSA) to test and give their stamp of approval to face masks that are capable of preventing the passage of the coronavirus. The CSA tests hockey face protectors, and helmets to ensure that they meet safety standards, and the CSA mark is placed on them to re-assure consumers of the safety of the product. Why is that not being done with the face masks being sold to Canadians.

One of the great scandals of the coronavirus epidemic, as yet unrecognized, is that tens of thousands or more of poor quality face masks -- some of which are totally incapable of preventing the passage of the coronavirus -- are being offered for sale to Canadians on the Internet. One has only to consult the numerous complaints in the ratings provided by purchasers of face masks -- on Amazon -- to realize that the millions of face masks from China, which western governments have rejected as being of a poor quality or of a material ineffective in screening out the coarnavirus, are now being sold to the public on the Internet. With Canadians now being advised by the federal, provincial, and municipal governments to wear face masks when out in the public, why are there not Canadian Standards Association (CSA) approved face masks to purchase? Also why is there not a government effort to ensure that fabric shops are open for Canadians who want to make their own face masks? And why has the garment industry in Canada not been engaged to make suitable non-medical cloth face masks, for approval and sale, to Canadians?

The lack of leadership and initiative at the federal government level is appalling. Other than devising ways to distribute billions of dollars in financial aid to victims of the coronavirus lockdown – to an ever-growing list of companies, social groups, and individual Canadians -- the federal government has done little. It has left the combatting of the coronavirus to the provincial and municipal governments, to medical personnel, first responders, and personal care workers on the ground, as well as to volunteer efforts by companies and individuals in devoting their own resources and support to the struggle against the coronavirus.

City of Ottawa: A health survey of coronavirus cases has revealed that the virus is present in all twenty-three city wards. Except for several long-care homes and retirement residencies, there are no outbreak clusters. The municipal health authority supports the relaxation of restrictions with the aim of achieving "some balance back in terms of employment and social connections" but cautions that the virus might take off again. Hence, the expressed need to maintain a social spacing of at least two metres when out in public, and to wear a face mask or face covering when unable to maintain a strict social spacing. On its part, the City of Ottawa extended the ban on social events, festivals, and cultural programming until the end of August. To date, the nation's capital, Ottawa, has had 1,849 coronavirus cases in total, 210 coronavirus-related deaths, and has 24 on-going outbreaks in institutions which comprises long-care homes and retirement residents, and several hospitals.

United Nations Politics: During the World Health Assembly virtual meeting at which the WHO Director-General Tedros, with the support of China, emasculated the Assembly resolution calling for an independent investigation of the response of WHO to the coronavirus situation in China, there was secondary issue playing out. Australia and the other developed countries, including Canada, tried to secure Taiwan the status of an observer at the World Health Assembly virtual meeting, China -- which regards Taiwan as being a province of China and denies that Taiwan is an independent country -- was adamantly opposed. The matter was settled by Director-General Tedros who refused to grant Taiwan an observer status at the World Health Assembly.

Terry Glavin -- a freelance journalist who writes on international affairs -- has drawn attention to that fact that China has gained control of four major U.N. agencies. Under Director-General Tedros, the World Health Organization (WHO) appears to be doing China's bidding, the U.N. Food and Drug Organization is controlled by its Director-General, Qu Dongyu – a former vice-minister of agriculture and rural affairs in China; and Chinese nationals occupy the top jobs at the U.N. International Telecommunications Union, and the International Civil Aviation Organization. As the Americans, under the Trump administration, have withdrawn from a direct involvement in the United Nations, the vacuum has been filled by China.

Friday, May 22, 2020

Court Deadlines Suspensions: The Justice Minister, David Lametti, announced this week that legislation will be introduced by the federal government to put timelines on court cases on hold until September. The postponed deadlines would apply to nearly two dozen different types of cases – divorce submissions and appeals, federal bankruptcy filings, business restructuring deadlines, pension dispute appeals, etc. The postponement is rendered necessary by the inability of courts to meet during the COVID-19 epidemic; although some courts have met with public health protections in place, and in other cases, virtual conference sittings have been held.

Provincial Debt: The heavy deficits being incurred by the provinces has attracted little attention in the media. However, an article in the *Financial Post* raises the prospect of what can be done if a province is on the brink of being forced into bankruptcy owing to the loss of tax revenues during the coronavirus and the heavy fixed expenses and coronavirus response costs being incurred. Even before the coronavirus pandemic struck, the provincial governments in Canada had a combined total debt of $853 billion, and now financial analysts are predicting weak economic growth during the recovery phase. It is expected that increased spending requirements will add another $64 billion to the provincial debt total through government borrowings. There are concerns being expressed about the credit rating of the provinces being reduced, without federal government financial support.

To aid the provinces, there is an existing Fiscal Stabilization Plan by which the federal government can lend monies to any province that experiences a revenue decline of five-percent or more in any year, in other than resource revenues. Manitoba has called on the federal government to set up an emergency credit agency to lend money at low interest rates to the provinces; and there is the Disaster Financial Assistance Arrangements program, which could be used to provide financial aid to the provinces if a pandemic were to be classed as a natural disaster. Moreover, at present the Bank of Canada is buying up provincial bonds to provide financially strapped provinces with some liquidity. Whatever happens, the expectation of financial analysts is that the federal government cannot, and will not, let a province go bankrupt. There will probably be a resort to massive federal loans with a demand attached that certain reforms be made, and austerity measures introduced.

Inadequate Border Closure: It turns out the ban on foreign travellers entering Canada has many exceptions. The ban, which saw the closure of Canadian airports in mid-March to international flights, with but four airports left open – Montreal, Toronto, Calgary and Vancouver – for the return home of Canadians and permanent residents from abroad, has not been strictly enforced. A National Post columnist, John Iveson, has revealed that during the height of the coronavirus epidemic -- while Canadians were isolated a home, facing heavy fines for more than 2 to 5 person meeting together in public (depending on the province), were forbidden to enter public parks, and were banned from crossing inter-provincial borders -- a total of over 269,500 flights arrived in Canada from abroad. What is surprising is that international flights are continuing to arrive in Canada as of mid-May with passengers, long after Canadians and permanent residents would have returned home on the special flights arranged for them.

Iveson has found that on just one day – Tuesday, May 19th -- sixty-three international flights arrived at the Toronto International Airport alone from the United States (5 flights), Europe (8), Shanghai (3), Beijing (1), Hong Kong (3), Ghana (1), Jamaica (1), and Ethiopia (1). Some flights were no doubt carrying cargo, but others were carrying passengers. Why are flights arriving with foreign passengers at this late date, with a ban still in place on foreign nationals entering Canada?

A major part of the problem is that the ban of foreign nationals entering Canada was never absolute. In late March, an Order-in-Council was issued by the Governor-General -- acting on the advice of the Queen's Privy Council (the Liberal Cabinet) – that provided for 19 exemptions to the ban on foreign nationals entering Canada. Among the exemptions were international students, non-Canadian family members of Canadians and permanent residents, and foreign temporary workers. The exemption granted the first two categories is beyond belief at a time when 90 percent of COVID-19 cases were then linked to foreign travellers entering Canada, and even today 20 percent of new cases are directly linked to foreign travel. Moreover, foreign seasonal workers were not needed in late March. A request made by Iveson to the Canadian Border Services Agency for the nationality of the passengers entering Canada since the ban of foreign nationals entering Canada, was refused.

At present, some 26,000 temporary seasonal workers have arrived in Canada, out of 35,000 who have applied to be admitted to work, under the exemption from the travel ban on foreign nationals entering Canada. Last year saw upwards of 45,000 admitted. With the seasonal workers required to be isolated for 14-days following their arrival, the federal government has provided a $50 million grant to farm organizations to cover that cost.

U.S. Border Closure: To date, no survey has been undertaken concerning the attitude of Canadians towards retaining the ban on foreign nationals entering Canada for an extended period, but a survey has been completed of the attitudes of Canadians to the re-opening of the U.S. border during the coronavirus pandemic. Attitudes varied, but overall there was a cluster of 83 percent wanting the border to remain closed to American visitors 'for the time being', and at the other extreme, five percent wanted the border to be immediately opened to enable families to be reunited and to speed the recovery of the economy.

A more detailed breakdown revealed that 52 percent were willing to allow a gradual re-opening of the border under strict conditions: that American visitors would have to wear face masks and follow the physical distancing policy, with a strict system of fines and a quick deportation of anyone breaking the regulations. Another 25 percent would add additional safeguards in demanding temperature checks, and assurances that American visitors had been free of any virus symptoms over the previous 14-days. (How that would be verified, remained unanswered.) Lastly, 23 percent of Canadians wanted the border to remain closed indefinitely to American visitors. What is particularly interesting is that 12 percent of Canadians surveyed indicated that they would consider visiting the United States soon after the border is reopened.

COVID-19 Mutations: Chinese health authorities investigating new outbreak of the coronavirus in Northern China – that has been linked to infected Russian travellers – have found that it is taking longer than the established five to ten days for symptoms of the coronavirus to appear in exposed persons. A two-week delay is being reported before symptoms manifested themselves, which is rendering the standard 14-day isolation insufficient. This has contributed to numerous clusters of family infections during the latest Chinese outbreak. Scientists are differing as to whether this is a mutation of the coronavirus, or merely the result of a closer observation of the nature of a virus infection than was possible during the pandemic.

Vaccines: The Canadian Press has reported that a potential vaccine developed by the Can Sino Biologics Inc. of Wuhan, China, will be tested at the Canadian Center for Vaccinology at Dalhousie University in Halifax. The testing program is a result of a partnership of the Chinese Can Sino Biologics with the Canadian Center for Vaccinology and the National Research Council in Canada. The partnership is being touted as ensuring the Canadians will have a ready access to the vaccine, if proven successful, and will facilitate a domestic production in Canada.

The vaccine has already been tested in China on 108 adults, and it has been found to produce antibodies and a response in T- cells which protect the body from pathogens. However, there were 'mild' or 'moderate' side effects: pain at the injection site, fever, fatigue, and headaches. The first Halifax trial will involve 100 individuals aged 18 to 55, to be followed by a second trial of 500 individuals between 65 and 85 years of age. The Canadian Centre for Vaccinology is dedicated to vaccine research, discovery and evaluation of vaccines, and researchers in the fields of bacteriology, molecular biology, virology, and immunology.

Indigenous Services Grant: The federal government announced additional funding for off-reserve Indigenous service organizations to aid these organizations to cope with the demands being placed on them during the COVID-19 epidemic. Earlier, the federal government has granted $15 million for that purpose, but the amount of the grant is now being increased to $75 million. The grant is targeted for Aboriginal Friendship Centres across Canada. Given that aboriginals living off-reserve have access to all of the emergency financial grants and services provided to Canadians by federal, provincial, and municipal governments during the COVAD-19 epidemic, it was not explained why Aboriginal Friendship Centres would need an addition $60 million beyond the original grant. At present there are 107 Friendship Centres across Canada that are dedicated to helping off-reserve aboriginals to access services that they need to succeed in living in urban settings.

Saturday, May 23, 2020

Post-Pandemic Government: The Ottawa Citizen has an article on how government should innovate in the workplace and in the delivery of programs and services to take advantage of the new ways of operating and thinking evident during the COVID-19 crisis. The innovators are looking at the pandemic experience with government workers working from home, via virtual conferencing and digital technology links, and are concluding that it opens the opportunity for governments to change the operating model to adjust to new digital realities. One can appreciate government rethinking how programs work, and for seeking to take full advantage of new technologies to more expeditiously carrying out departmental mandates and the delivery of government services to the public. Indeed, it should be a focus of any post-pandemic investigation.

However, those who want to fundamentally change the public service culture through eliminating its hierarchical management system of management, the office rules and regulations, and the structured accountability for the expenditures of public monies, and to put the emphasis on public servants working from home to implement programs, are letting their enthusiasm for digital technologies lead them astray. The assumptions being made are that working from home is equally productive, if not more productive, than working in an office environment – which has not been tested through comparing the productivity of public servants working from home during the COVID-19 pandemic to the production and standard of work when in the office environment. There is an assumption that a virtual system of meeting will work equally well as in person meetings, yet there is an the absence of any study of how well the virtual meetings of parliament and of public service units worked during the lockdown. Moreover, not all government files are online for ready access by public servants. Yet another assumption by our working from home enthusiasts is that the Public Service will become more diverse and representative of all regions of Canada if public servants can work from home wherever they reside across Canada. Actually, the elimination of the arbitrary designation of jobs as 'bilingual imperative', and the hiring of public servants strictly on merit to work in whatever language a particular job requires, would do much more for increasing diversity and regional representation in the public service than any other reform.

One must beware of innovators who want to overturn an office culture and system of administration that has worked remarkably well in both government and the private sector for almost two centuries, and to do so on the basis of a blind faith that having public servants working in isolation at home in a digital world, is the wave of the future. It would be far better to set up satellite offices for units that can function independent of headquarters, but to do so in maintaining a traditional office culture and hierarchical administrative structure that fits within the departmental org chart. The digital revolution can speed work, increase productivity, and facilitate records storage and retrieval, but it does not provide a viable means for discarding the traditional office structure and work culture.

Retail Workers: Among essential workers who are facing the threat of a COVID-19 infection at their workplace, are the grocery store and pharmacy employees. To date 500 of these essential workers have tested positive of COVID-19, and ten have died. The retail companies have sought to protect their workers by limiting the number of customers in a store, with directional arrows on the floor to keep shoppers from milling around, with plexiglass face shields for cashiers, with enhanced cleaning and disinfecting and, where obtainable, face masks and gloves for all employees.

The grocery store and pharmacy workers have benefitted from the pandemic lockdown. Almost 80 percent are part-time workers, but during the lockdown they were employed full-time and companies raised the base pay by $2.00 per hour. Whether the $2.00 per hour raise was in recognition of their dedication, or danger pay, or intended to keep employees from staying home and collecting the $500 per week CERB payment, is a moot point. However, for the first time, retail workers in grocery stores and pharmacies were well paid and employed in working a full week. During the COVID-19 lockdown, there has been no shortage of food, but food prices rose 3.4 percent during April. Based on scarcity or a particularly high demand, some prices have soared, such as the price of rice which rose 9.2% in April owing to Vietnam placing a ban on rice exports.

Lawyers: Sole practitioners and lawyers in small firms have seen their incomes plummet, some by more than 35 to 40 percent, with trial lawyers suffering an almost total loss of income with the courts being closed. Large law firms have reduced the pay of lawyers by as much as 20 percent or laid them off. The Law Society of Ontario has been encouraging lawyers to apply for the Canada Emergency Business Account loan. However, within the legal profession there are demands that the Law Society defer its $5,000-$6,000 annual fee and/or provide financial support to struggling lawyers.

Military Personnel: To date, 1,700 military personnel have been employed in providing medical assistance and personal care support in thirty long-care homes, mostly in Quebec. To date, 28 military personnel have become infected with COVID-19. Prime Minister Trudeau has responded to demands that the military personnel on duty in the long-care homes receive a hazard pay, and the Chief of Defence Staff, General Jon Vance, has confirmed that hazard pay will be forthcoming.

Contact Tracking: While individual provinces have been attempting to develop a contract tracing app -- some with more success than others – and the federal government has been promising support to the provincial efforts to develop a tracking app -- employees at a private high-tech company in Ottawa, Shopify, have volunteered to produce a suitable app, and have done so. They have developed a "COVID Shield" app which has been released as a free application for use by any government seeking to develop a COVID-19 contact tracking system. The app makes use of the "exposure notification" technology provided by Google and Apple, and it uses Bluetooth to collect and shares random IDs from nearby phones once the COVID Shield app is installed.

The COVID Shield data collection system is totally private as the sharing of the random IDs is voluntary, and only possible with a positive text result -- confirmed by a health-care professional -- that the smartphone owner has been infected with COVID-19. (This is an app that those who are concerned about personal privacy can embrace. As to this diarist, he would much prefer a smartphone app that automatically records the contact data on a central server, so that health authorities could act, as soon as infected person is identified, to trace the contacts who were exposed to the virus, to test them, and to isolate those who test positive. The maintenance of personal privacy in public spaces should not be a factor in combatting a deadly virus threat.)

Government Approval Rating: The latest public opinion poll shows that the minority Liberal government, and Prime Minister Trudeau personally, have benefitted politically through handing out billions of dollars in financial aid to Canadians, Canadians businesses and industries, and many Canadian organizations. Upwards of 58 percent of Canadians polled approve of the government, and 48 percent of Justin Trudeau, which are major improvements for both. What is more, 88 percent of the Canadians polled approve of the financial support measures introduced by the federal government.

Restoring Parliament: The Conservative Party has continued to call for a restoration of parliament, and an end to what they have called the "morning show" on which Prime Minister dispenses billions of dollars to grateful subjects on network television, which is recorded and posted later on social media. Andrew Scheer, the Leader of the Opposition has called for 'Parliament to be declared an essential service', and wants parliament to be recalled, in a reduced numbers format – a suggested 50 members in total -- based on party strength in the House of Commons, to restore parliamentary accountability and the functions of parliament. The Conservative opposition intends to submit a motion to parliament on Monday, declaring that parliament is an essential service, and ought to continue to fulfil its constitutional function.

That the Liberal Party, and its supporters in the NDP and Bloc Quebecois, do not appear to consider that a properly functioning parliament is an essential service for Canadians, boggles the mind! Andrew Scheer charges – and what he is saying is perfectly true -- that the Liberal government has announced hundreds of billions of dollars in new spending to address the economic distress caused by the COVID-19 lockdown, but has not provided parliament with any formal financial update. Under the present arrangement, the House of Commons in formed into a Special Committee of the House to deal with matters relating to the COVID-19 epidemic that meets one-day per week in the House of Commons with 32 members sitting in the House who comprise a proportionally reduced representation from each party; and there are two days a week of a virtual conference meeting of all 388 MPs.

In this system, the Liberal government has been able to pick and choose what questions they want to answer, and the Speaker has confined MPs to simply posing questions on programs and policies related to the coronavirus epidemic. The regular business of parliament in holding the government to account, and overseeing spending, and contributing to the government of the country, has been suspended. Even Liberal backbenchers have been deprived of any influence, as caucus is not meeting.

The Leader of the Opposition, Andrew Scheer has striven to make clear that the Conservative Party is not taking a stand on a partisan issue. ""This is about whether or not a country like Canada can have a functional Parliament during a crisis". What the Conservative Party is proposing is that the House of Commons return to its normal four-day in-house sittings, and its traditional functions, with a reduced representation by 50 members to conform to public health spacing within the House of Commons chamber, and with a reduced support staff. Moreover, he is demanding that all of the House of Commons committees be reconstituted to resume regular meetings via virtual conferencing if necessary, as part of the plan to restore a "normal parliamentary business cycle".

What the Liberal Party is now proposing is what is being called a "hybrid" model. It involves the continuation of a reduced proportional number of MPs present in the Commons chamber, but with a large screen on each side of the speaker to enable MPs outside of the House in their home ridings to follow and participate in the House of Commons business via a videoconference hookups. Moreover, the one-day in house sitting per week, and the two day virtual meeting of the entire House per week, will be replaced by a four day sitting of the reduced membership House with the two large screens and a video-conference hookup to enable MPs outside of the House to observe and participate in debate – at least in theory. The "hybrid system" proposed by the minority Liberal Party government needs to be fleshed out, and will need the support of the Bloc Quebecois and the NDP to be enacted over the opposition of the Conservative Party.

The Bloc Quebecois separatist party has been a strong supporter of the COVID-19 spending programs of the Liberal Party government. Apparently the Bloc Quebecois leader, Yves-François Blanchet, has been providing lists of demands to Prime Minister Trudeau in return for Bloc Quebecois support – demands no doubt based on making sure that any proposed program expenditure would be highly beneficial to Quebecers, in keeping with the separatist mantra: 'What's in it for Quebec'? A moment of supreme political irony occurred during a parliamentary sitting – as reported by Rex Murphy, a National Post columnist – when Blanchet threatened that the Bloc Quebecois would support the Conservatives in demanding 'a resumption of in-person sittings of the House of Commons five days a week', if the Liberal government did not meet the demands made by the separatist party. Needless, to say the demands being made by the separatist party were not revealed to the Canadian public. Whatever the demands were, they remained in the private confidences of two Quebec politicians: Trudeau and Blanchet.

The New Democratic Party (NDP) has made clear what it will demand for supporting the Liberal Party 'hybrid' parliament proposal. Jagmeet Singh, the NDP leader, is demanding that the federal government work with the provinces to provide a two-week paid sick leave to workers who become infected with the COVID-19 virus, and that more government support be provided for people with disabilities who are struggling during the coronavirus lockdown.

A *National Post* columnist, John Iveson, has noted that the two virtual conference sessions of parliament per week have not been working well. There have been technical problems, and the Speaker has been cutting off any opposition MP speakers who try to question the government on any subject beyond the immediate COVID-19 situation. Now, the Procedure and House Affairs Committee, which is dominated by a combination of Liberal, NDP, and Bloc Quebecois MPs, has proposed that members of parliament be able to vote electronically during the proposed video-conference hook ups when the reduced representation House of Commons is sitting.

Nonetheless, there are problems. A serious concern has been expressed that hackers might intervene and corrupt the voting process if MPS outside of the House of Commons are permitted to vote on government issues via the video-conference hookups. There is a continuing concern as well about how parliamentary procedures will be maintained with respect to points of order and privilege for sitting MPs. The Liberal Party House Leader, Pablo Rodriguez, was not available to reporters to question with respect to how the 'hybrid system' is envisaged as working in practice.

In one respect, the Liberals have expressed a willingness to meet two Conservative concerns. The reduced House of Commons will sit four days a week – with sittings extended into June and July – and the 'hybrid' sessions of parliament are to include a question period each day during which MPs can pose questions to cabinet ministers about non-COVID-19 issues. It is a positive move towards restoring parliament to its true function, but only minor step with no guarantee that answers will be forthcoming. There are nine parliamentary committees that will be meeting virtually to discuss matters related to the COVID-19 epidemic.

What is oddly unreal is that all parties agree that there are technical limitations to establishing a full visual conferencing parliament, which is a problem that does not exist for the smaller parliamentary committee virtual meetings. (Why is the Liberal government seeking to establish a video-conferencing system to supposedly enable MPS outside the House in their ridings across Canada, to participate in debates and parliamentary votes, when the technology currently available does not permit such a system to function properly?)

The fate of Canada as a parliamentary democracy, and the function of parliament, will be decided Monday when parliament reconvenes.

Personal Protective Equipment: On Friday, during the House of Commons virtual meeting, Dr. Theresa Tam, Chief, Public Health Canada Agency, was asked – by an NDP opposition member – if she had warned the Liberal government that the national stockpile of personal protective equipment was inadequate? However, before Dr. Tam could reply, she was cut off by the Liberal government Health Minister, Patty Hajdu, who involved the principle of cabinet confidentiality. What is confidential about a question pertaining to Canada's national supply of personal protective equipment? This episode provides yet another example of an on-going Liberal government coverup of an irresponsible action that has had terrible consequences for Canada's medical personnel, frontline responders, and personal care workers.

Sunday, May 24, 2020

Herd Immunity Strategy: To date, the Public Health Agency of Canada, and its Chief, Dr. Theresa Tam, have been emphasizing the need for Canadians to build up a 'herd immunity' to successfully combat the COVID-19. The emphasis has been on maintaining some form of lockdown and social distancing until a vaccine can be developed, and up to 60 percent of Canadian immunized to attain a 'herd immunity'. The potential vaccine developed by the Sino Can Biologics, and about to be clinically tested at Dalhousie University, appears to be what the PHAC is counting on for providing a vaccine. However, the federal government cannot simply base a public health strategy on the hope that at a successful vaccine will be quickly developed, and the fear of some highly speculative 'second wave' of infections.

Hopes that a 'herd immunity' would eventually be developed through large numbers of recovered COVID-19 cases having developed a natural immunity are proving rather forlorn. At Rockefeller University in New York, scientist have discovered that individuals who recovered from a milder COVID-19 infection that did not require hospitalization, do not have many antibodies in their blood. This finding suggests that the large number of infected cases will not serve as a basis for developing a 'herd immunity' capable of putting an end to the spread of the coronavirus. That long-term public health strategy appears to be a dead end. Without the natural production of a large number of strong, durable, and long-lasting antibodies in the blood of recovered cases, or produced by some future vaccine that produces that type of antibodies in large numbers, the 'herd immunity' strategy is a false hope. What is decidedly more promising is testing and isolation of infected persons, and the tracking, testing of exposed contacts and the isolation of those who test positive – a policy of containment.

Vaccine Strategy Concerns: More recently, Prime Minister Trudeau has shifted his position, and is now emphasizing the importance of a targeted testing to identify and contain outbreaks together with the maintenance of social spacing "so that the population at large won't be in a situation of having to go back into confinement". However, what is evident is that the continuation of a nationwide lockdown is not necessary – if it ever was -- and that the general strategy of maintaining a social distancing during the recovery phase will be unworkable once the economy is open again and social life resumes. It will not be possible to maintain a social spacing, at all times, in stores, factories, office buildings, and on public transit. A new approach is needed.

Another strategy, in which publish health authorities are putting their faith, is the development of a successful vaccine that, when widely distributed, will enable a 'herd immunity' to be developed.

In Britain, the Science Editor, Ian Sample, of *The Guardian* newspaper (May 22, 2020) has researched and prepared a much more astute evaluation of the COVID-19 situation with regard to the potential for developing a successful vaccine and alternative strategies available for normal social and work-related activities to resume, regardless of whether the search for a long-lasting vaccine is successful or not.

While Oxford University is recruiting volunteers for the second phase of testing for its potential vaccine, the Deputy Chief Medical Officer for England, Jonathan Van-Tam has declared that "We can't be sure we will get a vaccine". Among the potential problems are:

- that coronaviruses do not tend to trigger long lasting immunity. The example cited is the common cold, which is caused by human coronaviruses, but immunity fades so rapidly that one can become re-infected the next year. When researches at Oxford University analyzed blood from recovered COVID-19 patients, they found that the levels of antibodies responsible for long lasting immunity levels – the IgG antibodies – rose steeply in the first month of infection, and then began to fall. This raises the question of whether the several vaccines being tested to date are causing only a temporary rise in the level of antibodies. If a vaccine provides only a year of protection, then the COVID-19 virus will remain present within a large community:

- developing a proven vaccine can take years in dealing with a complex virus such as COVID-19, and the research is not guaranteed to be successful. An example cited is the search for an HIV vaccine which remains unsuccessful 30 years after the HIV was isolated; and

- the rate of a virus acquiring mutations can prevent the development of an effective vaccine as has happened with the HIV.

Even if a vaccine is not found that is 100 percent effective, there will be benefits from the research effort. One vaccine developed earlier at Oxford University does not prevent COVID -19, but it appears to prevent pneumonia from developing in a COVID-19 patient. Hence, it would greatly reduce the death rate from COVID -19. Yet, another research result is the newly developed drug, Remdesivir, which speeds the recovery of COVID-19 cases. In effect, if the effort to develop a vaccine fails, the strategy will need to shift to "reducing the serious outcomes of infection". Repurposed drugs may provide an antiviral treatment -- such as anti-body drugs that can be used to fight COVID-19 infections in patients.

Living with the Coronavirus: If the effort to develop a long-lasting vaccine fails, governments and peoples will have to adopt to a living with the presence of the coronavirus. David Heyman, a world-renowned medical epidemiologist, and professor at the London School of Hygiene & Tropical Medicine, maintains that governments will have to maintain an extensive system of monitoring for infections and the capacity for a swift outbreak containment – presumably through quarantining infected persons, the tracking and testing of contacts, and the isolating of contacts for 14 days and quarantining of those who test positive with the requisite medical attention and personal care support.

Based on the practical experience gained in the successful containment of the COVID-19 threat in Hong Kong, Yuen Kwok-yung, a professor of infectious disease at the University of Hong Kong, has taken a positive approach to the recovery period. He has advised the Hong Kong government that there is no need for any type of lockdown, and that social distancing can be relaxed, but only if people wear face masks in enclosed spaces on trains and at work. Concerts and cinemas can function, but only if people wear face masks and consume no food or drink during their attendance. In restaurants, tables need to be shielded from one another – presumably in booths with plexiglass dividers – and waiters need to follow strict rules – presumably of personal hygiene in washing their hands, in wearing masks and gloves, and disinfecting tables after use – to prevent the spreading of infections. The key factor, from a Hong Kong perspective, is the diligent and correct wearing of reusable face masks that are washable. Schools are open, with children wearing face masks, and desks have been equipped with a plexiglass surround on three-side, but otherwise are in the traditional spacing arrangement as both pupils and teachers are accustomed, and that children are habituated to and feel comfortable with.

Rather than focusing on modellings of a highly speculative second wave of infections, and undertaking a slow opening of the economy in phases – a difficult prospect given the complexity of social and economic integrations – Canadian governments at all levels ought to supply Canadians with a standard CAA approved face masks, put in place a mandatory requirement to wear a face mask in public with stiff fines for not complying, and proceed to open the economy as quickly as possible before irreparable damage is inflicted on Canadian businesses and industries. Such an approach in conjunction with the maintenance of a capacity to quickly test and isolate anyone showing flu-like symptoms and, if testing positive, a rapid tracking, testing and isolating of any contacts testing positive, will enable society to continue to function in the presence of the coronavirus. It is time for Canadian governments at all levels to act on the practical experience gained in combatting the COVID-19 threat, and to fully re-open the economy with the prescribed health protection protocols in place.

This is exactly the approach advocated by William Haseltine, a distinguished American researcher in cancer, HIV/AIDS, and human genome research. His position is that governments ought not to count on the development of a vaccine any time soon. That the best approach is to manage the disease in tracking infections, and strict isolation measures wherever virus outbreaks are found. Even without a vaccine, the virus can be controlled. He recommends that people wear face masks, wash their hands frequently, clean and disinfect common touch surfaces, and practice social distancing whenever and wherever possible.

Retrospective

The history of the coronavirus pandemic is still unfolding with some countries, inclusive of Canada, apparently on the road to recovery and other countries just beginning to suffer its devastating impact. What is evident, as of the third week of May, is that the coronavirus pandemic in Canada is now entering a recovery phase. The diary entries covered in the present work -- COVID CANADA, First Wave -- focus on the politics of the virus epidemic in Canada during the height of the pandemic, the origin of the coronavirus threat and the evolving science, and the economic impact of the virus on Canada, within the broader framework of the worldwide pandemic. It covers the period from early March to May 24th, from the introduction of the coronavirus (COVID-19) as a real threat to the health and lives of Canadians, through the struggle of the provincial governments and public health agencies to contain its spread, and ends with the coronavirus spread apparently under control with the number of new cases dropping dramatically each day, but with some daily upticks.

The politics of the coronavirus epidemic in Canada has been treated in conveying and critiquing the response of the federal Liberal government to carrying out its duty and responsibility to protect the health and well-being of Canadians in the face of the threat of a deadly foreign virus. The science of the event has been covered in the advances yielded by scientific research in understanding the nature of the coronavirus, and its contagiousness, as well as the struggle to contain the spread of the virus and to develop a vaccine, and the toll exacted by the virus in sickness and deaths. The economic impact of the virus epidemic has been covered in setting forth the financial aid programs that were introduced, and the massive expenditures that were made, by the Canadian federal government in responding to the economic and social devastation wreaked by the coronavirus.

Canada is now entering the recovery stage, but the struggle against the coronavirus may well go on for another year or more, with periodic upticks, until a vaccine can be successfully developed to inoculate a majority or more of the population. Hopefully, the precautions being taken to curtail the spread of the coronavirus, will spare Canada a second wave of coronavirus infections this coming fall.

Lessons Learned

During the course of the spread of the coronavirus worldwide, and the epidemic in Canada, much has been learned about the novel virus, and mistakes have been made, as well as lessons learned in how to protect a community from a deadly pathogen, the vulnerabilities of any society that relies on a global supply chain in times of crisis, and the role of ideology in influencing the response of government to a national crisis. Among the lessons learned are:

1) **That whenever there is a deadly virus outbreak anywhere in the world, the borders of Canada ought to be closed immediately to foreign travellers from the country concerned and from any other country where outbreaks occur.**

By the time Canada closed its borders to foreign nations on March 18th, with the exception of American travellers, and on March 21st to American visitors, the coronavirus had been raging in Iran and Italy during February, and as of early March had made inroads into most of the countries of western Europe, was already present in the United States, and travellers had introduced the coronavirus into the Canadian community in Ontario, British Columbia, Quebec, and Alberta.

The slowness in closing the border was a major error, and was attributable to two factors: First, misinformation from the World Health Organization (WHO) that mistakenly maintained that the novel coronavirus could not be transmitted from human to human; that the virus outbreak in Wuhan, China, presented a low threat to other countries; and that closure of borders was not necessary and would be too disruptive of global relations. A second factor was the globalist Modern liberal mindset of the federal Liberal government of Prime Minister Justin Trudeau that believes in 'open borders' and 'the free movement of peoples' and was reluctant to close Canada's borders to international travellers. Yet another factor was the political correctness stance of the federal Liberal government in not wanting to stigmatize any racial or ethnic group by singling out citizens of a particular country, or countries, as potential carriers of a deadly virus by banning their entry to Canada.

Rather than close Canada's borders to international travellers, the Liberal government, on the advice of the Public Health Agency of Canada, took the position that, in an era of global travel and trade, the coronavirus would enter Canada anyway. Hence, a public health policy was instituted that was based on slowing the spread of the coronavirus to prevent the public health system from becoming overwhelmed. There was no concern on the part of the federal Liberal government, or any concentrated effort, to prevent the coronavirus from entering Canada.

Common sense, a concern for protecting the health and lives of Canadians, and an observation of what was happening in other countries, should have dictated a different policy. In slavishly following the advice of the WHO, the Liberal government of Justin Trudeau resisted all demands from the Conservative Party Opposition, medical personnel, and members of the public, to close the border of Canada during the month of February and early March. By the time, the border was closed, the coronavirus was already becoming established in-community in several Canadian provinces and was no longer traceable exclusively to contact with a traveller from an infected country.

Not only did the federal Liberal government act too late in closing the Canadian border, but international students were exempted from the travel ban and allowed to continue to enter Canada. (The previous year, 2019, there were 640,000 international students studying in Canadian post-secondary schools. Why international students were exempted from the border closure has never been explained. Allowing international students to freely enter Canada and to disperse to colleges and universities across the country was, and is, a recipe for spreading the coronavirus within the Canadian community.)

The south-east Asian countries in close proximity to China closed their borders to travellers from China as soon as they were aware of the deadly virus outbreak in Wuhan, China, and to international travellers as soon as the coronavirus spread to other countries. Moreover, they immediately introduced and enforced public health protocols – the wearing of face masks, hand washing hygiene, social spacing, and disinfecting common-touch surfaces and urban contagion areas. In doing so, the Asian countries were able to limit the introduction of the coronavirus into their communities, and to keep their respective numbers of coronavirus cases and related deaths, remarkably low. In Canada, the Nunavut Territory -- in the far north -- closed its borders to all travellers, including their fellow Canadians from the south, and insisted that returning residents be quarantined in airport hotels in Canada outside of the Nunavut Territory and be tested, with only those testing negative being permitted to return home. The Nunavut government was active in establishing and financing the quarantine hotel accommodation system for detaining and testing its returning residents, and Nunavut has not had a single coronavirus case.

2) **That Canadians and Permanent Residents returning to Canada ought to have been quarantined in airport hotels and tested for a coronavirus infection, and those who tested positive ought to have been placed in a mandatory hotel quarantine and provided with medical care and those testing negative ought to have been ordered to self-isolate under a strict supervision.**

A two-week quarantine is required to allow symptoms to develop, which are not evident for up to four days after contacting the virus, and testing is required to identify asymptomatic virus carriers who show no symptoms. However, the federal government neglected to institute such a policy. Instead, the Liberal government relied on airline personnel to refuse to board international travellers for flights to Canada who were showing symptoms of a coronavirus infection, limited international flights to four airports – Montreal, Toronto, Calgary and Vancouver, and simply handed out pamphlets to returning Canadian and Permanent Residents upon their arrival in advising them to self-isolate for fourteen days and to contact public health authorities if they became ill with coronavirus symptoms.

Eventually, a follow-up phone contact system was instituted by the federal Public Health Agency whereby new arrivals from abroad were contacted by phone to ensure that they were self-isolating at home, a system of fines was instituted, and the RCMP was empowered to lay charges against anyone failing to self-isolate and to ticket and fine the recalcitrant, and there was a provision for the imposing of a jail term for repeat offenders. However, no fines were levied, and no charges were laid by police after making personal contact, in following up on failed phone contacts. The violators were simply warned about the danger they posed to others and were encouraged to remain in self-isolation. The police effort focussed on educating the violators and on persuasion.

The persuasion approach was yet another example of the discipline adverse mentality of the Modern liberal Canadian establishment in failing to take command and to impose and enforce government regulations to protect the health and lives of Canadians during a deadly pandemic. Tens of thousands of returning Canadians and Permanent Residents -- a significant number of whom may well have been carriers of the coronavirus -- were permitted to return home unimpeded. Those who chose to intermingle socially within the Canadian community and refused to voluntarily self-isolate, were free to do so with impunity.

3) That Canadian expatriates living abroad ought to have been told to stay where they were, and to self-isolate in the country where they were living.

As of the spring of 2020, there were three million Canadians living abroad, and so many of them were returning to Canada, along with Canadians and Permanent Residents returning from travelling abroad, that by early-March the Public Health Agency and the Minister of Health -- under criticism for failing to institute a testing and quarantining system at the four international airports -- admitted that it was no longer possible to do so. Moreover, the situation did not change appreciably even after foreign travellers and American visitors were banned on March 18th and March 21st, respectively.

In effect, the argument presented by the federal Public Health Agency and Minister of Health was that the sheer number of Canadian expatriates, Canadians, and Permanent Residents, re-entering Canada from abroad would have overwhelmed any testing and quarantining system put in place, and hence no effort was made to establish a testing and quarantining system at the four international airports in service. However, Australia by closing its borders at an early date to international travellers and Australian expatriates living abroad, and limiting the number of planes allowed to carry Australians and Permanent Residents home each week, was able to establish a viable testing and quarantining system at its international airports to limit the exposure of Australians to the deadly coronavirus.

4) That the novel coronavirus (COVID-19) is a highly contagious and potentially deadly disease of which much has become known, but of which much remains unknown.

When China reported to the World Health Organization (WHO) -- on December 31, 2019 – that there was an outbreak of a mysterious 'pneumonia' in Wuhan, China, little was known about the virus which appeared to have originated in the Wuhan wet market. As of early January, the unknown virus was identified as a coronavirus; and on January 23, 2020, the City of Wuhan was placed under a strict quarantine by the Chinese government. Subsequently, in early February, Chinese researchers worked out the DNA genome of the novel coronavirus and found that it was related to the RNA (ribonucleic acid) family of viruses, inclusive of the SARS virus (Severe Acute Respiratory Syndrome) and the MERS virus (Middle Eastern Respiratory Syndrome), and Ebola; and that the novel coronavirus had been transferred from bats to humans, probably through an intermediate animal, such as the pangolin. The novel virus was named COVID-19 (or SARS-CoV-2). Initially, the WHO reported that the new virus was not transmitted by human to human contact; that the threat to other countries was low; and that there was no need to disrupt global relationships by closing borders. In Canada, the federal Liberal government adhered to the advice of WHO despite the fact that during February the novel coronavirus was present in South Korea, Taiwan, Japan, Singapore, Vietnam, and Japan, and by early March was raging through Iran and Italy, and present in Spain, France, Germany, Britain, and the United States. Yet, the Liberal government of Canada remained reluctant to close the Canadian border to international travellers. It was only in March 2020 that the WHO issued a report advising that the coronavirus was highly contagious and potentially deadly.

In early March, there were 118,000 coronavirus cases in 114 countries, yet the federal Liberal government did not close the Canadian border to international travellers until the United States closed its borders to European travellers on March 13th – the United States having earlier closed its borders to travellers from China. Moreover, as of March 18th, when the Canadian border was closed to international travellers, it was reported that 82 percent of the coronavirus cases in Canada were directly traceable to contact with a traveller from abroad who had transmitted the disease into Canada.

Given the highly contagious nature of the coronavirus, it is essential that borders be closed to travellers from countries suffering a virus outbreak, and that quarantine restrictions be enforced on citizens returning home from those countries. For Canada, the closure of the border came too late. By that time, the coronavirus was already well established within Canada with 18 percent of the new cases traced to in-community transmission. In just over a month after the border closure, there were 45,354 coronavirus cases in Canada, and 2,464 deaths. It soon became apparent that long-term care homes were hotspots with severe and widespread outbreaks among the elderly residents, and with a significant number of cases among personal care workers on staff, owing to a critical shortage of personal protective equipment, the close contact, and the sharing of common facilities.

By that time, reports out of China confirmed the Canadian experience that the coronavirus severely impacts the elderly with patients over 80 years old having a 14.8 percent chance of dying, versus a death rate of but 2.3 percent in the general population from the disease. Where the novel respiratory virus is concerned, it is believed to be spread primarily by droplets in saliva or nasal discharge when an infected person coughs, sneezes or breathes; that the droplets can remain active for three hours to three days on different surfaces for transferal; and that the maintaining of a two-metre – six foot -- physical spacing is necessary to prevent its spread. (The two-metre spacing rule is based on earlier studies of the dispersal of cold virus droplets.)

The general symptoms are a high fever/high temperature, persistent coughing, and a severe shortness of breath. In severe cases, patients would develop Acute Respiratory Distress Syndrome – generally among the elderly and those with a suppressed immune system – in which the virus spreads into the lungs, develops into pneumonia, and fills the lungs with fluids which makes breathing very difficult, if not impossible. Hence, severe cases need to be placed on a mechanical ventilator to push oxygenated air into their lungs. In addition, to respiratory failures, the coronavirus can cause blood clots, strokes, and cardiac issues.

That was the general state of the 'scientific' knowledge about the novel coronavirus during the height of the coronavirus pandemic in Canada during March and April. There was no vaccine, although research efforts were under way worldwide to develop a vaccine. Oddly enough, the WHO was advising against the wearing of face masks, except for medical personnel and support workers in direct contact with an infected person.

In the Canadian provinces, schools were being closed by mid-March. However, by that time it was known that children were not particularly susceptible to the coronavirus; yet, based on experience with the cold and flu viruses, medical authorities feared that children would be super spreaders of the virus. But that has not proved to be the case. There have been very few cases reported of children conveying the coronavirus into families; although that may be due to children being isolated at home from an early date. Yet, few children have been reported as becoming infected by the coronavirus anywhere in the world, and when children have become sick, their cases have been quite mild. Perhaps, their general immunity may be related to some of the childhood vaccines that children have received for other viruses.

It is known that a thorough washing of the hands with soap – an advised 20 seconds – will destroy the fatty tissue membrane surrounding a coronavirus droplet and will deactivate the virus; and that exposure of the virus to a hand sanitizer of more than 20 percent ethanol will produce "a near 100 percent reduction of infectivity".

One promising area is the development of drugs to treat patients suffering from a coronavirus infection. To date, one existing drug, Remdesivir, has been found to reduce the severity of coronavirus infections and to speed the recovery of patients.

5) **That the elderly, and individuals of all ages who have underlying health problems or a suppressed immune system, are the most severely affected by a coronavirus infection and more likely to succumb.**

In Canada, as of April 15th, there were 29,000 coronavirus cases, and 1200 coronavirus related deaths. During the initial phase of the pandemic, upwards of 94 percent of the deaths were among Canadians over sixty years of age.

The major outbreaks were situated in long-term care homes for the elderly. More generally, the cases requiring hospitalization were among the elderly, as well as individuals of all ages who were suffering from diabetes, heart diseases, cancer, a respiratory illness, or who had a suppressed immune system. Among healthy individuals under 50 years of age, those who have become sick have experienced only mild flu-like symptoms.

Ultimately, the virus spread was confined mostly to major urban areas, the most severe outbreaks continued to occur in long-care homes but were concentrated in the homes with poor health care standards, and younger people accounted for more of the new cases, with the elderly comprising 70 to 75 percent of the cases overall. As of May 24th, there were 84,699 confirmed coronavirus cases in Canada, but during May the number of new cases dropped downward from close to 1,825 per day to less than one thousand daily.

6) That the traditional public health protocols employed to limit the spread of flu viruses are equally effective in limiting the spread of the coronavirus without the need for a national lockdown.

The south-east Asian countries, although highly exposed to the novel coronavirus that originated in China, did not resort to national lockdowns. Upon the coronavirus outbreak in China, travellers from China were immediately banned from the various east Asian countries, and subsequently travellers from other countries were banned as the virus spread there. Otherwise, the Asian countries relied on the implementation of traditional public health protocols to protect their people. Large gatherings were banned, citizens were told to practice a one-metre social spacing, to wear face masks, and to practice a frequent hand washing, as well as to disinfect common-touch surfaces. Medical personnel and health care workers were provided with personal protective equipment. Government workers sprayed urban public areas with a disinfectant where there were clusters of infections. The wearing of face masks was universally practiced. In South Korea, reportedly upwards of 90 percent of the population wore face masks during the pandemic in that country.

In some Asian countries, schools were closed but there were no lockdowns of business and industry. All governments instituted a program of screening and testing individuals who showed coronavirus-like symptoms, and those who tested negative were ordered to self-isolate and those who tested positive were quarantined. All contacts within the previous 48 hours were tracked down and tested in the same process thorough a government tracking app downloaded on all smartphones. The tracking app was also used to keep track of the movements of the infected individuals in quarantine, and any individual who did not have a smartphone was given one to facilitate the enforcement of the self-isolation and quarantine restrictions.

The Asian countries and Hong Kong were able to gain control over their coronavirus outbreaks without a national lockdown, and they did so in a relatively short period of time compared to Canada. Moreover, they experienced only a fraction of the coronavirus cases and deaths experienced in Canada where the Liberal government delayed in closing the Canadian border to foreign travellers, and the provinces resorted to imposing provincial lockdowns as their primary weapon in controlling the spread of the coronavirus. In utilizing a more traditional approach to combatting a virus pandemic, South Korea, which has a 20 percent greater population than Canada, has had only one-fifth of the number of coronavirus cases, and only 8 percent of the number of deaths that have occurred in Canada -- as of mid-April when South Korea was entering its recovery phase and Canada was still in the throes of the coronavirus pandemic with the number of cases and deaths continuing to rise.

The Asian countries have proven that the enforcement of elementary public health protocols, in conjunction with the employment of smartphone app contact tracing, testing, and the strict quarantining of those who test positive, and an enforced self-isolation of those who test negative, is highly effective in halting the spread of the coronavirus without a national lockdown.

The federal Liberal government had many early warnings of the need to combat the threat that the novel coronavirus posed to Canadians, and the 'tools' required were readily available in Canada and cost little. However, the federal government totally failed to take note of the warnings. What is more in an unbelievably naïve and short-sighted act, the federal government shipped Canada's national stockpile of personal protective equipment and ventilators to China in early February to aid the Chinese in containing the coronavirus, which resulted in an ongoing critical shortage of personal protective equipment and ventilators during almost the entire period of the coronavirus pandemic in Canada. It was a critical error in grossly underestimating the coronavirus threat to Canada that was compounded by the slowness of the federal Liberal government in turning to domestic companies to produce the badly needed personal protective equipment and ventilators, and in doing so only after efforts to obtain an immediate replacement of the equipment in the global market were unsuccessful.

What was lacking was an activist Canadian federal government willing to take command, to provide direction to Canadians as to what was required of them. What was lacking was a federal government, and Public Health Agency of Canada, with a long term commitment and a sense of duty and responsibility to taking action to protect the health and well-being of Canadians in the face of a virus pandemic – an activist government committed to limiting the exposure of Canadians to a foreign virus threat through an immediate and early border closure, to imposing and enforcing the testing, self-isolating, and quarantining regulations on Canadians and Permanent Residents returning from abroad, and to taking steps to ensure that personal protective equipment was readily available in the national stockpile for use by Canadians when needed. Had that been the case, there would have been no need for Canada to undergo the social and economic disruptions of a national lockdown, nor consequently to expend billions of dollars on massive government financial aid packages in providing social assistance and support for workers forced into unemployment by a national lockdown.

7) That smartphone tracking by public health authorities is the most effective way to trace individuals exposed to the coronavirus and to trace the virus spread pattern.

Smartphone tracking has proven to be a highly efficient and effective system for tracking contacts with an infected person so that they can be notified of their exposure, be tested, and advised to self-isolate if testing negative, or quarantined if testing positive. Smartphone tracking can also be used to compile aggregate data to map the pattern of virus spread and identify clusters of cases. The system was first introduced in Singapore and South Korea and has since been widely adopted in Europe. There are two systems of smartphone tracking: a public system monitored by public health authorities with an open app that everyone is required to have on their smartphone, and which a public health authority uses to contact individuals that were exposed to a coronavirus case; and a private tracking system with an app available for voluntary download by anyone who wants to participate in the coronavirus tracking system. Under the private smartphone tracking system, individuals who voluntarily download the app, and subsequently become sick, or test positive for a virus infection, are responsible for informing contacts, or they can turn over their smartphone to a public health authority to trace the contacts who have voluntarily download the app for tracing contacts.

The mandatory smartphone tracking system introduced in Singapore and South Korea proved remarkably effective in tracing contacts, but there are concerns about the effectiveness of a voluntary smartphone tracking system. For the private, voluntary smartphone tracking system to work effectively, a vast majority of the population must voluntarily download it, and infected persons have to ensure that contacts are informed of their exposure. Civil libertarians and privacy commissioners object to a mandatory smartphone tracking system administered by a public health authority as being an invasion of the privacy of smartphone users in enabling their movements to be traced. Another argument is that the identification of virus spread patterns might stigmatize a particular ethnic or racialized community through identifying high-risk places. Hopefully, Canada will adopt a compulsory smartphone tracking system administered by public health authorities, in putting the health, safety, and well-being of the entire country above any personal privacy and political correctness concerns.

8) That the wearing of face masks in public is a highly effective means of preventing the transmission of the coronavirus, and that face masks ought to be worn at all times in public and not just when a two-metre social spacing cannot be maintained.

In various countries, the widespread wearing of face masks – the N-95 respiratory mask and even cotton face masks – has been highly effective in preventing the spread of the coronavirus. Indeed, the wearing of a face mask is the ultimate social spacing protection as it prevents the transmission of the coronavirus from one individual to another.

The wearing of face masks needs to be made compulsory in public, and particularly so in any areas of the country where there are coronavirus outbreaks through in-community transmission. The compulsory wearing of face masks is also the singularly most effective way of preventing individuals who are asymptomatic from becoming super-spreaders of the coronavirus in circulating within society.

The widespread wearing of face masks in conjunction with a general two-metre social spacing rule, hand hygiene, the disinfecting of common-touch areas, and the spraying of common areas where there is a cluster of infections, has been highly effective in several Asian countries in preventing the spread of the virus and keeping the number of coronavirus cases quite low.

9) That ideologues in a minority government, under a charismatic leader, will often take advantage of a national crisis to seize absolute power to gain control the apparatus of government and the Treasury to impose their ideology and social vision on society; and that is the case with ideologues of the Left as well as the Right.

In March 24th, when parliament reconvened an omnibus draft bill was submitted to parliament by the Liberal government to secure approve of a number of major government emergency spending programs to provide financial assistance to Canadians who had lost their jobs in the coronavirus lockdown. However, the emergency spending bill was found to contain a clause that granted the Finance Minister an unlimited power to raise taxes, borrow, and spend monies, without parliamentary approval until December 31, 2021 – a period of twenty-one months. In effect, it was an effort by the Liberal Party to establish an absolutist government in Canada independent of parliamentary control and oversight. The minority Liberal government bill was opposed by all of the Opposition parties, and the clause was removed, enabling all parties to provide an unanimous support for the financial aid package in aid of unemployed Canadians.

Defeated in its first grasp at absolute power, the Liberal Party government, with the support of the New Democratic Party, subsequently managed to emasculate parliament by imposing a 'virtual system' of government whereby a reduced representation of members of parliament would meet once a week as a COVID-19 Committee to debate and vote on government spending programs, with two days of sessions per week for all members of parliament to meet through a virtual hookup. It is a system that severely limits the time available for debate, confines questions to COVID-19 concerns, and prevents parliamentary committees from functioning, while depriving parliamentarians of their rights, powers, and prerogatives.

Through political partisanship, parliament has been put in the position of being a rubber stamp for approving, in a one-day session, multi-billion-dollar spending initiatives without any time to scrutinize the bills. Government spending programs are being announced by the Prime Minister in a TV 'morning show' setting that bypasses parliament. The virtual parliament system has effectively established Prime Minister Trudeau as a benevolent despot with a rubber stamp parliament approving of his dispensing of largess to the masses. The virtual system of government has made a mockery of parliamentary government and of representative democracy in Canada.

Through his indulging in a highly-partisan, Machiavellian political manoeuvring, Justin Trudeau has shown that he has no respect for parliament, or parliamentary democracy. Previously, he has stated his admiration for the Chinese Communist dictatorship, which one suspects is based on envy of its ability to impose its vision on society without the impediment of a parliamentary Opposition.

Modern liberals are 'progressives' who believe that the values they advocate puts them in the vanguard of history in the making of a better world; and that they alone, because of their 'progressive' values and policies, are entitled to hold political power and to guide Canada into a promised utopia of 'world peace, equality, and prosperity for all'. Given such a mindset, it is only natural that Modern liberals regard any political party, group, or individuals, that opposes them as being 'reactionary' and motivated by some base motive.

Modern liberals are present and future oriented, are continually motivated to gain and to hold political power to pursue their social agenda and are willing to promise and spend whatever government monies it takes to woo the electorate. They continually disparage and denigrate conservative values – ironically, the traditional value on which Canada was built – and they denounce Conservatives as being 'old fashioned' for upholding patriotism, love of country, pride in national achievements, and reverence for Canada's history and military heritage. They categorize Conservatives as being 'reactionaries' for wanting to maintain Canada's traditional cultural and social values, and for their respect for religion belief, and they seek to brand Conservatives as 'closet racists' for rejecting open borders and wanting to limit immigration to levels that the Canadian economy can sustain. Conservatives are held to be 'stupid people, who just don't get it' for refusing to embrace 'Modern liberalism' and join the Liberal crusade to 'save the world' through embracing pan-nationalism, social egalitarianism, open borders, and the free movement of peoples, goods, services and capital, as well as identity politics, a political correctness that places limits on free speech, and an environmental zealotry for transitioning immediately to a totally green economy, regardless of the costs.

From a disparaging and denigrating of Conservatives and a resentment of the Conservative Opposition in parliament, it is but a short step to having contempt for the institution of parliament itself, and for parliamentary democracy. In taking advantage of a national crisis, the Liberal Party minority government, with the support of the New Democratic party, has emasculated parliament through a sordid political coup. Parliamentary government has been replaced by a virtual system of government, and presidential-style TV 'morning show' announcements of government policy and programs by the Prime Minister. That transformation has been affected without any substantive negative comment or outrage expressed in the media. Instead of being denounced as a travesty of parliamentary government, and of representative democracy, the Presidential-style government has been welcomed by the Press.

The Fourth Estate is relishing its new prominence. The elected representatives of the people in parliament have been bypassed, and supplanted by a press gathering that is being addressed directly by the

Prime Minister, Justin Trudeau, during his TV 'morning show' with only the media enjoying access to a question period each day. Canada has lost its tradition of parliamentary government with nary a whimper. The country is being ruled by a benevolent despot bestowing government largesse on whomever he favours and whatever causes he supports, both domestically and internationally.

10) That under the guise of providing financial assistance to Canadian men and women who have lost their job due to the coronavirus lockdown, Prime Minister Trudeau has introduced a massive social assistance spending program.

Under the guise of providing financial assistance to Canadian men and women who have lost their jobs during the pandemic, Prime Minister Trudeau has established open-ended social assistance spending programs that are open to all applicants. It is but a reflection of his social egalitarian ideology which he articulates as ensuring that "no one get left behind'. The Trudeau government has universalized the Canada Emergency Response Benefit (CERB) wage subsidy program for the unemployed, and has turned it into a guaranteed income program by introducing a 'look the other way' payment policy that issues payments to each and every applicant without verifying their eligibility under the program parameters. Moreover, the Liberal government has included in its mammoth omnibus financial aid bills – which were supposedly aimed at providing support for unemployed workers and support for businesses suffering a closure or drastic revenue loss during the coronavirus lockdown – a number of special multi-hundred-million-dollar financial grants to various communities within Canada in promoting the social agenda of the Liberal Party.

Economists in reviewing the massive cost of the supposedly temporary universalized CERB program, are expressing concerns that it might become a permanent, highly costly, and unaffordable, guaranteed annual income social assistance program. What is equally concerning is that the Liberal government has rejected any effort by the public service to flag or investigate obvious cases of fraud. Moreover, international students and foreign seasonal workers have been made eligible for CERB payments with 'no proof of status' required to show whether they have worked for any period of time in Canada, or whether they are presently in Canada or have left and are simply having the money deposited into a Canadian bank account.

Moreover, Conservatives are expressing a fear that the $2,000 per month payment to part-time workers is overly generous and will prove to be a disincentive for them to return to part-time work as the economy re-opens. For Conservatives, the way in which the CERB is being administered by the federal Liberal government not only raises serious economic and management concerns, but a moral concern in that it encourages fraud and, where part-time workers are concerned, it undermines the work ethic.

On the other hand, the Prime Minister has shown a definite anti-business bias in the programs established to provide financial assistance to businesses. The financial support programs for businesses have strict eligibility requirements, and most are in the form of loans that are repayable. Moreover, the financial support provided for large companies – such as potentially the oil and gas companies, and the airlines, under the Large Employer Emergency Finance Facility (LEEFF) -- consists of loans at a prohibitive rate of interest, repayable within five years, with companies applying for a loan having to report on how they will be net carbon emissions neutral by 2050. It is a blatant imposition of the Liberal government green energy ideology on Canadian companies seeking emergency financial assistance during a pandemic that has devastated their industry through no fault of their own.

11) **That the federal Liberal government under Prime Minister Justin Trudeau has failed to show any sense of fiscal responsibility in establishing open-ended social assistance programs that have caused the national deficit to soar out of control.**

Rather than targeting financial assistance benefits to the men and women who lost their jobs during the pandemic, the Liberal government has universalized the Canada Emergency Response Benefit (CERB) program in making payments to anyone who applies. As of late May, the CERB program alone has expended $41 billon dollars to 8.25 million recipients. (In contrast, the Canada Emergency Wage Subsidy (CEWS) payroll payment program – intended to encourage employers to keep their workers employed -- has paid out only $7.9 billion to companies under the eligibility rules.)

Where the CERB wage subsidy for unemployed workers is concerned, the Liberal government deliberately did away with the conventional screenings of applications, ignored the eligibility criteria governing the CERB program as authorized by parliament, and has provided opportunists and criminal elements with an open invitation to fraud. Prime Minister Trudeau claims that in order to get financial assistance quickly to Canadians, his government was willing to accept that "one or two percent' of the CERB payments might be based on fraudulent claims. However, the Public Service has reported that CERB payments are being made to upwards of 200,000 recipients who may be defrauding the program under the open-ended, pay all applicants without question system established by the Liberal government. Over the four months duration of the CERB program, the payments to 200,000 claimants who are suspected of engaging in fraud, will amount to $1.6 billion; yet nothing is being done to investigate these cases. The Liberal government is maintaining that it will undertake to recover the money that has been 'mistakenly paid' when income tax returns are filed, which supposes that the fraudsters pay income tax and can be located.

As of the late May, the new financial assistance programs of the federal Liberal government have accounted for an expenditure of $146 billion in payments to Canadians negatively impacted by the coronavirus lockdown. The Parliamentary Budget Officer has estimated -- as of the end of May -- that the federal government deficit may reach $260 billion by 2021. It will be the highest Canadian deficit on record. In 2019, Canada paid $23 billion in interest payments to service the national debt, and that debt is now soaring out of control with the Liberal government of Prime Minister Justin Trudeau making no effort to rein in costs.

12) **That the coronavirus pandemic has revealed the dangers inherent in relying on global markets for basic necessities; and that Canada ought to institute a national economic policy – a good Tory Conservative policy – to ensure that Canada has a domestic production capacity to supply personal protective equipment, medical supplies and testing equipment, critical drugs, and basic**

foods, as well as energy supplies, in the event of any future worldwide crisis – war, famine, drought, or a virus pandemic.

During the coronavirus pandemic, the global market was a 'wild west' with needed supplies unobtainable, or exorbitantly priced, with substandard products being sold in the global market, and purchased products often not being delivered owing to transportation problems with ports and airports being closed down or with restricted access. Moreover, the economy was damaged by a flooding of the global market with cheap oil during a pricing dispute between OPEC and Russia which contributed to the downward plunge of Canadian oil prices, which was compounded by the impact of the shrinking of the local market demand during the lockdown period. In Canada, it was the Ontario Conservative government that took the initial action in turning to domestic companies to manufacture personal protective equipment and ventilators that were in a critically short supply in hospitals and long-term care homes, owing to the federal Liberal government having sent Canada's national stockpile of that equipment to China in early February. And it was the Ontario government that acted to introduce legislation against price gouging in critically needed supplies and equipment.

The coronavirus pandemic illustrates the need for Canada to institute a policy of national economic development to ensure the well-being and security of supply of basic necessities in times of international crises – war, famine, drought, or pandemics. Canada ought to review the extent of its involvement in the global trade system on a cost and benefits analysis and on the basis of strategic national concerns, and ought to abandon the current Modern liberal fetish for 'universal free trade'.

Canada ought to strive for a self-sufficiency in the production of medical supplies, drugs, testing kits, basic foods, and energy, to protect Canadians from future shortages and exposure to the vicissitudes of the 'wild west' of global markets. Moreover, Canada's national interests ought to be primary in any trade negotiations. What is needed are trade agreements based on quid pro quos with clearly defined economic and social benefits for Canadians, rather than simply opening up the Canadian market to foreign countries in assuming that 'free trade' will yield substantial benefits to Canada. The movement of manufacturing and services offshore has shown the fallacy of that argument. Moreover, the coronavirus pandemic has shown the danger inherent in relying on a global supply chain for basic needs in a free trade system.

13) **That whether or not a successful vaccine can be developed and widely-distributed, that the spread of the coronavirus can be stopped, and outbreaks brought under control, by traditional flu epidemic public health protocols, without the need to develop a 'herd immunity'.**

To date, the federal Public Health Agency has been fixated on developing a 'herd immunity' to stamp out the coronavirus. The concept is that it can be done by a vaccination of upwards of sixty percent of the population – when, and if a proven vaccine has been developed -- or by the development of a 'background immunity' when upwards of sixty percent of the community have become infected with the coronavirus and have developed a natural immunity with antibodies having been produced by their immune system. However, the effectiveness of a 'background immunity', if it can ever be attained, will depend on the antibodies being produce by the immune system retaining their strength over a long period – for at least a year or more. It has yet to be determined whether that is the case with the coronavirus. The fallacy of relying on a 'herd immunity' approach to control the spread, and eliminate the coronavirus is that both the vaccination and background immunity approaches are potential long-term solutions. They do nothing to address the immediate practical problem of stopping the spread of the coronavirus within society.

However, the traditional flu epidemic public health protocols have proven successful in preventing the spread of the coronavirus, as was the case during the Spanish flu pandemic of 1918-1919 when doctors were dealing with another highly contagious, unknown, and deadly virus. In response, the public was warned to practice a physical distancing and avoid crowds, large public gatherings were banned, the public were advised to wear cotton face masks, and to cover their mouth when coughing, to avoid the use of common drinking cups, to wash their hands before eating, to sterilize dishes with boiling water, and to stay at home when feeling ill. Churches and many businesses were closed, and the number of persons permitted on streetcars and admitted to grocery stores was limited. The sick were quarantined in their home, or in hospital if severely ill. These public health protocols were highly successful in curtailing the spread of the Spanish flu virus in the cities where they were enforced by municipal government edicts. Moreover, the cities that maintained the public health protocols in place following the decline of the Spanish flu pandemic, were spared the second wave of virus infections that followed in many areas.

The question is: why did the Public Health Agency of Canada neglect to provide Canadians with a similar public health advice and direction -- based on the Spanish flu experience -- during February and March 2020 when Canadians were faced with the threat of the onslaught of yet another unknown foreign virus? Instead, the federal government and the Public Health Agency of Canada advised Canadians simply to 'stay home' and self-isolate, to maintain a two-metre social spacing when out in public, and to wash ones hands with soap and water or to use a hand sanitizer after contact with outside common surfaces. It was a passive approach to the coronavirus threat by the federal government, which left it up to the provincial public health care systems to deal with the wave of coronavirus cases. While the federal government public health authorities remained rather passive and fatalistic, it was the provincial governments, and provincial and municipal health agencies, that promulgated public health regulations and provided health care advice for the public in addressing the immediate problem of curtailing the spread of the coronavirus.

14) **That Canadians may have to live with the presence of the coronavirus for some time to come, but that it can be kept under control and outbreaks can be readily suppressed.**

With the provincial lockdowns being gradually lifted in phases, in a cautious re-opening of the economy, there is a palpable fear among the public that a second wave of coronavirus infections will break out as the lockdowns are relaxed. As of late May, most of the provinces are re-opening retail stores, businesses and workplaces under strict public health protocols, with the opening of indoor dining restaurants, bars, gyms, and sporting events that bring large numbers of people together, to follow in a later phase. Daycare centres are re-opening, and elementary schools in Quebec, but most provinces are waiting to the fall to re-open their schools.

It appears that the education ministries intend to provide both in-school classes as well an on-line learning option, with restrictions on the number of students in a classroom to enforce a physical spacing of the students. Parents will have the option of whether to send their children to school, or to keep them home in accessing the online learning available.

There is a public pressure on the federal government to keep the Canadian border closed to international travellers, inclusive of American visitors. With the coronavirus surge in the United States appearing to have peaked in its New York area epicentre, there are hotspots developing in the American south, south-west and north-west. It appears that the securing of a proven vaccine is still a long way off, yet the dramatic fall in new infections in Canada, and the decline in coronavirus patients in Canadian hospitals, is an encouraging sign that Canada has passed through the worst of the coronavirus pandemic. It provides grounds for hope in moving into the recovery stage.

Epidemiologists are becoming convinced that the coronavirus will be present within communities worldwide for some time to come, perhaps for several years. However, they are convinced that coronavirus outbreaks can be managed, and the coronavirus kept under control, through tracking infections, testing contacts, and the imposition of a strict 14-day self-isolation on those testing negative and a quarantine on those testing positive. More generally, controlling the spread of the coronavirus will require individuals, whether working, shopping, or socializing, to continue to wear face masks at all times, and to observe public health protocols in practicing a frequent washing of hands, and social spacing whenever and wherever practicable while avoiding large gatherings, and that these personal efforts will need to be supplemented by a commitment from businesses, employers, retailers, and schools, to the disinfecting of common-touch surfaces, and the enforcing of the wearing of face masks, hygiene rules, and social spacing within their premises.

What is indisputable is that although the number of new coronavirus cases is declining daily, and there has been a reduction in the severity of the sickness among coronavirus cases, COVID-19 remains an ever present threat to reassert itself if Canadians relax their adherence to public health protocols.

Note: The commentary in this Retrospective provides an overview of the lessons learned in recording and analyzing developments in the politics, science, and economics of the coronavirus pandemic in Canada up to May 24th, 2020. Subsequent developments -- and the commentary and analysis thereof -- have been recorded in a second volume of diary entries spanning the period from May 25th through to July 31st, inclusive.

Index

Index: Temporary Programs

March 2020

BCAP: Business Credit Availability Program – a federal government loan and loan guarantee program available to small- and medium-sized business owners to help cover their operating costs while revenues are temporarily reduced owing to the coronavirus pandemic.
  introduction (March 25th), 56
  program, 56, 246-247
  focus & eligibility, 56, 247
  $12.5 billion loan fund, 56
  immediate funding, 56

CEBA: Canada Emergency Business Account – provides an interest-free emergency government loan of up to $40,000 to help small businesses and not-for-profits to cover unexpected business-operating expenses incurred with the impact of the coronavirus pandemic.
  introduction (March 25th), 56
  program, 56-57, 203
  emergency loan, 56
  $25 billion in funding, 56
  tax deferral, 296
  applicants, 203
  eligibility (initial), 295-296
  eligibility broadened to include self-employed, 295

CERB: Canada Emergency Response Benefit – provides a monthly $2,000 payment for up to four months to workers who have lost their job through the impact of the coronavirus pandemic; recipients must re-apply each month for the benefit.
  introduction (March 25th), 53
  earlier wage subsidy proposal, 71
  purpose, 53, 76
  monthly $2,000 payment, 53
  four-month duration (initially), 172-173
  fully computerized payments system, 76-77, 79
  activated April 1st, 80 (program backdated to March 15th)
  eligibility (initial), 53, 76
  $40 billion projected cost, 200
  administrative integrity compromised, 80, 240, 242
  no applicants screening, 265
  potential fraud concern, 297
  eligibility extended, inclusive of seasonal workers, 94
  becoming a 'universal basic income', 203
  claimed inequities, 172-173
  work disincentive for part-time workers, 180, 203, 230
  number of applicants, 180, 203
  mounting costs, 180, 200
  CERB fraud, 240-242
  extent of fraud, 265-267
  potential fraud costs, 188-189

Auditor-General concern, 298
double dipping with EI, 242-243
public service morale problem, 266
acceptance of fraud losses (Liberal government), 266
necessity argument, 266

April 2020

CEWS: Canada Emergency Wage Subsidy – a payroll wage subsidy paid to companies who recall workers laid off due to the coronavirus pandemic, with the individual wage subsidy payments made on a sliding scale based on the regular pay of each recalled worker.

legislation passed (April 11th), 67, 94
initial announcement (March 26th), 67-58, 94
initial proposal, 77
program, 67-68, 171, 277
open to all companies, including not-for-profits and charities, 67-68
eligibility terms, 68
payments to companies that apply, 68
payroll wage subsidy must go to recalled employees, 68
initial coverage period (twelve weeks, March 15th- June 6th), 230
$73 billion initial estimate, 200
few initial applicants, 171
small businesses qualifying problem, 68, 171-172
broadening of eligibility for small businesses, 67-68, 276-277
new program cost projection ($83 billion, early April), 200
estimated $75.9 billion in payments made (early May), 200
benefitting 1.7 million recalled workers (early May), 230
over 130,000 company applicants (early May), 230
coverage period extended (May 15th) from June 6th to August 29th, 276
further loosening of eligibility requirements, 276
viewed as a recovery stimulus for companies, 230

CECRA: Canada Emergency Commercial Rent Assistance – provides commercial rent relief for small business tenants, during the coronavirus pandemic, through paying 50 percent of their monthly rent in the form of a forgivable loan to landlords who agree to 'reduce the rent by 25 percent' (actually forego collecting 25 percent of the rent), who agree to accept a payment of 25 percent of the rent from their commercial tenant as payment in full from the tenant, and who agree to refrain from evicting the small business tenant paying the reduced rent levy.

need for a commercial rent relief program, 68
announced (April 25th), 158
commercial rent relief program, 158-159, 256-257
benefit for retail store tenants, 159
joint federal-provincial funding, 158,
forgivable loan to landlords (terms), 159
eligibility (initial), 159
projected $2 billion cost, 159, 256
low response from landlords, 257
reasons for, 257-258
broader eligibility introduced, 256

CESB: Canada Emergency Student Benefit – provides financial support to recent high school graduates and post-secondary students who are unable to find work due to the impact of the coronavirus pandemic to help them finance their education when returning to school.

Announced (April 22nd), 130
submitted to parliament (April 29th), 179
student jobless benefit, 137, 179
monthly payment structure, 179
duration (May-August), 179
$9-billion projected cost, 179
payments increased (NDP demand), 179
extra earnings incentive (Conservative demand), 179-180
work disincentive concern, 180, 203
open to all post-secondary Canadian students, 180

(In announcing the projected CESB program on April 22nd, Prime Minister Trudeau mentioned that it would include a $5,000 bursary for students who volunteered to work in an essential job during the coronavirus pandemic. (133-134, 179-180). Subsequently, the $5,000 payment for student volunteer work was moved into a new separate program, the Canada Student Service Grant program, and a contract was let to the WE Charity of Toronto to manage the new student volunteer work program.)

May 2020

LEEFF: Large Employer Emergency Financing Facility – provides large employer companies, who can demonstrate a need for greater liquidity, with access to loans to help in minimizing layoffs and in sustaining their business and investment activities during the coronavirus pandemic.

announcement (May 11th), 243
projected large company loans, 243
oil industry financial need, 244
earlier low interest loans promise, 243
program, 243-244
federal government 'lender of last resort', 243
unlimited multi-million-dollar loans, 246
loan restrictions on management, 243
loans structure, 246
existing bank investment in oil industry, 245
program politicization, 244-246
environmental commitment requirement, 244
high interest rates, 246
short repayment term for unsecured portion of loans, 246
a poison pill for oil industry, 246
continuation of a policy of strangling the oil industry (Liberal government), 245
program activated (May 20th), 245
an inadequate and belated large company financial aid program, 243-246

Existing Student Employment Program

SWWP: Student Work Placement Program – provides assistance, in cooperation with potential employers, for students to secure a part-time or summer job, and provides a wage subsidy to employers who place students in 'quality work placements' to provide them with paid employment and experience in their field of study.

program administered by Employment and Social Services Canada, 136
wage subsidies paid to employers who hire students, 136
higher payments for employing visible minority, disabled, and female students, 136-137

international students eligible, 136-137

Index: General

Airports/Airlines (Canada)
voluntary self-isolation, 98
visual screening only, 18-19, 48
criticism of screening, 43-48, 322-323
no testing or quarantining, 43-44, 322-323
proposed quarantine, 61, 98
proposed fines, 61
lax enforcement, 61-62,
four airports designated, 19, 24
domestic flights sick ban, 65
Quarantine Act powers, 98
taxi driver vulnerabilities, 173
air traffic decline, 173, 296
airport financial losses, 173
airline financial losses, 206, 273
no direct airlines aid, 273
vs U.S. direct aid, 176, 273-274
airline job losses, 174, 206, 272
support from CEWS, 206
recovery prospects, 206
virus protection (planes), 174-176
South Korean airlines, 175-176
virus protection (airports), 175, 296-297
South Korean airports, 175-176
airlines indebtedness (global), 274
airplane seat spacing, 297

Bank of Canada
crisis response, 9
bond purchases, 64, 104, 138

Banks (Big Six)
mortgage relief, 62

Border Closures (Canada)
14-day isolation rule, 6, 11
open borders bias, 20
political correctness factor, 20
federal rejection of, 19-20, 23
Ontario view, 13,17
Alberta view, 17
British Columbia view, 22-23
Conservative demand, 20, 30-31,195
public demand for, 195, 306
travel ban needed, 195
N. American Influenza Plan, 169, 170
failure to implement, 170
travellers from China, 194-195
ban on foreign travellers, 17, 24, 27
exemption: seasonal workers, 41-42,
    305-306
exemption: international students, 41,
    305-306, 321
four designated airports, 19
Americans exemption, 24-25, 27
border closure delay, 196-197
Trudeau defence of delay, 197
Canada/US border closure, 27
border closure extension, 256, 289
Northwest Territories, 46
Nunavut, 46, 322
returning travellers, 48
Canada-Mexico-US Act, 169-170
criticism of government, 102
inadequacies of, 170, 304-305, 322-323

Border Closures (Global)
Italy, 4, 6, 19
South Korea, 115
Taiwan, 115
United States, 16, 20
Australia, 20
Britain, 16
European Union, 16, 22, 35, 45
Denmark, 22

Canadian Military Aid
ready to aid, 63
Long-Care Homes (Ontario), 261
Long-Care Homes (Quebec), 261, 310
sickness among military, 310

China
virus threat, 3, 36
cases/deaths, 3-4, 10, 39-40
death rates, 4
quarantines, 3, 60, 66-67
strict lockdowns, 3, 15
recovery, 75

Conservative Party
pandemic response, 20, 30-31
McKay, Peter, 30
O'Toole, Erin, 30
Lewis, Dr. Leslyn, 31
Sloan, Derek, 31
Parliament essential, 119, 122, 311-312

Coronavirus (COVID-19)
novel virus, 3, 7, 324-325
Wuhan, China 3-4, 38
early view of, 4-5, 38, 40
symptoms, 3,5, 325

'low risk' claim, 14
elderly vulnerability, 10, 326-327
age factor, 248
Wuhan lab origin, 282
contagiousness, 12-13
impact on children, 13, 326
asymptomatic carriers, 13, 67
flattening curve, 13-14
early advice (other governments), 13
social distancing, 13
general advice (Federal government), 13
soap & water, 12
spreading ratio key, 13
pathology, 38-39
quarantining, 39
no vaccine, 39
genome mapping (China), 177
COV virus DNA family, 177
canine detection, 181
questioning lockdowns, 184-188
inflammatory syndrome, 209-212
future evolution theories, 222
mutations possible, 306
new outbreaks preparedness, 222-223

Coronavirus Cases (Canada)
modelling, 7
questioning of modelling, 233
traveller transmission, 6-7, 21, 27, 196
importation from, 196
cruise ships, 8, 196
first case (January 26th), 37,
first death (March 8th), 10, 196
first in-community transmission, 196
in-community transmission, 27, 66, 196
early infection rate, 61
hospitalizations, 76, 231-232
elective surgeries delay, 70
confirmed cases (March), 4, 7, 11, 21, 25,
    27, 40, 47, 54, 66, 75, 197
deaths (March), 27, 40, 47, 66, 75-76, 197
testing (March), 76
cases (April), 99-100, 116, 125, 16, 197
deaths (April), 99-100, 116, 161, 197
April epicentres, 99
long-care homes, 99
flattening of curve (mid-April), 125, 201
confirmed cases (May), 196, 259
daily cases descending (May):
    1,825 high, 757 low, vi
daily cases record high:
    May 3: 2,760 cases, vi
downward trend (early May), 208, 214

Maritimes (early May), 209
lessons not learned, 233-234
practical measures, 234
provincial cases (mid-May), 260-262
provincial deaths (mid-May), 260-262
cases (mid-May), 263
deaths (mid-May) 263
Indigenous peoples' cases, 262-263
drop in new cases (May), 263
deaths (mid-May), 259
daily cases low (mid-May), 259
cases (late May), 300
deaths (late May), 300

Coronavirus Cases (Global)
China, 3, 15-16, 66
Iran, 3
Italy, 3, 6, 8, 66, 75, 188, 290
South Korea, 3, 114-116
Spain, 4, 22, 125, 126
United States, 4, 66, 75-76, 256, 289
U.S. global percent (mid-May), 289
age factor (New York), 248
February situation, 3-4
global modelling, 4
global travel, 8
United Kingdom, 2, 9
global cases, 4, 8, 12, 75-76, 100, 207
global deaths, 8, 12, 75-76, 100, 207
death rate, 4
early inaction (Europe), 22
Denmark, 22
Europe, mid-March, 22
potential contagion, 22
Taiwan, 32
April epicentres, 100
number of countries (May), 207
Brazil: cases & deaths, 227
Eastern Europe surge (May), 264
U.S. cases soaring (May), 289
U.S. deaths soaring (May), 289
Sweden, 298-300
Africa: cases & deaths (March end), 72

Coronavirus Impact (Canada)
initial business response, 10
provincial leadership, 16, 76
on workforce, 75
on retail sector, 75
on airline traffic, 200
on economy, 200
growing fiscal deficit, 53
increasing national debt,

unemployment claims (March), 77
unemployment levels (March), 77
job losses (March), 106
job losses (April), 297
reduced work hours (April), 297
on tourism industry, 130-131
on real estate, 159-160, 258
on municipal debt, 138, 189, 265
on farmers & ranchers, 139-140, 206
packing plant closures, 140
on child immunizations, 177-178
on renters, 259
apartment rents, 259
massive layoffs, 180
economic sectors impact, 180
manufacturing decline (April), 184
job losses (April), 228
reduced hours workers, 228
unemployment rate, 228
hardest hit sectors, 228
food sales increase (April), 184
transmission by travelers, 196
social distancing, 224
seafood market collapse, 268-270
court postponements, 303-304
essential retail workers, 309
lawyers, 310
total provincial debts (May 22nd), 304
provincial debt problem, 304

Coronavirus Impact (Alberta)
confirmed cases, 7, 209
deaths, 209
packing plant closures, 140
testing, 209

Coronavirus Impact (B. C.)
confirmed cases, 7
first death, 10, 196

Coronavirus Impact (Ontario)
initial response, 26-27
lockdown, 26
Ontario modelling, 83
death rate benchmark, 84
cases 7-8, 66, 83, 161, 191, 207
deaths, 66, 83, 161, 191, 207
hospitalizations, 191
patients on ventilators, 191
intensive care patients, 191
domestic PPE supply, 86
lockdown extension, 84
long-care homes, 10, 99

high infection rate, 99
'hospital teams' support, 99
testing, Ontario rate, 99

Coronavirus Impact (Quebec)
initial impact, 7, 27
cases, 99, 113, 161, 207, 229
deaths, 99, 113, 161, 207, 229
½ Canadian deaths (May), 229
long-care homes, 99
Montreal epicentre, 229
high infection rate, 99
processing plant closures, 140
job losses, 181

Coronavirus Impact (Saskatchewan)
La Loche outbreak, 213-214

Drug Treatments
remdesivir, 201, 317
potential, 317
reducing impact strategy, 317

Excess Deaths,
concept, 237
British Columbia, 237
New York City, 237

Emergency Measures Act (Canada)
rejection of, 41, 45-46, 50, 52
Conservatives for, 45
terms of, 46, 49-50
Conservative rationale, 46-47
provincial enactments, 46, 65-66
too late to implement, 98
War Measures Act memory, 98

Employment Insurance (EI)
initial claims, 47, 53
lockdown claims, 79-80
new payments system, 80
no applicants screening, 240-241
heightened fraud risk, 241
international students, 241-242

Face Masks
shortages, 45, 81, 84
effectiveness, 43, 114-115, 152-155,
330-331
domestic production, 22, 71, 155
purchases, 213, 224-225
China gift to Canada, 64
China quality problem, 64
China export ban, 225
N-95 mask efficiency, 225

new material (China), 67
South Korea, 114-115, 152
Spain, 202
Europe, 202
controversy, 291-292
Public Health rejection, 290
Public Health reversal, 290
face masks effectiveness, 152
supplies from U.S., 86, 87

Face Shields
government orders, 72
domestic production, 89,138
3D printer production, 182

Federal COVID-19 Response
initial response, 3, 18, 23-25, 39-40, 44-45
slow-the-spread strategy, 5, 14
border closures, 23, 27
ad hoc approach, 24, 200
self-isolating policy, 23-25
failure to quarantine, 36-37
crisis management failure, 38
lack of direction, 44
globalist outlook, 60

Financial Aid Programs:
Omnibus Bill: (March 25th),
announcement, 52, 77
initiatives, 33-34, 53-57, 172-173,
246-247
see Index: Programs, BCAP, CEBA,
CERB
projected $82 billion cost, 73

Financial Aid Programs:
Omnibus Bill: (April 11th),
earlier announcement, 55, 94
initiatives, 67-68, 73
see Index: Programs, CEWS,
projected $71 billion cost, 73
extension, 67-68

Financial Aid Program:
CECRA, 158-159, 256-258
announced (April 25th), 158
projected $2 billion cost, 159
see Index: Programs,
CECRA,

Financial Aid Program:
CESB, 179-180
announced (April 22nd), 179
projected $ 9 billion cost, 179

see Index: Programs, CESB,

Financial Aid Program:
LEEFF, 243-246, 295-296
announced (May 11th), 243
see Index: Programs, LEEFF,

Financial Aid Projects (targeted)
initial spending, 9
Indigenous communities, 34, 108-109,
Indigenous, Inuit & Metis students, 133
Indigenous Services, 307
farm aid, 104, 106, 200, 212
Seafood Stabilization Fund, 160
vaccine research, 180
food processing, 212
Agri-Recovery, 212
surplus food purchase, 212
dairy products purchase, 213
aid for seniors, 215, 248-251
fishing industry, 267-268
research institutions, 280
Income Tax postponement, 280

Fiscal Deficit
soaring, 57, 200, 230
pre-pandemic record $27 billion deficit, 71
projected $200 billion deficit
(March 30th), 71
projected $292 billion (mid-May), 230

Globalism
Liberal globalist mindset, 320
supply chain problem, 90
growing rejection of, 163, 221-222,
223-224
food security concerns, 165-167, 212
global 'decoupling' need, 157-168
national energy policy need, 167
domestic supply need, 85
energy self-sufficiency, 219-221
drug supply problem, 252

Hajdu, Patty
Health Minister
initial response, 9
no border closure, 19, 23,27
vs Conservatives, 20
no emergencies act, 46
defence of China, 108

Illegal Migrants
Roxham Road issue, 28-29
view of PM Trudeau, 29, 55

banning of, 54
Liberal concern for, 58-59
American troops, 54-55

International Students
border closure exemption, 41
travel difficulties, 198
numbers of (2019), 198
concerns, 198-199

Italy
lockdown, 6
cases, 15, 45, 75, 188
deaths, 5,8, 45, 75, 188
border closure, 19, 185-188, 194
recovery, 289-290

Lessons Learned
Retrospective, 319-340

Liberal Government
open borders commitment, 196
power grab attempt, 49, 53, 331
absolutism, 49, 239
agenda, 50, 270
information access, 52
unrestrained spending, 52
pre-pandemic deficits, 70-71
ignored Keynesian theory, 71
escalating national debt, 71
criticism of, 70, 72, 74, 102-103, 216-217, 234
discipline adverse, 32-33
neglecting oil industry, 73-74
grants to WHO, 204
foreign takeovers problem, 125
ad hoc government, 134-136, 270
'hands off' recovery approach, 147-148
pre-pandemic deficits, 70-71
soaring federal deficit, 200
reliance on WHO, 233
CERB fraud acceptance, 266
necessity defence, 266
lack of leadership, 302, 329
by-passing parliament, 311
globalist outlook, 320

Liberal Press
bias, 30, 33, 145, 216, 333-334
praising Trudeau, 74

Lockdowns
China, 3, 5, 15-16,67
Italy, 6
France, 25

Ontario, 26-27, 47-48, 84
Quebec, 27, 202
unnecessary, 184-185, 187-188, 278-280
other countries, 187
comparative statistics, 188
need to lift (Europe, early May), 202-203
cost to Canada, 300-301
alternatives to, 300-301, 315-316

Long-Care Homes
vulnerability, 10
major outbreaks,
British Columbia, 10
Ontario, 10, 99
Quebec, 99,
outbreak hotspots, 99, 131
high infection rates, 99
Ontario 'hospital teams', 99
City of Ottawa, 109-110
staff wage supports, 112-113
military support, 131, 214
staff shortages, 132-133, 208
Ontario testing, 137
vaccinations not updated, 199
soaring infections, 207
percent of deaths, 207
Ontario response, 208
private homes problem, 229
Quebec dire situation, 208
B.C. outbreaks, 232-233
cases in Ontario
cases in Quebec,
military support, 261, 310

Medical Services
hospital situation (April), 109
plight of private practitioners, 109

Medical Supplies
from China & India, 92
swabs from Italy, 92
need 'global decoupling', 92
'national strategy' needed, 92, 117
Insulin example, 92-93
drugs from India, 117

Modern liberalism
values & beliefs, 199, 270-272, 332-333

Modern liberals
discipline adverse, 57, 266
globalist mindset, 20, 51, 223-224, 320
ideology, 270-272
open borders bias, 20, 35-36

political correctness, 20, 143-144, 320
crave power, 50
agenda, 51-52, 332-333
denigration of Conservatives, 332-333
managerial inadequacies, 74
La La Land mentality, 30, 71
no fiscal responsibility, 57
free spending, 266

National Debt
projected $962 billion (mid-May), 264
percent of GDP, 264
debt service charges, 264
$64 billion added (May 22nd), 304

National Emergency Stockpile
purpose & organization, 285-286
PHAC responsibility, 285

Newspapers (Canada)
job losses, 206-207
factors, 206

Oil Industry
market collapse, 9-10, 217
economic crises, 75-74
no federal aid, 73,
financial needs, 96
contribution to Canada, 97
global oil production, 97
an economic driver, 97
oil well remediation, 107
financial aid promises, 217
rumoured $15 billion aid, 107, 115, 244
carbon emissions decline, 107,
global production cuts, 124-125
potential recovery driver, 129-130
shutdown oilsands (Greens), 217-220
contributions to Canada, 219
carbon emissions cuts, 247
LEEFF: a poison pill, 246
investment withdrawals, 247
petrochemicals, 251
China threat, 251-252
industry recovery, 290-291

Parliament
initial suspension, 17-18
smaller representation, 17-18, 93
emergency sessions, 118
Liberal 'virtual' proposal, 119, 121
Conservative proposal, 119, 122
virtual sessions problem, 121-122

emasculation of Parliament, 123-124, 276
rubber stamp Parliament, 136
Conservative recall demand, 239, 311
an essential service, 311-312
restore parliamentary democracy, 239-240
government by 'experts', 274-275
lacks experience (ministers), 275
lack of leadership, 275
virtual parliament bias, 312
Liberal 'hybrid' proposal, 312
Bloc Quebecois position, 313
NDP position, 313
virtual parliament problems, 313-314

Personal Care Workers
PPE shortages, 128-129
staff shortages, 11-12
pay supplement, 225, 260

Personal Protective Equipment
shipments to China, 59-60, 81, 198
national stockpile depletion, 86-87, 198,
    314, 328-329
Liberal cover-up, 314, 315
critical shortages, 7, 44-45, 59, 60-61, 66
parliamentary investigation, 285
national stockpile purpose, 285
Public Health Agency obfuscations, 285
Public Health Agency mandate, 286
ventilators, 40-41, 42, 71-72, 88-89
N-95 face masks, 42, 45, 81
Algonquin College loan, 59
global situation, 72, 85
efforts to purchase (global), 14, 84
exorbitant prices (global), 84
domestic suppliers, 22, 64, 71-72, 84, 86,
    89-90, 155, 182
distribution concern, 182-183
excessive purchases, 73, 85
faulty products (China), 64, 85, 301
national standards needed, 301-302, 317
failed global supply chain, 84-85, 87,
    90-91
a 'Wild West', 91
American export ban, 85-86
excessively massive orders, 86-87
non-fulfilment of global orders, 87
domestic supply needed, 86, 91
face mask sterilization, 89-90

Phoenix Pay System
earlier mismanagement, 77-78

Post-pandemic Government
   innovation theories, 308-309

Public Health Agency (Canada)
   initial response, 5, 7-10
   initial policy, 4-5, 13-14
   reliance on WHO, 5-6
   modelling, 14
   poor airport screening, 18-19, 43-44, 48
   quarantining proposal, 61
   lack of enforcement, 61-62
   criticism of approach, 108, 321
   herd immunity focus, 149
   Immunity Task Force, 149-150
   herd immunity problem, 142-143
   parliamentary investigation, 192
   revelations, 192-195
   preparedness failure, 193
   lack of threat awareness, 193
   no early warning system, 197
   mandate failure, 197
   open borders commitment, 196
   ignored SARS experience, 156, 197
   national stockpile dereliction, 198

Public Health (Ontario)
   initial assessment, 8
   health protocols, 10

Public Service
   response, 11-12
   office closures, 73

Quarantine Act (Canada)
   powers, 61-62, 98
   adoption, 98

Quarantine
   China, 3, 66-67

Recovery
   herd immunity concept, 142-143
   herd immunity strategy, 148, 189, 315
   variolation controversy, 142
   vaccine delays, 149
   antibody levels concern, 315
   WHO position, 149
   'background pool', 149
   impracticality of, 142-143, 150-151
   Immunity Task Force, 149-150
   disease pathology research, 152
   a different strategy, 153-155
   work return fears, 171
   tourism corridors (Europe), 176

provincial leadership, 139
phased approach, 178-179
provincial precautions, 202
Ontario plan, 178-179, 190-191, 229, 254-255
Quebec plan, 181-182, 202, 229
continuing virus threat, 189
long-care homes battle (mid-May), 201
elsewhere under control (mid-May), 201, 259
Alberta plan, 191-192, 202
Manitoba, 202
recovery in Germany, 126-127, 215, 235
restaurant social spacing, 251, 300
indoor spacing problem, 113-115
CEWS recovery factor, 230-231
hospitalizations, 231-232
elective surgeries renewal, 231-232
health protocols, 234
practical approach, 247-248
cottage visits dispute, 251
childcare support need, 281
contact tracking need, 288
re-opening borders (Europe), 288-289
Italy, 290
Oil industry, 290-291
City of Ottawa, 302-303
living with COVID-19, 317-318

SARS Pandemic (2002-2004)
   earlier deaths/death rate, 4
   health protocols, 156-157
   impact, 156-157
   deaths (global), 156
   deaths (Canada), 156
   symptoms, 156
   experience ignored, 156

Schools (Elementary)
   schools closed (mid-March), 26, 326
   Quebec re-opening, 238-239, 259
   Ontario re-opening plan, 292
   school days missed, 293
   social promotion system, 292-295

Seasonal Workers
   essential workers, 104
   border ban exemption, 41, 305-306
   employment areas, 41
   14-day isolation, 42, 105
   better approach needed, 105-106
   problem in securing, 42, 106

numbers admitted, 41, 306
countries of origin, 41
Liberal government policy, 42
existing legislation, 42

Second Wave
fears, 235
false alarms, 235

Serology Testing
new developments, 151
process, 151-152

South Korea
pandemic response, 114
early border closure, 115
testing kits, 16, 115
contact tracking, 115
low case numbers, 116
low death numbers, 116
no lockdown, 114

Spanish flu (1918-1919)
total cases, 156
deaths, 4, 156
death rate, 156
health protocols, 4, 156-157
impact, 156

Sports Leagues
problems faced, 111-112
government grants issue, 235-236
early events, 236-237

Student Job Creation Project
WE Charity proposal, 134

Taiwan
pandemic response, 31-32
smartphone tracking, 31
borders closures, 32
low case numbers, 32
low death numbers, 32
no lockdown, 32

Tam, Dr. Theresa
Chief, Public Health Agency
initial response, 5
border closure rejection, 23, 168
not in 'the playbook', 169
'individual responsibility', 23
reliance on provinces, 26
voluntary self-isolating, 2, 169
criticism of, 102, 143-144, 170
rejecting face masks, 102, 152

Immunity Task Force, 149-150
testing preference, 157
on airport screening, 169
close links to WHO, 197
face masks rejection, 290
face masks reversal, 290

Testing
swab shortages, 158
Spartan Bioscience Cube, 71, 94, 151, 158
new developments, 40, 64,
defective testing kits (China), 65
problem (Europe), 65
swab testing process, 65, 95
nasal swabs, 65
PCR lab analysis, 65
daily testing target, 157
number of tests, 208
positive test rate, 191
drop in positives (early May), 208
number of tests (early May), 213
Canadian testing target, 213
telephone triage, 58, 69
testing kit shortages, 137
in provinces, 47
in Ontario, 43, 191, 289
food processing plants, 214
testing booth concept, 224

Testing, Rapid Blood
process, 81-82
accuracy/global use, 82
BTNX Inc. (Canada), 82
American company, 82
Health Canada refusal, 83

Tracking Systems
process, 161
importance of, 161-162
in Canada, 162-163
smartphone tracking, 163, 329-330
public vs private, 226-227
civil liberties concerns, 163-164
Tory conservative view, 164-165
app development efforts, 310
privacy concerns, 310-311
South Korean system, 115

Travel Ban Exemptions
Americans (initially), 24-24, 27
Canadians abroad, 25
Canadian Expatriates, 25
international students, 41, 305-306
seasonal workers, 41-42, 305-306

Treatments (patients)
antibody injections, 205
limitations of, 205-206
drug Remdesivir, 201
emergency treatment, 201
speeds recovery, 317

Trudeau, Justin
Prime Minister
TV addresses, 18, 57, 135, 216, 332
border closure rejection, 19
quarantining of refugees, 28
illegal migrants view, 29
craves power, 50, 332
personal domestic agenda, 51, 270-271, 277
ignoring parliament, 50-51
La La land mentality, 70
conflict of interest, 100-101
dependence on WHO, 103-104
defence of WHO, 103-104, 107
provincial lockdowns,104
defence of China, 107-108
criticism of, 102, 103, 116
a benevolent despot, 136
no fiscal responsibility, 200
massive social spending, 334-335
WHO grant ($650 million), 204
Canadian Treasury view, 204-205
popularity of, 216, 311
U.N. personal agenda, 269-270
'new world order', rhetoric, 272, 277
Modern liberal mindset, 270-272

United Nations (Fund Raising)
Africa & Latin America focus, 227
concerns, 227-228
different approach needed, 228

United Nations (GAVI)
fund raising goals, 62
Third-World vaccinations, 62
vaccination programs, 254
vaccine distribution issue, 252
nationalist view, 252-253
internationalist view, 253-254

United Nations (Politics)
investigate WHO calls, 282, 303
WHO response, 282-284
Chinese influence on, 183, 303
China financial aid, 283
Chinese retaliation, 283

U.N. Security Council Seat
Liberal campaign, 68-69,72, 269
sordid blackmail aspect, 69
questioning of, 69
high cost of, 69
jaunts by Prime Minister, 269
government priority, 270
agenda driven, 270
government motives, 269-270
Trudeau ideological agenda, 270-271

United Nations (WHO)
misleading advisories, 183, 204, 233, 320
death rate prediction, 4
travel advisory, 11
vulnerable groups, 11
pandemic declaration, 12
testing & quarantining, 14
belated contagion warning, 127, 184
reversal of diagnoses, 184
rejection of face masks, 108, 153
criticism of, 101-102,107
parliamentary investigation, 103, 183
WHO second wave warning, 263

United States
modelling, 4
border closures, 16, 20, 21
coronavirus response, 16, 20, 21, 138
cases, 4, 66, 75-76, 125, 256, 289
deaths, 75, 125
worst afflicted (mid-April), 125
testing (April), 96

Ventilators
critical need for, 88
over-the-top orders, 89
production problem, 88
health policy, 88
domestic orders, 71, 88
orders (March 30th), 72

Vaccine Developments
early research focus, 9
first financial aid, 9-10
vaccine research, 9,
$1-billion research fund, 148
German progress (Pfizer), 131
Oxford University, 176, 317
worldwide research, 176
University of Ottawa, 176-177, 205
Canadian research, 176-177
potential problems, 316-317

future access, 228
Moderna trials, 280-281
distribution concerns, 284
patent property rights, 284-285
Can Sino vaccine effort, 306

Robert W. Passfield is the author of *The Upper Canadian Anglican Tory Mind, A Cultural Fragment* (2018).

Website: www.passrob.com

www.ingramcontent.com/pod-product-compliance
Lightning Source LLC
Chambersburg PA
CBHW051710020426
42333CB00014B/923